FORENSIC PSYCHIATRY

FORENSIC PSYCHIATRY
(Psychiatry and Law)
Indian Perspective

S Nambi

MBBS MD (Psychiatry) DPM
Professor and Head
Department of Psychiatry
Sree Balaji Medical College and Hospital
Chennai, Tamil Nadu, India

Past President
Indian Psychiatric Society
Formerly, Professor of Psychiatry
Madras Medical College/Institute of Mental Health
Chennai, Tamil Nadu, India

JAYPEE

JAYPEE BROTHERS MEDICAL PUBLISHERS

The Health Sciences Publisher

New Delhi | London

Jaypee Brothers Medical Publishers (P) Ltd

Headquarters
EMCA House
23/23-B, Ansari Road, Daryaganj
New Delhi 110 002, India
Landline: +91-11-23272143, +91-11-23272703
+91-11-23282021, +91-11-23245672
E-mail: jaypee@jaypeebrothers.com

Corporate Office
4838/24, Ansari Road, Daryaganj
New Delhi 110 002, India
Phone: +91-11-43574357
Fax: +91-11-43574314
E-mail: jaypee@jaypeebrothers.com

Overseas Office
J.P. Medical Ltd
83 Victoria Street, London
SW1H 0HW (UK)
Phone: +44 20 3170 8910
E-mail: info@jpmedpub.com

EU GPSR Authorised Representative
Logos Europe, 9 rue Nicolas Poussin
17000, La Rochelle, France
Phone: +33 (0) 6 67 93 73 78
E-mail: contact@logoseurope.eu

Website: www.jaypeebrothers.com
Website: www.jaypeedigital.com

Inquiries for bulk sales may be solicited at: jaypee@jaypeebrothers.com

Forensic Psychiatry (Psychiatry and Law)

First Edition: 2014

Reprint: **2026**

ISBN: 978-93-5090-625-5

Printed at: Samrat Offset Pvt. Ltd.

Dedicated to

The beloved caregivers
of the mentally disabled

PREFACE

It is my long-term dream to write a book on Indian Aspects of Forensic Psychiatry. The forensic psychiatry books are available mostly from the West and they are totally different from our legislation, civil and criminal procedures. Hence, there is an urgent need for practising psychiatrists, postgraduates in psychiatry, and other law enforcing and judicial officers to know the Indian Perspective of Forensic Psychiatry.

There is an increasing awareness regarding mental health in our population. Along with this, comes an increasing involvement of psychiatry with the law, which forces into focus our attention on the relationship between the psychiatry and law.

I trust this book would enlighten the mental health professionals, some basic concepts of the legal aspects of psychiatry.

I take this opportunity to convey my deepest gratitude to Professor O Somasundaram, who has been an inspiration in taking up the subject.

I owe a lot to Dr Shanthi Nambi, for her continuous support and encouragement for assisting me in this task. I also sincerely thank Professor V Palaniappun, Dr Priya Shivashankar and Dr Swetha Purkanti, for their endeavors in this book.

My thanks to Ms J Sujatha and Ms I Ram Gowri.

S Nambi

CONTENTS

1 Chapter

Forensic Psychiatry in India

Legislation forms and integral component in the implementation of mental health care. It has long been known that there is a dynamic relationship between the concept of mental illness, treatment of mentally ill and the law. Because of the increased awareness about the rights of the mentally ill and increased activities of the civil rights movements and the consumer protection groups, there is a possibility of increased litigation centre on psychiatric practice in India. Hence, mental health professionals should have a better understanding of the medicolegal aspects related to mental health problems.

Psychiatrist have a unique role among medical specialist regarding the law, because they have regular contact with legal issues, lawyers and courts whether they like it or not, psychiatrist must regular confront sensitive legal issues. Psychiatrists often get caught in the middle between what may be legally right and what may be ethically right; because of this interface with the law. Psychiatrist would treat mentally ill persons need to have an understanding of fundamental legal issues and the typical problems they will face as practitioners.

In enacting laws for the mentally ill, a recurring dilemma is the conflict between the freedom bestowed in the individual and restraint to be imposed on him for his own and other's protection.

It is universally accepted that the persons, who are mentally ill, require different sets of rules in relation to their rights, responsibilities and liabilities. Not only the society should be protected from the mentally ill, but also, such people should be given care and concern of the society. Of course, the emphasis has varied from time to time and from region to region. It has depended on the state of prevailing knowledge (and ignorance) and the values of the society.

Three fundamental assumptions about the mind are responsible for special consideration about the mentally ill.

- The mind is innocent and does not know the difference between the right and wrong. (Mental sub-normality may also fall in this category)
- The mind is diseased, i.e. insane
- The mind is (temporarily) absent, i.e. automatism.

It is painfully noted that there are mentally ill persons who:

- Cannot grasp the situation, circumstances and the reality
- Cannot understand the consequences of their action (or inaction).

This abnormal mental state is likely to:

- Harm the interests of the other persons, by causing injury to the individual and/or destruction of the property.
- Jeopardize the interests of the affected person also.

FORENSIC PSYCHIATRY

During the British rule in India, few mental asylums were established and mostly with the aim of removing the poor mentally ill patients from human visibility. The British also brought about written laws and the Indian Lunacy Act promulgated in 1912. They also brought the so called Modern Systems of Medicine in the country and with it came modern trends in psychiatry.

There is an increasing awareness regarding mental health in our population. Along with this comes an increasing involvement of psychiatry with the law which forces into focus our attention on the relationship between the psychiatry and the law.

In the present age of increase in crime, many a times a criminal pleads "not guilty" by virtue of being insane and the psychiatrist has to appear in the court and testify as to the soundness of mind and to advice about criminal responsibility of the defendant. This is only one of the circumstances when a punishment comes into contact with law.

Patients who require the expertise of a psychiatrist and those who may harm themselves or the society, those who cannot look after the welfare of their family or property, who may turn not to be dangerous if they Act upon their abnormal thinking. Their management often requires taking away their basic civil rights involving freedom, activity and residence. According to existing laws in force such restraints can be imposed only through a due process and thus it is imperative that the psychiatrist be familiar with these.

Spouse of mentally ill patients may drag the psychiatrist into court to offer evidence in matters of divorce. The institution of marriage is now under great stress and with the resultant increase in divorce rate; the role of psychiatry is also expected to assume a large proportion. There is now an increase awareness of rights in our democracy, which results in increase in litigation. Civil rights movements and consumer council are gaining more and more importance in our day-to-day life.

Forensic psychiatry is comparatively a new upcoming and a developing field in India. The definition of forensic psychiatry as provided by the American board of forensic psychiatry and the American academy of psychiatry and law is as follows:

"It is a subspecialty of psychiatry in which scientific and clinical expertise is applied to legal issues in legal context, embracing civil, criminal, correctional or legislative matters. Forensic psychiatry should be practiced in accordance with guidelines and ethical principles enunciated by the profession of psychiatry."

Thus, forensic psychiatry operates at the interface of two non-related disciplines viz psychiatry and law. It will be interesting to know the extent of dimensions as well as the influence of one system on the other, their respective roles and professional sensitivity. The forensic psychiatry has to offer his professional expertise to the criminal justice system, whenever required, for decision making in the greater interest of the society. While offering his expert service he has to keep in mind that he has to be objective, honest and impartial so that full justice is done in the interest of the society.

The scopes of forensic psychiatry in India, the legal provisions as are available in relation to psychiatric patients, their implications, benefits and drawbacks. The training of undergraduate and postgraduate medical students in forensic psychiatry viz, the role of psychiatrist report, presentation in the court when called upon, etc. and research in forensic psychiatry.

In future the psychiatrist can offer valuable expert service for the welfare of the society at large, safeguard his own interests as well as that of the patients.

Mental illness and diagnoses and treatment of the mental illness have been well documented in *Ayurveda*.

The institution of mental asylum, was a British concept, the first lunatic asylum was established in Kolkata in 1787. The purpose of these asylums was not the care and treatment of the mentally ill but to shut him up in places far away from towns to rid the society of his presence, while at the same time protecting him against himself. Mental health legislation was first enacted in India in 1858 based on the two English Acts of 1853. Law relating to the custody of lunatic and management of their estates was introduced in India. This Act was modified in 1883 and more elaborate instructions and guidelines for admission and treatment of lunatics were outlined. The central supervision of the mental hospital was established in 1906. This was brought out in the form of Indian Lunatic Act of 1912. In 1920, the names of all lunatic asylums were changed to mental hospitals and the control of mental hospitals was shifted from prison authorities to civil surgeons.

A draft of the Mental Health Act was prepared in 1949 by Indian Psychiatric Society. After repeated attempts the bill was passed by the Rajya Sabha, in 1986 and Lok Sabha on 19th march 1987. The Act got the president assent on 22nd may 1987, it became an Act no.14 of 1987. The central and state mental health rules were framed in 1990 and with effect from 1st April 1993, the Act came into force but the real implementation of this Act came into existent only after the unfortunate incident of *Erwadi tragedy*.

There is a momentum gained recently in India, in the relation between psychiatry and law. Though Mental Health Act 1987 has lot of positive qualities, there are lot of criticisms against it. Hence, the Government of India is already in the process of bringing out a new Mental Health Act. The Mental Health Care Act of 2012 Draft has already come and this new Act is going to be enacted most probably during 2012. The ministry of health, Government of India has already set up a committee to formulate the first mental health policy for India and this committee is already in the process of preparing it. Like, the new Mental Health Act, the Mental Health policy, the first of its kind in India is to be put into action in the near future.

Apart from this the care and protection of the children Act, i.e. the Juvenile Justice Act 2000 as already been implemented. The disabilities Act 1995 which is aiming at giving equal opportunities, protection of rights and full participation of the disabled including the mentally disabled is already in function. In 2000, there is a new addendum to the Disabilities Act namely the National Trust for Welfare of persons with Autism, Cerebral Palsy. Mental retardation and Multiple Disabilities Rules, 2000 provides quality care of all the disabilities.

Recently, the Government of India has come out with the Working Draft of the Rights of Persons with Disabilities Act, 2010. The Rehabilitation Council of India Act, 1992 improves the quality care and protects the welfare of all handicapped persons including persons suffering from mental retardation.

The Narcotic Drugs and Psychotropic Substances Act, 1985 (NDPSA) and its amendment in 1988 provides regulations and punishment of persons handling narcotic drugs. The Protection of Women from domestic violence Act, 2005 protects rights of women who are victims of domestic violence. Apart from this the various acts concerns with marriage and divorce in India the Family Court Act 1984 and the protection of the Human Rights Act in addition to the mental health acts protects the rights of the mentally ill persons. The Section 309 of IPC states that the attempted suicide is illegal and punishable. Attempted suicide is considered to be "A cry for help", "An act of despair" and "A disease of hope." The mental health professional and the Indian psychiatric society is fighting to remove this anomaly. It is learnt the law commission of India is also recommending the Government of India to remove this section.

Mental health professionals, postgraduate in psychiatry, lawyers, police officers and judicial officers are all expected to know the basic mental health legislation in India. The forensic psychiatry in India is to focus three areas:

- Active training of postgraduate in forensic psychiatry
- Research activities and
- Better understanding and implementation of the mental health legislation.

The other important area in forensic psychiatry, i.e. prison psychiatry is yet to be developed in its expected line of functioning.

The practice of psychiatry anywhere in the world is influenced by four overlapping spheres of:

1. The moral, ethical, legal and professional duties of the psychiatrist to provide care to his patients.
2. The right of self determination of patient to receive or reject care.
3. The ethical codes and practice of professional organization and
4. The decisions, direction of courts, regulatory authorities and legislature.

This practice applies to India also. Finally, we have to understand that the majority of psychiatric patients do not require any intervention from the law and can be managed comfortably in day-to-day practice without any clinical legal conflict like in other specialties (Dutt, 2001).

SUGGESTED READING

1. Bhujang. The Mentally Ill and the Law. Universal Publishing Corporation, 2003.
2. Mental Health Care Act, 2010, Ministry of Health & Family Welfare, Government of India, New Delhi.
3. Nambi S. Legal Aspects of Psychiatry—Indian Perspective, 2009. Manashanthi Mental Health Care Publications, 2008.
4. Sethi BB. Need for Growth of Forensic Psychiatry. Indian Journal of Psychiatry. 1984;26:1.
5. Shah LP, DLN Murthy Rao Oration. Indian Journal of Psychiatry, 1994; 34.
6. Trivedi JK. The Mental Health Legislation: An Ongoing Debate. Indian Journal of Psychiatry, 2001;44:2.
7. Working Draft of the Rights of Persons with Disabilities Act, 2010, prepared by Centre for Disability Studies. NALSAR University of Law, Hyderabad, India.

Chapter 2

Quality Mental Health Care in Private and Government Psychiatric Hospital—Legal Issues

Mental health forms an important component of health. Mental Health Care delivery in India gaining a momentum in the recent past. Almost every aspect of life in the modern days is regulated or affected in some way by law. All civilization in the world have enacted laws to regulate human behavior so that the weakest can live freely and enjoy all his human rights. There is a dynamic relationship between the concept of mental illness, the treatment of the mentally ill, and the law.

In the Indian context, many acts are directly related to mental health. Among them, the Mental Health Act, 1987 is a major legislation and it is supposed to be operational in 1994 in all States of the Indian Union, but only after the *Erwadi tragedy*, many states started implementing in the real sense. The Act replaces the Indian Lunacy Act, 1912.

Legislation is an expression of the society with regard to the way it views and cares for the mentally ill persons. It has long been known that there is a dynamic relationship between the concepts of mental illness, the treatment of the mentally ill and the Law. Social systems, through laws set boundaries of acceptable or mentally competent persons entitled to take an active part in the social, economic, and political life of the community. Those people found to fall outside these boundaries and definitions are generally considered mentally incompetent or "insane", treatment programmes also have a legal component in that they are often controlled by laws on admissions and discharge, or on the use of treatment methods or therapeutic drugs, this is likewise the case, where psychiatric services are a part of social programmes for the sick and the handicapped, however, it is recognized that "an access to effective treatment and rehabilitation, and would guarantee full protection of the individual's rights. Mental Health Administrators and Legal Experts have been searching for such model for many years. Searching for a model law is like searching for the end of a rainbow: the goal, although, eminently attractive can never be attained. In short, "Model legislation of universal applicability for Mental Health Problems is an illusion, at times, even a dangerous illusions."

The development of mental health is chiefly influenced by larger developments in the society. The WHO Expert Committee on Mental Health in its 1955 report was critical of the Mental Health Laws of its day are as follows:

"Most of the existing Mental Health Legislation is unsatisfactory, although, in some countries, laws based on outmoded concepts of mental abnormality when interpreted liberally can be made to work fairly well in practice. The greatest

single weakness is that purely legal consideration is given too much weight and medical considerations too little" (WHO, 1955).

PRIVATE PSYCHIATRIC PRACTICE AND MENTAL HEALTH LEGISLATION IN INDIA

WHO (Curren and Harding, 1978) suggested that "Consideration be given to the need to provide effective management policy and quality control standard for all psychiatric facilities regardless of whether the institutions are publicly or privately owned".

The encouragement for the Private Psychiatric Practice by Government is not much appreciable. To quote: NHRC report (1999) "The Present Mental Health Act 1987 is not very friendly towards the Private implementation of the Mental Health Act 1987, because of many reasons including discrimination in the licensing procedure, the interference of the visitors and inspecting officer, and the difficulties in the admission and discharge procedures. At times, the new Act is even interfering with the basic rights of the persons, who want to have Private psychiatric care.

Many consider the present Mental Health Act is merely a Mental Hospital Act and not much caring about Government Hospital Psychiatry or Community Psychiatry.

Human Rights Abuse in Psychiatric Hospitals

Human rights commissioners found "appalling and unacceptable" conditions when they visited several psychiatric hospitals in India.

They include filthy living conditions, leaking roofs, overflowing toilets, eroded floors, and broken doors and windows. Most of the patients visited were in pyjamas or naked.

Some were penned into small areas of residential wards, where they were left to sit, pace or lie on the concrete floor all day. Children were left lying on mats on the floor, some covered with urine and faeces. Physical restraint was commonly misused; many patients were observed tied to beds.

At least, one-third of the individuals were people with epilepsy or mental retardation for whom psychiatric institutionalization is unnecessary and confers no benefit. They could well return to live in the community if they could be provided with appropriate medication and a full range of community-based services and support systems.

What is Essential for Mental Health Legislation?

Mental Health Legislation arose from the "asylum" model of western colonies, which did not have a concept or tradition of "asylum" almost wholly inappropriate to the rural/agrarian communities of these countries.

The care of the mentally ill operates in many countries under the extra-judicial "informal" system, which seems to work as well.

Legislation needs to go from its concern with the "Right of freedom" to the "Right to treatment".

Legislation should be such as to take advantage of all possible available resources, not to hinder these and avoid complex, wasteful procedures.

Legislation should take into account the move from the large mental hospitals, private nursing homes, and the Community, and should integrate mental health with General Health Care.

Mental Health Act, 1987; the positive and negative qualities and remedies "there are a lot of positive changes made in the Mental Health Act, 1987 inspite of which there were difficulties in implementing it. The Mental Health Act, 1987 was said to be complicated and arduous, overtly legal in approach and promoting instutionalization and stigmatizing and isolating psychiatry from other medical branches. There is a broad definition of mental illness, which makes the law liable to be abused.

The regulation of involuntary admissions is present, however, it is very stringent and promotes instutionalization. Human rights of the patients have not been adequately addressed. A single regulatory body, which should have regulatory as well as promoting functions is what is needed instead of the multiple checks that are present in the current Act. No provisions for emergency treatment are present, which may be required in our country. A separate category of non-protesting patients can be introduced, which will broaden the scope of Mental Health Care and promote deinstitutionization.

In view of the shortcomings of the Mental Health Act, there is an overwhelming consensus for a completely New Act and not mere amendments to the existing legislation. It is important that the New Act is not overtly legal and provides power to those, who treat mental disorders and is progressive and reflects the trends of the modern world.

The Mental Health Act, 1987 has three components:

- The Core Act, 14 of 1987, effected from 1/04/1993
- The Central Mental Health Authority Rules, 1990
- The State Mental Health Authority Rules, 1990

The second component can be amended or modified only through parliament legislation.

The second component can be modified only by Central Government, but the third component, i.e. State Mental Health Authority, the Tamil Nadu State Mental Health Rules can be revised or modified by State Government in exercise of the powers conferred by the provision to Subsection 2 of Section 94 of Mental Health Act, 1987.

The Tamil Nadu Government has taken initiative in this regard; in coordination with State Mental Health Authority, the Tamil Nadu State Mental Health Rules, 2005 draft has been finalized and waiting for approval in the Assembly.

The State Mental Health Authority in other States, the Mental Health Professionals, and the Indian Psychiatric Society. State branch should initiate this change in state mental health rules, which will facilitate effective implementation of Mental Health Act, 1997.

PRIVATE PSYCHIATRIC PRACTICE AND MENTAL HEALTH LEGISLATION IN INDIA

Prior to independence, Mental Health Care was delivered only through Government Mental Hospital in India. We should not underestimate the services rendered by the Government Mental Hospital in the care of the mentally ill India. No doubt, the vast majority of the mentally ill in India are taken care of by these state hospitals. Today, we are witnessing the advent of psychiatric hospitals and nursing homes in the private sector also. In India, today after the enactment of Mental Health Act 1987, a psychiatrist in private practice is facing much more medicolegal problems than his counter part in government service. In this "era of privatization, the attitude of the government and legislation in India towards the private psychiatric care is not one of institutionalization. The government facilities are burdened with problems of infrastructure, poor maintenance of buildings, inadequate trained staff, and poor statures of service, very poor hygiene and absence of good work culture. These facilities generally lack a sense of commitment." (NHRC report on quality assurance in Medical Health 1999). Of course, the Government Mental Hospitals are taking care of the bulk of the mentally ill persons free of cost as a welfare measure, whereas, the private institutions are catering to the need of affluent population mostly.

The encouragement for the private practice by the government is not much appreciable. To quote: NHRC report (1999) " The present Mental Health Act, 1987 is not very friendly towards the private psychiatric facilities." The private psychiatric hospitals and nursing homes are apprehensive regarding the implementation of the Mental Health Act 1987, because of many reasons including discrimination in the licensing procedure, the interference of the visitors and inspecting officer, and the difficulties in the admission and discharge procedures. At times, the New Act is even interfering with the basic rights of the persons, who want to have private psychiatric care.

LICENSE OF PSYCHIATRIC HOSPITAL AND NURSING HOMES

The spirit behind the need for regulating the Mental Health Care in India is to be appreciated. There should be same standard for both the government and the private psychiatric hospitals, whereas a psychiatric nursing home with a licence under section 8 of Mental Health Care, 1987, the government can establish or maintain a psychiatric hospital without any licence. This is definitely against the WHO principle. Some private psychiatric practitioners even claim that there need not be a licence for establishing and maintaining a psychiatric hospital or nursing home alone. Because the practicing psychiatrists are basically medical practitioners with a post graduate qualification in psychiatry and are already governed by the codes and ethics of Medical Council of India, Consumer

Protection Act, and Private Nursing Home Act, where is the need for one more licence permitting them to practice psychiatry.

It is not clear in the Mental Health Act, whether a private practicing psychiatrist can have separate special centres without licence. For example, De-addiction Centre, Geriatric Mental Health Centre, Rehabilitation Centre, Daycare Centre, Half-way Home, etc. The nongovernmental institutions will be required to strictly follow the rules laid down by the Act, whereas the governmental institutions need not be in all aspects. This discrimination and step motherly attitude towards private psychiatric care is definitely against the global principles on Mental Health Care delivery.

Admission and Discharge Procedures

There is no problem for admission on voluntary basis in the private hospitals. Hence, the psychiatrists in private practice should encourage voluntary admission. It is necessary that procedures should be simplified not only for admission, but also for discharge. The procedure should be made easier and prompt at the request of the patient. As per Mental Health Act, 1987, the private psychiatrists face problems in the involuntary admission and admission through reception and detention orders. Sometimes, to discharge a patient from the psychiatric nursing home or to get extension of treatment period, the medical officer in-charge of the private psychiatric institution should constitute a medical board in which two medical officers should be there out of which one should be a government psychiatrist. This makes the discharge procedure a difficult task and the private psychiatrist has to depend upon a government doctor for his day-to-day administration of the psychiatric nursing home.

As per the Mental Health Act, 1987, the mentally ill person can be admitted in a private psychiatric hospital and nursing home through magistrate's reception order or a detention order for a mentally ill prisoner, if the patient or his relative wish to do so, after giving an assurance to adhere the rules laid down by the private institution. The judiciary can also order a mentally ill person to be admitted in a private psychiatric hospital or nursing home at the request of their relatives or guardian. They have to give the undertaking to meet all the expenses in a private hospital. If the bed is available, the medical officer in-charge of a private hospital cannot refuse. This is the Magistrate Order.

The Role of Inspecting Officer and Visitors

The another disturbing interference in running a private psychiatric hospital is the role of inspecting officers and visitors. The inspecting officer is appointed by the government. He may be a non-medical person also. He may enter and inspect any private psychiatric hospital or nursing home at any time. He may interview the patients and go through the case records. Similarly, five visitors are appointed by the government out of which two are social workers. The definition of social worker is not clearly mentioned in the Act. Hence, government can appoint anybody for this post. This nonmedical, at times, qualified persons also visit the private psychiatric hospital at least once a month. He or she can examine the mentally ill persons, their mode of admission and the certificates issued. The provision of appointment of visitors as found in some Nineteenth Century Law and also in the Indian Lunacy Act, 1912, has been retained in the Mental Health Act, 1987.

The mentally ill person and his relative want to have the psychiatric treatment to be confidential for many reasons, but the entry of the nonmedical personnel into private psychiatric hospital and examining the patients and their case records is definitely a violation of the patient's fundamental rights. This may amount to the breach of confidence. The UN Commission on Human Rights (1983) recommended that every Mental Health Institution should be inspected by higher competent authorities. Inspection of institution by higher competent authority is not equal to inspection of patients by unqualified persons. "The inspection or visit by the nonmedical persons or even outside medical persons in a private psychiatric nursing home goes against the fundamental rights of a citizen or a member of his family and the disclosure of his psychiatric illness to the knowledge of public may amount to indignity."

The practicing psychiatrists who maintain or plan to establish private psychiatric hospital or nursing home are highly apprehensive about the partiality of the Mental Health Act towards them. Law does not enforce implementation; it needs public and professional support to get fruitful results. The Mental Health Act 1987, needs to be amended to encourage the private sector to enter the field of Mental Health Care. More private psychiatric hospital and nursing homes should emerge not only to improve the quality of care, but also to minimize the stigma and discrimination attached to mental illness.

The Indian Psychiatric Society in 2000 made some recommendation on Mental Health Legislation to the Government of India.

Recommendations of the Indian Psychiatric Society on Mental Health Legislation, 2000:

1. Since the Mental Health Act, 1987 is not based on any Mental Health Policy and plan of the Government, the Government of India is urged upon to declare its Mental Health Policy and the plan and programme based on the said policy.
2. Mental Health Act, 1987 be repealed by a new Mental Health Legislation based on—
    a. Mental Health Policy of the Government.
    b. Modern concept of psychiatry.
    c. Basic statutory structure of mental health legislation as laid down in the guiding principles and alternative approaches recommended by the WHO in 1978.
    d. Principles, guidelines and guarantees for the protection of persons detained on grounds of mental ill health or suffering from mental disorder adopted by the UN in 1999.

3. Among others, the following changes should be made:
   a. Inconsistencies between the provisions made in different sections and subsections of the Act must be corrected and the rules made under Act must be consistent with the provisions of the Act and all the rules (including rules regarding aid to mentally ill persons) must be framed before the Act is given effect to.
   b. The expression "Mentally Ill Person" should be redefined as suggested by the WHO expert committee on mental health, 1955. A single Mental Health Act covering both mentally ill and mentally retarded persons are most useful form of legislation. Minimum qualifications of all mental health personnel mentioned in the Act and Rules should be clearly stated in the definition.
   c. Mental Health Authority should function in an advisory capacity and Licensing Authority should function in the administrative capacity. Members of the Mental Health Authority should have special knowledge in mental health legislation and mental health services. The function of the Mental Health Authority under a separate Mental Health Unit or Directorate Division in the Ministry of Health should include:
      - Promoting mental health programmes
      - Compiling educational materials
      - Coordinating with other bodies to increase human resources in the field of mental health.
   d. Adequate funds should be provided for proper functioning of any forum or authority constituted under the mental health legislation and for execution of all the provisions made under the said legislation.
   e. All "Mental Health Services" including residential establishment for the mentally retarded should be required to obtain licence under the Mental Health Act and the consideration be given to the need to provide effective management policy and quality control standards for all mental health facilities, regardless, of whether these facilities are publicly of private owned.
   f. Voluntary admission to any medical facility should be made informal as in English Mental Health Act, 1983.
   g. Change of status from voluntary to involuntary and vice—the medical officer in-charge of the psychiatric facility should do versa.
   h Forms should be prescribed for all orders passed under the Act and its use should be mandatory.
   i. Violation of the Human Rights of the mentally ill persons at any place or by any person or authority should invite action by the Human Rights Commission.

Although, amendment of clauses would take lesser time than replacing the Act by a new one, the Indian Psychiatric Society feels that not only large number of amendment are necessary in almost every section of the Act and every clauses of the Rules to remove the inconsistencies in the present Act and Rules, and any change of policy as recommended above would call or further changes in the Act and the Rules. Drafting of a new bill would be much easier than large scale amendments of the existing Act.

THE MEASURE TO IMPROVE QUALITY OF MENTAL HEALTH IN INDIA

The Central Government has taken special consideration and sanctioned funds to improve quality of Mental Health Care in India.

The Central Government sanctioned Rupees Fifty Lakh for many medical colleges and rupees one to three crores to all the State Mental Health Hospitals to improve the infrastructures.

District Mental Health Programme (DMHP) is extended to many districts. This will reduce the congestion in tertiary care hospitals treating major mental disorders without much complication and common mental disorders can be recognized and treated by District Mental Health Programme Team and Primary Care Physicians. Again, this will improve the quality of Mental Health Care.

Ways to Improve Implementation of Mental Health Act

1. The public
2. The consumers (caregivers of the mentally ill)
3. Judicial officers
4. Police officers.

Awareness campaign to the public can be carried out through popular lectures, propagation through media, observation of Mental Health week and programmes in schools and colleges are to be arranged. Awareness campaign to the consumers (caregivers) can be carried out through.

Awareness programs for caregivers, enlightening the rights of the mentally ill, and their duties and responsibilities as a caregiver (relative) of the psychiatrically disabled and other legal implications.

Judicial and police officers are to be sensitized through awareness programmes about Mental Health Authority, the admission and discharge procedures, and the legal aspects of mental disorders.

Care for the wandering mentally ill should be provided through increased awareness among police officers and involvement of NGOs. Wandering mentally ill should be admitted in Institute of Mental Health and taken care of.

State Mental Health Rules should be modified as per the need, availability of resources, and in order to ensure the efficient implementation of Mental Health Authority.

Solving Mental Health Problems

Over the past half century, the model for Mental Health Care has changed from the institutionalization of individuals suffering from mental disorders to a community care approach backed by the availability of beds in general hospitals for acute cases. These changes are based both on respect for the human rights of individuals with mental disorders and on the use of updated interventions and techniques. A correct objective diagnosis is fundamental for planning individual care and choice of appropriate treatment. The earlier, a proper course of treatment starts, the better the prognosis. Appropriate treatment of mental and behavioural disorders implies the rational use of pharmacological, psychological and psychosocial interventions in a clinically meaningful and integrated way. The management of specific conditions consists of interventions in the areas of prevention, treatment and rehabilitation.

Suggestions and recommendations to improve quality of Mental Health Care as promulgated by the Declaration of Caracas in November, 1990.

The Legislators Associations, Health Authorities, Mental Health Professionals and Jurists assembled at the Regional Conference on the restructuring of psychiatric care in Latin America within the Local Health Systems Model—

1. That the restructuring of psychiatric care on the basis of primary health care and within the framework of the local health systems model will permit the promotion of alternative service models that are community-based and integrated into social and health care networks.
2. The restructuring of psychiatric care in the region implies a critical review of the dominant and centralizing role played by the Mental Health Services delivery.
3. That the resources, care and treatment that are made available must:
   - Safeguard personal dignity and human and civil rights
   - Be based on criteria that are rational and technically appropriate.
4. That national legislation must be redrafted if necessary, so that:
   - The human and civil rights of mental patients are safeguarded
   - The organization of Community Mental Health Services guarantees the enforcement of these rights
   - Strive to ensure that patients remain in their communities.
5. That training in Mental Health and Psychiatry should use a service model that is based on the community health care and encourages psychiatric admission in general hospital in accordance with the principles that underlie the restructuring movement.
6. That the organizations, associations, and other participants hereby undertake to advocate and develop programmes at the country level that will promote the restructuring desired and at the same time that they commit themselves to monitoring and defending the human rights of mental patients in accordance with national legislation and international agreements.

To this end, they call upon the Ministries of Health and Justice, the Parliaments, social security and other care providing institutions, professional organizations, consumer associations, universities and other training facilities and the media to support the restructuring psychiatric care, thus assuring its successful development for the benefit of the population in the region.

SUGGESTED READING

1. Dalal PK, Pargaokar A, Kala AK. Mental Health Legislation in India—short comings and solutions International Conference of SAARC Psychiatric Federation, in Agra, 2005.
2. Indian Psychiatric Society—recommendation of Mental Health Legislation, 2002.
3. Mental Health: New Understanding, new hope. WHO—The World Health Report, 2011.
4. Nambi S. Mental Health Act, 1987—an evolution presented in the Indian Psychiatric Society, South Zone Conference, Mangalore, 1994.
5. Nambi S. Private Psychiatric Practice and Mental Health Legislation in India. Paper presented at the First Annual Conference of IAPP, New Delhi, 2000.
6. The Mental Health Act, 1987 (14 of 1987). Universal Law Publishing Company (private), New Delhi, 2004.
7. Verma VK, Verma SK. Mental Health Legislation in Ten Asian Developing Countries—the practical need for change. International Digest of Health Legislation, 1984;35(2).

3 Chapter

Ethical Issues in Psychiatry

The word Ethics is derived from the Greek word "Ethikos", which refers to which is customary. Ethics may be defined as the "Moral Principles" that determine the rightness or wrongness of particular acts or activities.

WHAT DO WE MEAN EXACTLY BY ETHICS

a. A set of rules laid down by government
b. Socially imposed rules
c. A set of principles
d. A person ought to do.

Ethics is the science of norms of behavior for any group; a code of conduct designed by a group of person in a particular society, it provides a frame work to guide one's own behavior in a particular setting.

They are relative and changing with time, ethics means moral duties, this duty cannot be unilateral.

"Will maintain the utmost respect for human life from the time of conception"—code of medical ethics. If so how about MTP?

Day-to-day ethical problems in psychiatry: Often the ethical practice is considered limited to obtaining informed consent and to follow major precepts as enunciated under ethical guidelines, but ethics is much more than that, it is an approach and is operative all the time a psychiatrist is interacting with the patient. Main constituents of psychiatric evaluation are history taking, examination, diagnosis, treatment and prognosis.

Doctors of medicine yield too much power of influence over their patients and if the power is not restrained then its misuse is very likely. It is precisely for this reason, that Hippocratic Oath was emancipated in the 5th century BC. The present day medicine was not satisfied with the Hippocratic Oath and hence a new type of ethics was evolved on the basis of present day philosophy prevalent in the western culture. The purpose of ethical guidelines is to safeguard the patient as well as physician. A doctor is a healer and he provides relief.

There are two Theoretical Bases in the Formation of Ethics

Utilitarian Theory

The fundamental aspect of this theory is to produce greatest amount of happiness to the greatest number of people. We in India are generally practicing this pattern.

This theory envisages that one should study carefully the needs of the people and then device policies or laws to produce greatest benefit to maximum numbers. This theory leads to paternalistic behaviour. The physician acts as a parent and does what he feels right for the patient. The words of the great physicians are not to be questioned.

Autonomy Theory

Modern Western ethics is based on autonomy theory, which implies that relationship between two people should be based on equality and every decision should have the consent of both. "Sharing of decision is the concept behind this theory."

Though often ethics, morals, and laws are used interchangeably, they are not the same. Morals are derived from religious and cultural practices of a given group and were unchangeable and any deviance from them evokes guilt. Laws are framed by states to regulate behavior of the people. The Laws are rigid and the violation will lead to punishment. Ethical guidelines are evolved by professional groups or amongst their own members.

American Psychiatric Association evolved ethical guidelines in 1970; later World Psychiatric Association evolved ethical guidelines in 1977. These are known as Hawaii Declaration. The Indian Psychiatric Society developed approved ethical guidelines in 1989 during the Cuttack Conference.

Ethical guidelines are not static and they should continue evolving with time, it is not only logical, but also ethical that most patients should be given a standardized treatment which should fulfill minimum required treatment for the condition, so, it is very essential to follow the guidelines prescribed by the respective countries psychiatric society.

For example, Psychiatrists in India are expected to follow the guidelines prescribed by the IPS guidelines for various disorders.

Psychiatrists need to be careful about the spoken words. Loose talk could be avoided and they should be careful to avoid improper explanations regarding etiology.

Moral Issues on Psychiatry

Psychiatry has been traditionally non-judgmental and it has assiduously tried to avoid moral issue. A time has now come when moral dimension of behavior should be an important area of study. We need not sit on judgment on our patient's morals, but we need to be sensitive to moral issues in management of patients. Treatment of individuals should involve assessment of values and the deficiencies in values or conflict with morals should be focus of therapy. Morality and values should form a part of psychiatric treatment and research in future.

Some values of ethical considerations when treating patients with schizophrenia in the modern medical practice have changed profoundly over the last few decades. Chief among these is truthfulness, specifically, whether physician should tell patients the truth when they have a potentially fatal illness such as cancer.

Just decades ago, it was thought that they should not, but now, it is thought that they should. The extent to which this value of truthfulness is now given priority is reflected by the current widespread ethical consensus that generally doctors should tell patients the truth, even when this may cause forceable additional harm to patients.

The following are some of the conflicting ethical issues in managing persons with schizophrenia.

- Telling of truths and persons with schizophrenia who are paranoid.
- Psychiatrists usually choose to initially withhold certain types of knowledge because if they disclose everything right away, they run the risk of patients never returning and therefore not receiving adequate care. Ethically, the degree to which a psychiatrist withholds information may disrespect patient's autonomy and may even be regarded as lying by omissions. The gains from psychiatrist sharing partial truths may not be evidence based.
- Supporting the "Risky ambitions of patients with schizophrenia".
- Asking a patient with schizophrenia whether he or she wants to write psychiatric advanced directives.
- Persuading patients with schizophrenia to involve their family members.
- Just as it may be ethically justifiable to encourage a patient with schizophrenia to continue taking his/her medication, a psychiatrist may also have some ethical obligation to try to persuade the patients with schizophrenia to involve his or her family more in his/her care. This may be considered coercive, but in the end, it will probably help their patient to have better quality of life.

The current consensus is that the value of respecting a patient's autonomy generally should prevail. It emphasizes the role of the patient in medical decision making. Psychiatrists, however, should always carefully consider what moral weight should be given to the values of doing good and avoiding harm which were given more weight in the past, when psychiatrist generally were more paternalistic. This particularly be the case when treating patients with schizophrenia, since, these patients decision making capacities are likely to be impaired.

ETHICS AND LAW

Both Ethics and Law are required to optimally regulate the behavior of both the therapist and the patient to achieve the therapeutic goal of maximum reduction of suffering. The therapeutic relationship should be based on trust and mutual respect. It should be a duty-based collaborative engagement wherein patient participates to help his therapist arrive at the best possible solution to his problem. The patient and the therapist should treat each other as natural allies and not be adversaries. They should be employed in the best interest of the patient and also the society. Psychiatrists should fulfill their dual responsibilities honestly and fairly. Law must be ethical and be continuously updated. Ethics on the other hand must respect the legal boundaries.

ETHICAL ISSUES IN PSYCHOTHERAPY

In contrast to routine clinical practice, psychotherapy should be considered as a special situation especially in our setting where there is no much distinction between psychotherapists per se and psychiatrist. Whenever a client approaches a psychiatrist and if he thinks that psychotherapy could be an appropriate treatment modality, or if the client requests for psychotherapy in the light of his competence, the therapist should obtain informed consent. This should include providing information to the client as to what is psychotherapy, what is expected out of the patient, what is expected from the therapist, what are the limitations of the therapy and therapist, fees involved, alternative modalities of treatment along with efficacy of each in condition, which the client is suffering from. After an informed consent is obtained, the therapist along with the client should draw a therapeutic contract, with Do's and Don'ts for either of them. Throughout the therapy and during drawing the therapeutic contract, therapist should be aware of the confidentiality issues and also make the client aware about the exceptions to the confidentiality issues. Similarly, the therapist should be aware of the boundaries and boundary violations and try to work in the limits of the boundaries. However, if boundary violations occur, steps must be taken to minimize the harm. Whenever therapy ends, it should be in congenial environment with the scope for the client to seek treatment again if he desires so or an opportunity to be referred to someone else. The dignity of the patient has to be kept in mind by the therapist. Confidentiality has to be maintained. If necessary, the family may be involved. The relationship has to be strictly professional. The patient may develop dependency on the therapist and this should not be used for prolonging treatment.

Managing Difficult Behavior

To do List

Acknowledging limits: Personal as well as professional limits must be acknowledged.

- Limit setting
- Documentation
- Avoiding argumentative stances
- Handling intimidation
- Seeking help
- Redressal from others
- Termination.

Not to do List

- Permitting a patient to run errands or do other small favors for the therapist.
- Non-therapeutic contact outside of the therapist's office.
- Hiring the patient or using the patient as an unpaid volunteer.
- Giving or accepting a valuable gift or loan.

- Using data from a therapy session (such as inside knowledge of a good investment) for personal gain.
- Spending time—and wasting the patient's money and time—talking about the therapist's problems.
- Disclosing personal problems or intimate details of personal life, such as illness, family situation or sexual experience.
- Dressing seductively.
- Repeatedly touching or hugging the patient, or worse engaging in sexual advances or interaction.
- Addressing the patients with a past name.
- Promoting the therapist's religious belief system.
- Promoting involvement in a social/political cause that the therapist is fond of.
- Patient joining the therapist in an investment or business venture.
- Encouraging patients to engage in cult-like behavior with the therapist as *guru*.
- Ignoring mounting unpaid bills for treatment.
- Offering not to charge or to greatly reduce the fee for sessions, even when the patient can afford the cost.
- Over-charging well to do patients.

ETHICAL ISSUES IN PSYCHIATRIC RESEARCH

About 450 million people are estimated to be suffering from neuropsychiatric condition (WHO) World Mental Health Report, 2001. These disorders are present either alone or in addition to one or more physical disorders. Apart from being widely prevalent, they are universal and there are no consistent differences in the prevalence between developed and developing countries. While no group is immune to mental disorders, the risk is higher among the poor, homeless, the unemployed, and persons with low education, victims of violence, etc. These factors influence the prognosis of the disorders through inequities in case detection and access to treatment that makes the treatment gap wider in developing countries.

However, over the past half a century, research, improved diagnostic reliability, clinical research in pharmacological and non-pharmacological interventions have let to better outcome in people with Mental Health Problems. This makes research in Psychiatry highly imperative which has to follow basic ethics.

MENTAL ILLNESS AND VULNERABILITY

People with mental illness are vulnerable on several accounts. Certain factors have been mentioned above. Added to this is the stigma and social detachment that accompanies the diagnosis of mental illness and leads to a sense of powerlessness to the client and the client's family. However, the public health consequences of mental illness create a high ethical imperative to perform scientific studies on etiology, management, and prevention in this vulnerable group, in order to find out effective interventions.

ETHICAL ISSUES IN RESEARCH IN PEOPLE WITH MENTAL ILLNESS

There has been considerable concern about the ethics of advancing scientific knowledge at the expense of the individual safety and interest of people with mental health. Many of these concerns pertain to research in humans in general, but particular concerns relate to the inexactness of psychiatric diagnoses and the validity of research findings. The use of coercive techniques of unproven efficacy on people with psychiatric conditions, the use of medication-free intervals and placebo control studies, interventional and observational research in the Prodromal phases are some of the abuse of psychiatric research. The validity and capacity to consent in the psychiatrically-ill patient is also under much debate. Concerns have been expressed on the ethics of research in developing countries, particularly, when done solely for regulatory approval elsewhere.

Should Research be done in people with Impaired Decisional Capacity?

People with mental illness are presumed to have poor decisional capacity. Cognitive dysfunction and symptoms shown to be associated with impaired decisional capacity are not unique to schizophrenia and may occur with other forms of illnesses also. Studies have shown that people with schizophrenia are able to give informed consent and retain the related information across time. Their decision making capacity may improve significantly with educational remediation.

Methods of scientific research should not infringe on the rights of the mentally ill. This is all the more important when research is combined with clinical care. The "therapeutic misconception" (inability to differentiate between the treatment arms such as use of placebo) is likely to occur when research trials are conducted in treatment centers and by their usual treatment teams. Older age, lower education, and worse health placed people are at a higher risk for therapeutic misconception.

The cardinal principles of ethical research practices harp upon respect of the autonomy of the individual, maintaining confidentiality, truth telling, obtaining informed consent, protection of the vulnerable people and a belief in beneficence and non-malfeasance. The benefits and safety of the individual take precedence over scientific or monitory advantage. The principle of justice includes a fair selection of subjects so that all people who might benefit from the research are included.

These principles have gradually eroded over the years in all cultures due to health care fragmentation and academic pressures. Cultural issues have compounded these challenges of traditional ethical practices. Other cultural influences are the widespread utilization of alternative health care systems. This range from *Ayurveda, Siddha,* and *Unnani* traditions, where symptom removal is not necessarily the overt goal of treatment and diagnoses based on contemporary disease category is not the norm. Meanwhile, the predominant privatization of "Health Care in India" has led to the rapid growth of the model that uses profit at the bottom line rather than the need to generate reliable evidence or advance the interest of research participants. This has led to the eroding of public confidence in research in a Country where health care has already come under the ambit of Consumer Protection Act (COPRA).

REGULATION AND OVERSIGHT OF RESEARCH IN PEOPLE WITH PSYCHIATRIC DISORDERS

The ethical principles that guide research in human participants stem from guidance from various organizations. The earliest such attempt was the Nuremberg Code. The key elements of the Nuremberg Code are:

- The voluntary consent of the human subject is absolutely essential.
- The results of the research must be useful and unobtainable by other means.
- The study must be rationally based on knowledge of the disease or condition to be studied. This was backed by the Universal Declaration of Human Rights.

THE DECLARATION OF HELSINKI

The final revision of the declaration of Helsinki was adopted by the 56th General Assembly of the WMA (World Medical Association) in Seoul in October, 2008. It contains 35 clauses organized in three sections.

- The first section defines human research and stresses the obligation of the physician that the well-being of the individual must take precedence over other interest.
- The second section has laid down the general principles of medical research.
- The third section outlines the principles to be followed when research is combined with care.
- The Declaration acknowledges the need for research and the attendant risks, but stresses that all research are to benefit local communities as well as the research participant directly.

ETHICAL GUIDELINES AND REGULATIONS GOVERNING RESEARCH IN INDIA

The Ethical Guidelines for Biomedical Research on Human Participants of the Indian Council of Medical Research:

The eight chapters cover the general principles of ethics in relation to the Indian Cultural Values and Context, particularly, in the application of informed consent and the primacy of the individual autonomy.

The Drugs and Cosmetic Act and Rules

The Drugs and Cosmetic Act 1940, and the Drugs and Cosmetic Rules, 1945 regulate the import, manufacture, and sale of drugs and cosmetics in India. Schedule Y requires that all applications for clinical trial should confirm to the requirements of the Declaration of Helsinki.

Good Clinical Practices for Clinical Research in India

Good Clinical Practices (GCP) guidelines were developed keeping in mind the need for specific guidelines to encompass the design, conduct, termination, audit, and documentation of the studies involving human subjects in India to ensure uniform quality of research findings. It incorporates essential elements of schedule by as well as the ethical principles enumerated in the Declaration of Helsinki and the ICMR ethical guidelines.

Study Design

The scientific validity of research is an important prerequisite. Research that does not yield reliable results is unethical. One major contributor to such outcome is the poor research design. All research designs, however, appropriate are prone to bias, confounding and the effects of chance. Hence, the design should incorporate procedures specifically meant to eliminate such pitfalls. The design must be clearly described in a research protocol. The consolidated standards for reporting the results of randomized controlled trials (CONSORT Statement) are universally accepted as providing evidence-based elements in relation to minimizing bias.

Ethical Review

All research proposal involving human participants should be cleared by an appropriately instituted Institutional Ethics Committee (IEC), also referred to as the Institutional Review Board (IRB). It should be properly constituted as per the ICMR guidelines. The responsibilities of the IEC are:

- To protect the dignity and rights of the research participant.
- To follow the universal ethical values.
- To assist in the development and education of a research community.

All research should not only be scientifically valid, but also socially relevant. An important duty of the researchers and the members of the IRB is careful evaluation of the potential risk benefit ratio of research protocols. The ethical review should be done in formal meetings and the EC should not take decisions through circulation of proposals.

Further information is made available on the ICMR website (http://icmr.nic.in/icmrnews/compensation guide-pdf).

The Declaration of Helsinki requires that all trials should be prospectively registered in a publicly accessible database. Researchers should report any adverse events and amendments to the protocol to the IRBs.

Obtaining informed consent from subjects must be accomplished prior to performing the research activity and using only an IRB/IEC approved consent form. The protocol for the study should include reimbursements to participants that compensate them for reasonable expenses associated with study participation. The results of all research should be made publicly available within a reasonable period of time after the completion of the study.

Research misconduct means fabrication, falsification, or plagiarism in proposing or performing or reporting research results. Policies should be developed by the IRBs on how to proceed with such allegations, so as to ensure integrity of the study results. All researchers should declare any potential conflict of interest in the research protocol. The study proposal should provide details of arrangements made regarding continued access to care of the studied drug to participants, should it prove to be safe and effective.

All researchers should receive adequate training in research methodology and research ethics and should read a copy of the ICMRs bioethics guidelines and other relevant documents. They should have the requisite time, facilities, and personnel to safely conduct the proposed research.

ETHICAL ISSUES IN DEALING WITH PHARMACEUTICALS

Relationship with pharmaceutical companies: Most clinicians interacts with pharmaceutical companies and these companies provide inputs for most of our conferences and CME programs. There is another special factor in our country where large numbers of different firms sell the same medicine. The physician has to keep in mind that this inducement should not lead to unnecessary prescription of drugs. One could choose drug of any company depending on the cost and quality of product.

ETHICAL GUIDELINES IN DEALING WITH PHARMA INDUSTRIES

Guideline 1

Medical practitioner in general is expected to evolve as a professional for ultimate benefit and wellbeing of the patients.

Guideline 2

Psychiatrists as medical professional will always protect their patients from whatever is deleterious and mischievous.

Guideline 3

Psychiatrists need to decide about benefit of treatment to the patients is worth the cost to society.

While doing so, they also have a commitment to save resources for the benefit of society.

Guideline 4

Psychiatrist will maintain their professional uniqueness and credibility. Psychiatrist will avoid the misuse or overuse of medications in ways that may adversely affect patients.

Guideline 5

The running of professional bodies in psychiatry will not jeopardize the basic interest of profession and professional commitments to the patients and to the society at large due to support from pharma industry.

Guideline 6

a. While dealing with pharmaceutical representative, psychiatrist will be committed to the wellbeing of the patient.
b. Hence psychiatrist will not utilize his time with medical sales representative at the cost of the patient time.
c. They will always keep the professional and ethical outlook while dealing with medical sales rep.

Guideline 7

The psychiatrist as a scientific professional will always endorse the scientific views of the pharmaceutical drugs hence will always promote rational and appropriate use of them.

Guideline 8

a. By and large the psychiatrist should avoid accepting the expensive and personal gifts from Pharmaceuticals.
b. Gifts and inducements must provide value to the practice of medicine or pharmacy.
c. They have to be reasonable and promote professional education and efficacy.
d. If the gifts are intended to promote education or scientific character of doctor's practice, they need not be objected.

Guideline 9

The psychiatrist will be transparent in his alliance with the pharma industry and will always focus on ethical and regulatory standard.

The psychiatrist will not indulge in the practice of accepting funds for personal benefit of any kind.

Guideline 10

While developing therapeutic guideline, the psychiatrist will not get influenced by pharma industries.

Guideline 11

a. The psychiatrist will not get involved in the ghost writing practices that are commercially involved in increasing drug sale.
b. Psychiatrist will not choose to be hiked speaker and promote non-rational prescribing associated, in increasing drug sale by pharma.

c. The psychiatrist will avoid endorsing pharma products at personal level by allowing to use their photographs or focused comments in pharma newsletters or promotional pamphlets.

Guideline 12

a. Psychiatrists are not supposed to sell products out of the office unless the products are exclusively pertinent to the patient's care.
b. The psychiatrist should never give incentives to the patient to buy particular brand of pharma products.
c. In the case of patients getting carried away by pharma advertisements and thereby likely to have adverse health effects, the psychiatrist will guide the consumers in right direction.

Guideline 13

The psychiatrist as teachers and medical educators.

ETHICS AND MEDICAL PRACTITIONERS

We need to take into following ethical consideration for being medical practitioner. Our professional integrity must be our topmost priority.

- Human right consideration of patients.
- Pharma getting into social welfare for better community health and health oriented healthy guidelines.
- We must be sensitive to consumer concern.
- We need to strengthen guidelines to cut back on bribery in the form of gifts.
- Rejecting those pharma, which are identified as nuisance due to their unethical business.

Ethics in Elderly

Ethical Issues in the Care of the Demented

Impaired cognition in severe cases prevents the patient to understand his illness and treatment. Obtaining consent from a confused, early delirious state is not only unethical and illegal, nor is it proper to wait till the patient becomes fully delirious so that the procedure can be done without his consent.

In patients with dementia, it is necessary to confer with family members about the procedures. Physician should assist patients and family members in deciding when the treatment is likely to be futile.

Medication Use in Elderly

- More appropriate treatment is needed for this high risk population.
- It is highly unethical to drug them too much and drug them against their will.
- Elderly need minimum number of drugs with minimum side effect profile and regular monitoring. "Start Low, Go Slow" principle. Drugs with severe side

effect should not be used as a substitute for human attention and stimulating surroundings.

Genetic Testing to Identify Dementia

- It is an ethical dilemma.
- Genetic test to identify persons at risk for dementia without offering the promises of treatment continues to be an ethical dilemma.

Is it Ethical?

- Several genes are found to be associated with AD.
- The apolipoprotein—E4 allele is associated with high risk of AD.
- Can the information about the risk of developing AD be passed on to the patients and to the relatives? Is it ethical?
- Physician will need to be mindful of the psychological impact of the information.

Ethical Issues in the Care of the Demented

Ethical and legal issues frequently arise in the care of the demented and delirious. They are:

1. Reduced capacity to give informed consent.
2. Involuntary hospitalization.
3. End of life care and decisions.
4. Research protocols.
5. Diminished capacity due to cognitive impairment.
6. Informed consent for medical treatment.

Agreeing or declining depends on:

1. Information disclosure by the physician.
2. Voluntary participation by the patient.
3. Patient's competence.
4. Mildly delirious or demented are still capable of making informed decisions.

Ethics on Medical Education and Curriculum

Of late, the need for strengthening and consolidating curriculum of ethics in medical professional education has been strongly felt.

In response to this, the medical council of India has taken measures to revise the curriculum.

The suggested changes focus on:

1. The medical curriculum should be oriented towards educating students to take up the responsibilities of physicians of first contact. The medical graduate should be capable of functioning independently in both urban and rural environments.
2. Every effort should be made to provide educational experience that allows hands-on-experience in hospitals as well as in a community setting. For this

purpose, a comprehensive list of clinical skills that a medical graduate must acquire at the end of the course including internship has been prepared.

3. Maximum efforts should be made to encourage integrated teaching and to de-emphasize compartmentalization of disciplines so as to achieve horizontal and vertical integration in different phases.
4. Educational experience should emphasize health rather than only disease, and community orientation instead of only hospital orientation. Population control and family planning should also be given due emphasis.
5. Due importance should be given to teaching common problems of health and disease as well as National Programmes.
6. Every effort should be made to use learner oriented methods which would encourage cultivation of logical thinking, clarity of expression, independence of judgment, scientific habit, and problem solving abilities, self initiated and self-directed learning.
7. Reduction of didactic lectures (not more than 1/3rd of total teaching hours) and increasing use of active methods of learning such as group discussions, seminars, role play, field visits, demonstrations, peer interactions, etc, which would enable students to develop personality, communication skills and other necessary qualities.
8. Examinations should be designed with a view to assess not merely the knowledge but also practical and clinical skills, habits, and values which are necessary for a graduate to carry out professional day-to-day work competently.
9. Regular periodic assessment should be done throughout the course for internal assessment. The assessment need not be limited to written tests. It should relate to other items like record maintenance, participation in seminars and group discussions, clinical case studies, proficiency in carrying out practical/clinical skills or participation in project and assignments, event during vacation. These should be evaluated objectively and recorded.
10. Every medical institution should evolve institutional objectives which would be in consistence with the national goals and health policy. The institutional objectives should prescribe the attributes of their product.
11. Shift in the role of medical teachers from merely imparting knowledge to that of a facilitator and motivator of student learning.
12. Every medical college should establish a medical education unit of faculty development, preparation of learning resource materials and improved evaluation methods.

Ethical Issues in Certification

The psychiatrist cannot afford to be careless in issuing certificates regarding the patient's illness and treatment. The certificate may be used for some purpose other than that intended. This writer has come across remarks like "procured medical evidence", certificate under psychological pressure, etc. in legal publications.

Ethical principles include responsibility, professional competence, benevolence, moral standards, patient's welfare and confidentiality. The therapist should avoid sexual advance towards the patient. Treatment should not be denied in an emergency. A patient who refuses treatment has to be motivated to accept it. The psychiatrist has to be in tune with his cultural ecology.

OATH OF HIPPOCRATES

1. I swear by Apollo Physician and Asclepius and Hygieria and Panaceia and all the Gods and Goddesses, making them my witnesses, that I will fulfill according to my ability and judgment this oath and this covenant.
2. To hold him who has taught me this art as equal to my parents and to live my life in partnership with him, and if he is in need of money to give him a share of mine, and to regard his offspring as equal to my brothers in male lineage and to teach them this art—if they desire to learn it—without fee and covenants; to give a share of percepts and oral instruction and all the other learning to my sons and to the sons of him who has instructed me and to pupils according to the medical law, but to no one else.
3. I will apply dietetic measure for the benefit of the sick according to my ability and judgment; I will keep them from harm and injustice.
4. I will neither give a deadly drug to anybody if asked for it, nor will I make a suggestion to this effect. Similarly, I will not give to a woman an abortive remedy. In purity and holiness, I will guard my life and my art.
5. I will not use the knife, not even on sufferers from the stone, but will withdraw in favor of such men as are engaged in this work.
6. Whatever houses I may visit, I will come for the benefit of the sick, remaining free of all intentional injustice, of all mischief and in particular of sexual relations with both female and male persons, be they free or slaves.
7. What I may see or hear in the course of the treatment or even outside of the treatment in regard to the life of men, which on no account one must spread abroad, I will keep to myself holding such things shameful to be spoken about.
8. If I fulfill this oath and do not violate it, may it be granted to me to enjoy life and art, being honored with fame among all men for all time to come; If I transgress it and swear falsely, may the opposite of all this be my lot.

INDIAN PSYCHIATRIC SOCIETY ETHICAL GUIDELINES

A committee comprising of Prof JS Neki, Prof DN Nandi, Prof AK Agarwal, Dr VN Vahia and Dr JK Trivedi was requested to prepare the recommendations of the workshop. The committee prepared the following drafts recommendations, which has been approved by the Indian Psychiatric Society at its Annual Conference, January 1989, held at Cuttack.

Preamble

Ethics has been as essential part of healing art. Ethical guidelines have been prepared by International and National organizations for different groups of practitioners. Each country has its own social, economical, and psychological compulsion which might make it difficult to translate and practice ethical codes of other countries. Hence this body proposes following ethical guidelines for members of psychiatric profession in this country.

These principles are intended to aid psychiatrists individually and collectively in maintaining a high level of ethical conduct. They are not laws, but standards by which a psychiatrist may determine the propriety of his conduct on his relationship with patients, with members of allied professions and with the public.

Principles

1. *Responsibility*: As a practitioner, the psychiatrist must know that he bears a heavy social responsibility because he not only deals with disturbed human behavior but also has to contend with intimacies of life. As a scientist, he would serve the society through observation, investigation, and experimentation and well planned and ethically carried out research.
2. *Competence*: The maintenance of high standards of professional competence is responsibility of all psychiatrists in the interest of both the public and the profession. Psychiatrist are responsible for their own continuing education and should realize that their must be a life-time learning.

   As member of the profession, they will not violate ethical standards and when such violation comes to their notice, will take steps to correct it.
3. *Benevolence*: The interest of the patient and his health will stand paramount with them in their professional practices. Personal interest would find, but a secondary place. Financial arrangements will never contravene professional standards. Psychiatrists will always safeguard the interests of the patient and the profession.
4. *Moral standards*: They will at all times be responsive to the moral codes and expectations of the community they serve and will not let their behaviour in any way malign their profession.
5. *Patient's welfare*: They will not treat a case that does not clearly fall within their competence. The ones they accept, they will treat with the best of their ability and with the highest regards for the patient's integrity and welfare as also that of the communities in which they work.

   They will terminate the clinical or consulting relationship with the patient when it is reasonably clear to them that the patient is no longer benefiting from it.

   In case of referral, they will continue to feel responsible for the patient's welfare until the responsibility has been formally transferred.
6. *Confidentiality:* They will safeguard information about a patient that they have obtained in the course of their clinical work, teaching or research in order to safeguard the patient's interest and protect him from social stigma, discrimination and harm. They will treat this as a primary obligation and not

reveal unto others any such information unless certain ethical conditions are met or when there is clear and imminent danger to an individual or society and then only to the appropriate authorities or concerned coorporate-professionals. Confidentiality of the clinical records will be meticulously guarded and identity of the patients will not be revealed even in scientific communication. No data about the patient shall be ordinarily revealed to any agency without the consent of the patient or his family.

Recommendations

1. Every person who has attained the age of majority and who does not appear to have lost the ability of reason shall be assumed to be capable of giving consent.
   A patient should be taken up for medical evaluation and treatment with his consent. In case a patient because of his mental illness is unable to express valid consent, the psychiatrist may undertake to treat him with the consent of a person close to him who appears to be clearly interested in the welfare of the patient. The only exception to treating without consent would be in an emergency situation involving an immediate threat to the life or health of patient or others. For purpose of research, the consent shall be obtained on the lines indicated above after satisfying the following:
   a. The consent is entirely voluntary.
   b. The patient can withdraw the consent at any stage.
   c. Withdrawal of the consent shall not affect the interest of the patient.
2. The decision to hospitalize a patient will essentially rest on the consideration of his welfare and will also take into consideration legal and administrative constraints as well as its social appropriateness.
3. Psychiatric treatments shall be initiated only on clinical considerations and shall be in accordance with scientific knowledge and professional ethics. The patient's welfare should be the primary factor determining the choice of the treatment modality. Should the specific modality not fall within the competence of a psychiatrist he should refer the patient to a competent colleague. The termination of therapy also shall be determined on clinical consideration. Treatment should not be permitted to continue unjustifiably or for material consideration.
   All treatment should be humane and never punitive. No psychiatrist shall refuse to treat in an emergency.
4. Gifts and gratifications from patients under treatment should not be accepted.
5. Any kind of sexual advance towards any patients is unethical.
6. In case of doubt or in situations where unconventional treatment procedures are contemplated, a second opinion must be obtained.
7. It is unethical to force a contract upon a patient during treatment.
8. Even when a patient has been referred by a legal or administrative authority or by the employer, welfare of the patients will remain of paramount

consideration. The patient should be informed of the purpose of which he is to be examined.

9. Basic human rights of the mentally retarded should not be subjected to unethical abridgement. Due ethical discretion should be exercised when advising such procedures as sterilization.
10. In this interest of the patient and society, drug abusers who refuse to give consent may be treated with consent of their relatives. Effort has to be made to motivate them for accepting treatment voluntarily.

These ethical codes have to be implemented with sincerity. It is proposed that ethical committees may be formed at central and zone level. These committees should consider complaints either from public or from fellow professionals and then carefully investigate them.

BASIC PRINCIPLES OF MEDICAL ETHICS

Principle	*Description*
Beneficence	Applying one's abilities solely for the patient's well-being
Non-malfeasance	Avoiding harm to a patient
Autonomy	Respect for a patient's independence
Justice	Avoiding prejudicial bias based on idiosyncrasies of the patient's background, behavior, or station in life
Confidentiality	Respect for the patient's privacy
Veracity	Truthfulness with oneself and one's patients

ETHICAL PRINCIPLES FOR PSYCHIATRISTS

Principle	*Annotations*
Competent care	The psychiatrist must scrutinize the effect of his/her conduct on the boundaries of the treatment relationship
Honest dealing	Sex with a current or former patient is unethical. Information given by patients should not be exploited. Contractual arrangements should be explicit. Fee splitting is unethical

CONFIDENTIALITY

Restraint in release of information to third parties. Respecting colleagues adequate disguise of case presentations, disclosure of lack of confidentiality in non treatment situations. Sex with students or supervisees may be unethical.

Informed Consent

The history of the doctrine consent begin with the ruling of Justice Cordoza in New York in 1914, when volunteric consent became a legal requisite and its absence constituted grounds for punishment. The term informed consent was unheard of till 1957 when in a legal case in California, the court ruled that adequate information is required before consent can be obtained for any procedure. Informed consent became necessary in the practice of psychiatry from the early 1960s when legislation for electroconvulsive therapy was enacted by the 1970s, statutes had been enacted in the USA granting event involuntarily committed psychiatric patients, the right to refuse treatment including medication. (Roth, 1986).

The acceptance of patients for the treatment they receive is a cornerstone of medical practice. Before a patient can be given any form of treatment whether for a mental disorder or for a physical condition, valid consent is required. This is sometimes called real or informed consent.

Definition

The voluntary and continuing permission of the patient to receive a particular treatment based on an adequate knowledge of the purpose, nature, likely effects and risks of that treatment including the likelihood of its success and any alternatives to it.

Permission given under any unfair or undue pressure is not consent.

Informed consent is a legal theory in medical malpractice. It provides a patient with a cause of action for not being adequately informed about the nature and consequences of a particular medical treatment or procedures undertaken. This theory is founded on two distinct legal principles.

The first is the right of every patient to determine what will or will not be done to his or her body often referred to as the right of self determination.

The second principle emanates from the fiduciary nature of the doctor patient relationship.

When a patient gives informed consent to medical treatment, it means that the patient is knowing, competent, and voluntary. The physician must explain the treatment so that the patient understands its indications, risks, benefits, and alternative treatment. It is presumed that adult patients are competent to make such decisions for them. Although, only a judge can declare a patient incompetent, physicians often assess a patient's ability to make informed decisions about health care. The capacity is termed clinical competency or medical capacity.

REQUIREMENTS OF CONSENT

The doctrine of informed consent could be restarted as the doctrine of informed decision making leading to informed consent or informed refusal. The minimum standards of informed consent should include the following: (Dyer, 1988)

1. A fair explanation of procedures or treatment.
2. A description of expected benefits.
3. Disclosure of alternative procedures and their attendant risk, discomforts, and side effects.

4. Assurances that the person is free to withdraw consent and discontinue participation in the project or activity.
5. A statement that withdrawal will not result in loss of benefits to prejudice treatment.
6. The likely consequences of a failure to be treated at all.
7. An offer to answer any queries.

THE PRINCIPLES RELATING TO CONSENT LAID DOWN BY SUPREME COURT IN 2008

- A doctor has to seek and secure the consent of the patient before commencing a treatment.
- The consent so obtained should be real and valid, should be voluntary, and should be on the basis of adequate information concerning the nature of the treatment procedure.
- The adequate information "to be furnished by the doctor should enable the patient to make a balanced judgment as to whether he should submit himself to the particular treatment or not.
- Consent given only for a diagnostic procedure, cannot be considered as consent for therapeutic treatment.
- There can be a common consent for diagnostic or therapeutic procedures where they are contemplated.
- The nature and extent of information to be furnished by the doctor to the patient to secure the consent need not be of the stringent and high-degree (Supreme Court Judgment in the case of Samira Kohli versus Dr Prabha Manchanda, 2008).

SUGGESTED PRECAUTIONS TO GET INFORMED CONSENT

1. Do not take consent from relatives or attendants except in the emergencies or incompetent patient.
2. Discuss and explain the patients the possibility of additional problems which may come to light during a procedure when the patient is unconscious or otherwise unable to make a decision.
3. Take a consent to treat any problems that may arise and ascertain whether there are any procedures to which the patient would object or prefer to give further thought before you proceed.
4. Do not exceed the procedure to which consent has been given no matter how strong the temptation is.

The three essential elements to the doctrine of informed consent are:

- Competency
- Information
- Voluntariness

Competency

It is clinically useful to distinguish the terms incompetence and incapacity. Incompetence refers to court adjudication, whereas incapacity indicates a functional inability as determined by a clinician. (Mishkin,1989). Legally, only competent persons may give informed consent. An adult patient is considered legally competent unless adjudicated incompetent or temporarily incapacitated because of a medical emergency. Incapacity does not prevent treatment. It merely requires the clinician to obtain substitute consent. Treating an incompetent patient without substituted consent is the same as treating a competent patient against his or her will. Legal competence is narrowly defined in terms of cognitive capacity without taking into account of emotional and other behavioral aspects.

Competency is not a scientifically determinable state and is situation specific. The issue of competency arises in a number of civil, criminal and family law contexts.

The following four standards for determining incompetence were suggested:

- Communication of choice.
- Understanding of relevant information provided.
- Appreciation of available options and consequence.
- Rational decision making.

A valid consent can be either expressed (oral or in writing) or implied from the patient's action.

Information

A doctor is expected to convey all appropriate information in terms that the average patient would understand. Although, there exists no consistently accepted set of information to be disclosed for any given medical or psychiatric situation, as a rule of thumb, five areas of information are generally provided.

Diagnosis	Description of the condition or problem.
Treatment	Nature and purpose of proposed treatment.
Consequences	Risks and benefits of the proposed treatment.
Alternatives	Viable alternatives to the proposed treatment including risks and benefits.
Prognosis	Projected outcome with and without treatment.

Voluntariness

For consent to be considered legally voluntary, it must be given freely by the patients and without presence of any form of coercion, fraud, are duress that impinges on the patient's decision making process.

THERE ARE THREE SITUATIONS WHERE IT IS PERMISSIBLE TO GIVE TREATMENT WITHOUT CONSENT UNDER COMMON LAW IN UK

1. To an unconscious patient to save life, or prevent serious harm unless there is clear evidence that the patient did not want that treatment.
2. To a non-consenting mentally disordered patient to prevent behaviour causing serious danger to himself or other, e.g. an assultative psychotic patient may be given medication to prevent a serious escalation of violence.

3. To "incompetent" patients likely to be informal patients with a learning disability, organic brain disorder or severe depression.

THE COMMON CONSENT OPTIONS FOR PATIENTS LACKING THE MENTAL CAPACITY FOR HEALTH CARE DECISIONS

- Proxy consent of next of kin.
- Adjudication of incompetence, appointment of a guardian.
- Institutional administrators or committees.
- Treatment review panel.
- Substituted consent of the court.
- Advance directing (living will, durable power of attorney, and health care proxy).
- Statutory surrogates (spouse or court—appointed guardian).

INFORMED CONSENT—INDIAN SCENARIO

In India, most psychiatrist consider the right of treatment as their right and prefer to be the sole authority to decide the treatment of their choice rather than the patient choosing or refusing certain types of treatment. In the West, it has been observed now that a patient who is competent to make treatment choice cannot be treated by psychotropics or other treatment methods against his will except in emergency situations.

The right to refuse treatment is unheard of in this country. Yet there are instances when the patients or their relatives explicitly direct the psychiatrist against the use of ECT largely because of ignorance and the prevalent negative attitude against shock treatment. (Sayeed Akthur, 1998)

The concept of informed consent is not much understood by the patients as well as by the psychiatrist in India.

How often our patients informed of their rights at the time of hospitalization?

How many of our patients are told of the risks and benefits of psychotropic drugs and ECT?

How many of our patients know about the dreaded side effect—tardive dyskinesia?

In India, the "Ideology of Entitlement" is yet to be conceptualized. In India, even though, we do not get informed consent for the routine treatment, it is very much essential to get informed consent in the following situations:

1. Admission of a person to a psychiatric hospital on a voluntary basis
2. Procedures like ECT, psychosurgery and other invasive investigatory procedures like lumbar puncture, sphenoidal EEG, etc
3. Pentothal analyis (narco-analysis)
4. Drug treatment like disulfiram therapy and clozapine therapy
5. Administration of any research drugs (Drug trials)
6. Before screening an individual for HIV.

The Mental Health Act, 1987 mentions about the patient's or the guardian's consent for the purpose of research. This is found in Chapter 8, which deals with human rights. It is the right of patients to be informed and to know the purpose of the research and risks and benefits associated with it.

In India, many psychiatric patients may be influenced in the discussion making by one of the following factors:

- The patient is not accepting that he is suffering from any psychiatric illness; hence, there is no question of consent for treatment.
- Others feel that they have psychological problem but they need to control it themselves and no treatment can solve their problems.
- Some people have that problem, but they think the problems are supernatural in origin and thus appropriate treatment would be religious and magical.
- Some others may have prejudice against psychiatric drugs, ECT, but may not agree to give consent.
- Informed consent is "consent given voluntarily by a competent individual who has received the necessary information, has adequately understood the information and after considering the information, has arrived at a decision without having been subjected to coercion, undue influence or inducement, or intimidation".
- Informed consent is based on the principle that competent individuals are entitled to choose freely whether to participate in research or not and protects that individual's freedom of choice and respect for the individual's autonomy. It also protects the subjects' rights.
- Taking informed consent is a process and does not merely consist of a signature on the consent form. Informed consent is a communication process between the researcher and the participant and starts before the research is initiated and continues throughout the duration of the study. The investigator or his delegate must discuss all pertinent aspects of the study, answer any queries/ doubts, request consent and then if freely given, document it. The ultimate responsibility is the investigator's.
- Informed consent includes a verbal description and discussion of the details of the study including the process of randomization, the components of the study, and other details mentioned in Schedule Y and the ICMR guidelines, as well as a written information sheet containing all relevant information in simple, non-technical language in the participant's vernacular and given to the participant to keep. Adequate time must be provided for the participant to decide on participation. A separate informed consent form must be used to document consent.
- In case of illiterate participant, a witness is crucial and thumb impressions are allowed. All signatures should be dated and in case a date is forgotten on the day the consent is taken, it must be retaken on the next visit and dated, with a clear explanation, which is documented in the source document.
- The investigator must not date the consent at any point in time; this must be done by the witness in the case of illiterate participants.

- In the case of minors, proxy consent from a parent/responsible guardian is permitted and only the parent/responsible guardian may sign the informed consent form. However, it is mandatory that the minor provides assent (permission) to participate and if possible, this should be recorded in a separate assent form.
- If the participant is incompetent to provide valid informed consent and it is deemed ethically justified to include this person in research, then the proxy consent of a responsible family member/legal guardian and a witness must be taken. There should be an independent verification of the validity of the consent given.
- Each subject (or their representative) must be given a copy of the signed consent form. The original consent form should be filed in such a manner as to insure immediate retrieval when required by auditing entities, IRB, or sponsor monitors.
- Written documentation of informed consent is required. Therefore, obtaining consent from an authorized third party via the telephone is not acceptable.
- Obtaining informed consent from subjects must be accomplished prior to performing the research activity and using only and IRB/EC approved consent form. Written request for amendments to an existing consent form must be approved by the IRB/ECT Prior to implementation.

When an informed consent form to be signed by the patient in order to meet legal requirements, both the clinician and patient experience it as little more than a manipulation: clinical utility is absent and its legal value is dubious. On the other hand, when we understand that the criterion for informed consent derives meaning from a two-person process, the criteria can help build the doctor-patient alliance.

Quality care and the informed consent process are the wheel and axle of the vehicle of psychiatric inpatient diagnosis and treatment. The inpatient psychiatrist is legally mandated to obtain and document informed consent before administering all diagnostic and treatment interventions.

The doctrine of informed consent has been described as the cornerstone of a patient's anatomy. The role of the patient has been changed from that of a trusting and ardent follower of medical advice to that of an equal partner with the physician. This fact has to be kept in mind for today's and tomorrows psychiatric practice in India.

Confidentiality

"What I may see or hear in the course of treatment or even outside of the treatment in regard to the life of men which on no account must spread abroad, I will keep it to myself, holding such things shameful to me spoken about".

—Hippocratic Oath

Confidentiality refers to the right of an individual not to have communications that were important in confidence revealed to the third parties. It is derivative of *The broad right to privacy which guards against a variety of intrusions of an individual's freedom from unwanted attention.* The subtle of confidentiality, those within the circle may share patient's information, "those outside the circle require the patient's permission to receive the information."

Patients have a right to expect that whatever they tell their doctor will be held in confidence. However, modern medical practice, in which increasing numbers of health professionals are involved in treatment can threaten confidentiality. This is a particular problem in psychiatric practice where multidisciplinary care is the norm.

In UK, the General Medical Council (GMC, 1993) gives guidelines on professional confidence. This states that doctors must not disclose information about a patient obtained in a professional capacity to any third party even after the death of the patient. There are some exceptions to this. They are:

1. The patient or his legal advisor gives valid consent.
2. It is undesirable on medical grounds to seek the patient's consent, information may be given to a relative or other person.
3. The information is required by law.
4. In exceptional situations, disclosure in the public interest, e.g. where the patient or someone else would be at risk of death or serious harm.
5. For medical research, where this has been approved by a recognized ethics committee.

A doctor should always be prepared to justify the decision to disclose confidential information. When in doubt, it is sensible to discuss the matter with an experienced colleague or to seek advice from a professional body. It is good practice to obtain a patient's written consent to disclosure. The patient must be told exactly what will be disclosed and under what circumstances.

Confidentiality and privilege have specialized and distinct legal meanings. Confidentiality, in the context of a psychiatrist-patient relationship refers to the right of patients, to have their communications with the psychiatrist not be disclosed to outside parties without authorization and the correlative duty of a psychiatrist to ensure that those communications are not disclosed. In general issues of confidentiality arise outside of the court room or with the investigating police. Confidentiality is the privacy created typically by State Law that governs the psychiatrist-patient relationship.

Testimonial privilege issues arise inside the court room. When it applies, privilege operates as a limitation on the power of the court to compel a psychiatrist to disclose communications between psychiatrist and patient cloaked by the privilege. In India, as it is elsewhere this privilege communication is only a relative one. In cases, where the interest of the individual or of the society is of greater importance, this privilege may be ignored. The individual may waive it or judiciary may order the disclosure.

In one case, a patient had expressed his decision to kill his girl friend to a therapist, and the girl was not forewarned. The girl was actually murdered subsequently. It was held that the threat should have been informed to the potential victim and defense of professional confidentiality was not valid. Psychiatrists should have a working familiarity with the relevant statutes, rules, and cases law in their country that governs confidentiality and disclosure. The American Psychiatrist's Association's (APA, 1987) guidelines of confidentiality are explicit concerning disclosure of information by a psychiatrist. Following are the examples of statutory disclosure requirements:

- Physical evidence or suspicion of child abuse.
- Initiation of involuntary hospitalization.
- "Duty to Warn" endangered third parties or law enforcement agencies.
- Commission of a treasonous Act.
- Intention to commit a future crime.
- HIV infection.

The APA guidelines on confidentiality spell out some strict principles, e.g. confidentiality is essential to psychiatric treatment. A psychiatrist may release confidential information only with the authorization of the patient or under proper legal compulsion and

Ethically the psychiatrist may disclose only that the information which his relevant to a given situation. He/She should avoid offering speculation as fact. Sensitive information such as an individual's sexual orientation or fantasy material is usually unnecessary.

The issue of confidentiality in psychiatric practice has two fundamental components:

1. A patient has a right to privacy that should not be violated except in certain prescribed circumstances.
2. The health professionals are duty bound to maintain the confidence of their patients.

The concept of confidentiality, in case of the mentally ill has different connotations, in day-to-day practice and in relation to the patient's family, employees, and a delicate balance needs to be maintained in matter pertaining to disclosure of confidentiality about the mental illness of affected person.

The concept of confidentiality is basically an ethical issue. Every professional body of health professionals expects their members to maintain confidentiality. Another view is that there is an implied contract between the patient and the health professional that the later will maintain the confidence reposed by the former. Thus confidentiality is more than ethical and legal issue. The duty to safeguard closely the confidentiality of any communication that transpires in the course of psychiatric treatment is the cornerstone of the profession. This obligation of confidentiality is a fundamental concern of all the mental health professionals.

Recommendations

1. Therapist should maintain confidentiality.
2. Therapist can release the confidential information without patient consent which requires mandatory reporting by the law.
3. The information collected in the professional relationship must be submitted as evidence in a legal proceeding.

4. Therapist can breach the confidentiality if the client threatened the therapist for his life or files a case against the therapist.
5. For situations which require interpretation of law, therapist should seek legal advice.

CONFIDENTIALITY IN PSYCHOTHERAPY

In contrast to routine clinical practice, psychotherapy should be considered as a special situation especially in our setting, where there is no much distinction between psychotherapist per se and psychiatrist. Whenever a client approaches a psychiatrist and if he thinks that psychotherapy could be an appropriate treatment modality, or if the client requests for psychotherapy in the light of his competence, the therapist should obtain informed consent. This should include providing information to the client as to what is psychotherapy, what is expected out of the patient, what is expected from the therapist, what are the limitations of the therapy and therapist, fees involved, alternative modalities of treatment along with efficacy of each in condition which the client is suffering from. After an informed consent is obtained the therapist along with the client should draw a therapeutic contract with do's and don'ts for either of them. Through out the therapy and during drawing the therapeutic contract, therapist should be aware of confidentiality issues. Similarly therapist should be aware of the boundaries and boundary violations and try to work in the limits of the boundaries. However, it should be in congenial environment, with the scope for the client to seek treatment again if he desires so, or an opportunity to be referred to someone else.

The Indian Council of Medical Research Guidelines (ICMR, 2006)

The investigator must safeguard the confidentiality of research data, which might lead to the identification of the individual participants. Data of individual participants can be disclosed under the following circumstances.

- Only in a Court of Law under the orders of the presiding judge or
- There is threat to a person's life or
- In cases of severe adverse reaction may be required to communicate to Drug Registration Authority or
- If there is risk to public health, it takes precedence over personal right to privacy and may have to be communicated to Health Authority.

Therefore, the limitations in maintaining the confidentiality of data should be anticipated and assessed and communicated to appropriate individuals or authorities as the case may be."

"Confidentiality refers to the right of an individual not to have communications that were important in confidence revealed to third parties". It is derivative of *The broad right to privacy which guards against a variety of intrusions of an individuals freedom from unwanted attention.*

The subtle of confidentiality, those within the circle may share patient information; those outside the circle require the patient's permission to receive the information (Figure 3.1).

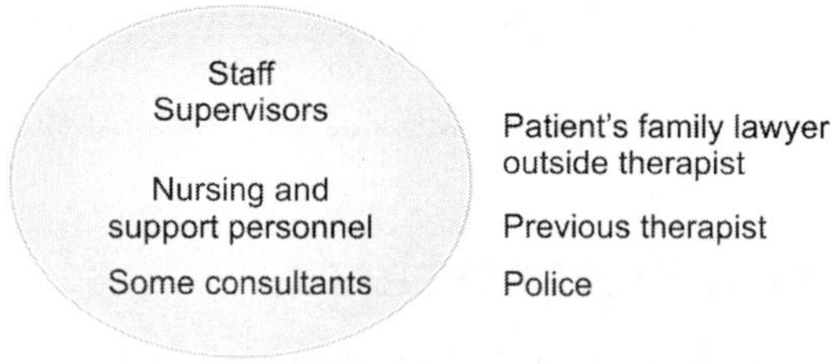

Figure 3.1: The Subtle of confidentiality

A. CHECK LIST FOR RELEASE OF INFORMATION TO THIRD PARTIES

1. Explore reason for request.
2. Determine extent of disclosure required.
3. Be certain that patient understand potential implications of data release.
4. Obtain written consent for disclosure, compliant with the HIPAA standards, if applicable.
   - Should specify the content of the material to be disclosed, e.g. history of outpatient treatment since 1995 or lifetime medication history.
   - Should be renewed for each subsequent disclosure.
5. Organize material to be released.
   - Whenever possible communicate in writing, not over the telephone
   - Reveal minimum necessary data
   - Stick to facts and first hand knowledge
   - Avoid psychodynamic material
   - Write letter as if patient will read it-patients often do.
6. Whenever possible, review letter with patient before it is sent.
7. When patient request falsification or omission:
   - Derive stance from incorruptibility
   - Side with healthier part of patient's ego
   - Discuss issues thoroughly with patient.

B. CHECKLIST FOR RELEASE OF INFORMATION WITHOUT PATIENT'S CONSENT

1. Determine if one of usual exceptions apply, including:
   a. Clearly acting in emergency situation and in patient's best interest.
   b. Patient incompetent and substitute consent not available.
   c. Patient incompetent and substitute consent obtained.
   d. Acting to hospitalize or commit patient.
   e. Acting to protect third parties.
   f. Required to report data by State Law.
   g. Sharing data will collaborative caregivers or supervisors.
2. Document efforts to obtain patient's consent and existence of exception.

3. Alert patient that information is to be released.
   a. Discuss basis for decision.
   b. Discuss impact on therapeutic alliance.
4. Reveal minimum necessary data, in writing if possible.
5. Repair alliance afterwards, focusing on how situation evolved and patient's feelings about it.

C. CHECKLIST FOR RELEASE OF INFORMATION FROM PATIENT'S RECORD TO THE PATIENT

1. Explore reasons for request.
   a. Identify fantasies.
   b. Be alert for delusional basis.
2. Determine whether one of the exceptions under HIPAA applies.
   a. Likely to endanger life or physical safety of patient or others.
   b. Information in record about third party and release likely to cause that person substantial harm.
3. Prepare patient for impact of disclosure.
   a. Discuss confusing, technical, or seemingly pejorative terms.
   b. Discuss possible impact on ongoing therapy.
4. Whenever possible, go over records together with the patient.
5. Use material revealed to advance therapy.
   a. Use as means of integrating past experience.
   b. Explore effect of fantasies confirmed or denied.
6. Do not alter or destroy records before patient sees them—potential legal liability.

D. CHECKLIST FOR REVELATION OF INFORMATION IN COURT PROCEEDINGS

1. If request is from patient, no privilege applies—handle as in checklist C, above.
2. If request is from party opposing patient, determine laws governing privilege in your locale.
   a. If no patient-doctor or patient-psychotherapist privilege exists, handle as in checklist B-3, B-4, and B-5.
   b. If privilege exists, determine if this case constitutes an exception or not.
3. When subpoena arrives, remember that it mandates your appearance only judge must still decide if privilege exists.
4. Consult with lawyer requesting subpoena to see what information is desired.
5. Notify patient and patient's lawyer of arrival of subpoena, giving them a chance to challenge it.
6. Consultation with your own lawyer may be useful.
7. If your testimony is inevitable, follow checklist C-3 through C-6.

NEGLIGENCE IN MEDICAL PRACTICE

Recently three doctors in Chennai city were arrested for alleged negligence. The news of arrest of the doctors appears to have agitated the minds of the medical practitioners creating apprehensions about the far reaching of implications of the event. Of course, the guilty should be punished, but there should not be indiscriminate condemnation of the profession as a whole. There is a feeling of insecurity generated among the medical practitioners in the recent day.

Doctors have several ethical, moral, and legal obligations in the performance of their duties. It is very important therefore that every doctor understands the nature of these obligations and then fulfills them. Further, all doctors should know about medical legal cases and the procedures to be adopted in them.

Lapses (advertent or inadvertent) committed by doctors give rise to legal liabilities. This may be either a criminal liability or a civil liability. Criminal liability arises when it is proved that doctors has committed an Act or made any omission which causes the patients death. Then under section 304 A of IPC, the doctor is punishable. Section 304A of IPC is a bailable offence. Civil liability arises in case of medical service rendered on payment of a fee, under section 73 and 74 of Indian Contract Act.

Negligence in medical practice is the breach of duty owed by a doctor to a patient to exercise reasonable care, resulting in some bodily, mental and in-turn some financial disability. Not doing what is requested to be done (Act of Omission) and doing what is prohibited to be done (Act of Commission) amount to negligence. To prove negligence it must be established that—

1. Doctor owed a duty of care to the patients.
2. The patient suffered damage as a result.
3. If no damage occurred to the patient, it is not considered to be negligence. Also, an error of judgment does not account to negligence.

The most important element in a case of negligence is that the patient must prove beyond doubt that the omission or by the physician was the direct cause of the harm.

A doctor has the following defenses against negligence:

1. Actual denial of negligence having taken place.
2. Delegation of duty for subordinate.
3. Contributory negligence by the patient.
4. Assumption of the risk of the patient.
5. Emergency of the situation.
6. A wrong that is independent of the contract (Tortfeasor).
7. A complete case cannot be tried again. (Res Judicata)

WAYS TO PREVENT NEGLIGENCE

Most negligence cases are due to very causes hence, medical practitioners should take precautions against these pitfalls.

1. Updating the knowledge through continuing medical education programme.
2. Maintain accurate and complete case records.
3. Obtain informed consent.
4. Guard against therapeutic hazards.
5. Practice with reasonable skill and care.
6. Never criticize another doctor.
7. It is advisable to have medical indemnity insurance.

In the wake of various litigations against doctors, they are forced to indulge in defensive practice. Hence, when they want to protect themselves, they should have a sound knowledge of the negligence in medical practice and way to rectify them.

A. CHECK LIST FOR PREVENTING NEGLIGENCE AND MALPRACTICE

1. Behavioral Approaches:
   a. Refrain from unprofessional behavior.
   b. Avoid exploitation of patient (sexual, financial, and dependent) and boundary violations.
   c. Maintain "open door" policy to avoid abandonment; send letters (with copies) signaling cessation of treatment, cancellation of time slot.
   d. Treat patients within area of competence; refer others.
2. Technical Approaches:
   a. Establish a clear treatment contract.
   b. Acknowledge limitations and avoid statements implying promises.
   c. Exercise care regarding informed consent and its documentation; remember memory loss from ECT as a factor and renegotiate information about medication at point of clinical stabilization or discharge form hospital (See Section E below).
   d. Maintain a position of therapeutic disinterested impartiality; resist giving premature advice.
   e. For legalistic acting out:
      - Remain calm
      - Avoid struggle in the legal arena
      - Actively confront and interpret clinically
      - Extract maximum therapeutic benefit from the event
      - Reach out to victims and affected parties in suicide or homicide; consider attending funeral.
3. Documentation Approaches:
   a. Record factual details, especially forensically sensitive events, e.g. emergencies.
   b. Describe in detail the basics for clinical judgment, especially in sensitive areas.
   c. Think out loud for the record, especially for calculated risks and indications for non-routine interventions.

   d. Anticipate forensically significant events, (e.g. commitments, possible suits) and write record with clarity from viewpoint of future readers.
   e. Maintain a professional tone throughout record.
   f. Correct errors and omissions in transparent, current-time manner.
4. Consultative approaches: Participate in peer review, private review, private supervision, retrospective review; seek specific colleagues, advice in complex, risky, or unusual areas.

B. CHECKLIST FOR RESPONDING TO CHARGES OF NEGLIGENCE AND MALPRACTICE

1. Maintain calm and perspective under an aggressive approach of attorneys; resist dynamic formulation of suit at outset.
2. Obtain legal advice.
   - Use collaborative approach with attorney.
   - Inform attorney with absolute candor of all relevant data, including uncertainties, ambiguities, and omissions.
   - Assist attorney in selection of expert witnesses; weight witnesses' renown and experience, personal knowledge of patient or clinician (or both), and similar theoretical viewpoint.
   - Surrender only requested records and only through your attorney.
   - Avoid discussions with plaintiff's attorney; refer to your attorney.
   - Never alter the existing record.

CHECKLIST FOR TREATING PATIENTS DURING LITIGATION

1. Avoid increasing caseload or administrative responsibilities, if possible.
2. Avoid electively treating patient suing you.
3. If inevitable:
   - Obtain consultation actively.
   - Attempt transfer to alternative facility.
   - Remain alert for inevitable counter transference difficulties.
   - General—
     – Avoid seeing the patient as enemy
     – Remain the clinician
     – Use record for clinical and risk management purposes only.

CHECKLIST FOR OBTAINING INFORMED CONSENT

1. Provide sufficient information concerning
   - Nature of procedure or treatment
   - Risks and benefits of procedure or treatment
   - Risks and benefits of alternatives
   - Risks and benefits of no treatment.
2. Simplify language so that laypersons can understand.
3. Offer opportunity to ask questions.

4. Test patient's understanding after process is completed.
5. Reeducate as needed according to gaps in knowledge detected by testing.
6. Consider presence of factors that might impair voluntariness of consent.
7. Assess patient's competence to offer consent (see Chapter 5, Action Guide).
8. Document all relevant factors.
   - Patient's consent, either by patient's signature or clinician's note in chart
   - Material disclosed
   - Patient's understanding
   - Voluntariness and competence.

GUIDELINES FOR SECLUSION AND RESTRAINT OF MENTALLY ILL PERSONS

Nature of mental illness may make a person deny and make him inaccessible for treatment. These situations at times can be detrimental to the safety of patient and others. Mentally ill patients have the right to refuse treatment and/or transport if they are of legal age and are competent. Competence is defined as the capacity or ability to understand the nature and effects of one's acts or decisions. A person is considered to be competent until proven otherwise. There are situations, however, in which the interests of the general public outweigh an individual's right to liberty:

1. The mentally ill person is likely to commit self-harm or suicide.
2. The mentally ill person poses a threat to the community because of his dangerousness due to the mental illness.
3. The mentally ill person presents a specific threat to innocent third parties.

Certain medical, traumatic and psychological conditions can cause incompetence and behavior that interferes with the ability of hospital personnel to care for the patient or that threatens the physical well-being and safety of the patient or others. In the above-mentioned conditions, the hospital personnel may be authorized the use, if reasonable force upon or toward the person of another without the other's consent. Verbal threats are a legitimate reason for restraint. The following is a guideline for the use of seclusion and restraints in the hospital care setting.

Indications for Seclusion and Restraint

- Behavior or threats that create or imply danger to the patient or others.
- Safe and uncontrolled access for medical procedures.
- Involuntary evaluation or treatment of incompetent.

Procedure for Seclusion

1. Seclusion should always be resorted only with the permission of the psychiatrist or medical officer.
2. Reason for seclusion should be recorded in the case sheet of the patient.

3. As far as possible, seclusion and restraint should not be practiced together. If practiced, the patients should be continuously monitored by the staff members.
4. Seclusion cannot be indefinite. The patients should be reviewed on daily basis and should be removed from seclusion at the earliest sign of improvement.
5. Secluded patients should be constantly monitored by the staff nurse and attendant. Staff nurse should monitor and check the patient at least once an hour, where as concerned attendant should check the patient every half an hour.

Procedure for Restraint

1. Care should be taken not to aggravate or worsen pre-existing injuries or medical conditions.
2. Attempt to control the patient with verbal counseling should be tried first.
3. The least restrictive means of control should be employed. Preferably by delirium sheets or securing the limbs with restraining pads.
4. Only "reasonable force" may be used when applying physical control. This is generally defined as the use of force equal to, or minimally greater than, the amount of force being exerted by the resisting patient.
5. Restraints should not interfere with the assessment or treatment of the patient.
6. The decisions to restrain a patient should be endorsed by a psychiatrist or medical officer on duty.
7. Do not remove restraints once applied, unless the patient becomes quiet and calm. If blood circulation becomes compromised, the benefit of removing the restraints must be weighed against crew safety.
8. Restraints should be individualized and accord as much to the patient as the situations allows. Attempt to accommodate patient comfort or special needs whenever possible.
9. Ensure that enough help is available to insure patient and provider safety during the restraint process; optimally, five people should be available to apply full body restraint (one for each limb and one for restraint application). Communicate the restraint plan to all the persons involved in the process.
10. Assure that the patient's clothing and personal belongings have been searched for weapons.
11. Whatever method used for restraining the patients, it should be ensured that normal blood circulation is maintained, no abrasions are caused due to restraining methods and patient's basic needs like feeding, and drinking water, bowel and bladder movements should be attended.
12. The restrain should not be practiced indefinitely. The patients should be continuously monitored and restrain should be removed as the earliest sign of improvement.

Pediatric Considerations

Always make efforts to involve the parents when restraining children.

Pregnancy Considerations

Pregnant women should be restrained in a semi-reclining or left lateral recumbent position.

Precautions

1. Be aware of items at the place or medical equipment that may become a weapon.
2. Make sure that the place is safe before approaching the patient.
3. Patients that are actively throwing convulsion should never be restrained.
4. The patients should be restrained in the prone position only as a last resort and only with continuous monitoring.
5. Restraining a patient's hands and feet together behind the patient (hog tying) is not allowed.

Documentation Requirements

1. The need for the seclusions or restrain and the nature of the emergency situation should be recorded in the case sheet.
2. The need for treatment should be explained to the patient in their language (regardless of competence).
3. The fact that patient refused treatment or was unable to consent to treatment should be mentioned in the case sheet.
4. Evidence of the patient's incompetence to refuse treatment should be made in the case sheet.
5. A note should be made in the case about failure of verbal control in diffusing the situation.
6. Continuously assessment of blood circulation (distal to the restraints) and the patient's ability to breathe should be monitored and mentioned in the case records.

SUGGESTED READING

1. Agarwal AK. Ethics in Psychiatry. Indian Journal of Psychiatry. 1994;36:1-5-11.
2. Agarwal AK, Gupta SC. Ethical issues in Psychiatry. Souvenir of the Annual Conference of Indian Psychiatric Society and World Psychiatric Association held at Jaipur, 1993, 1998.
3. Appelbaum PS. A: Health information infrastructure and the threat to confidentiality of health records. Psychiatric Serv, 1998;49:27-28;33.
4. Appelbaum PS. Privacy in psychiatric treatment: threats and responses. Am J Psychiatry, 2002;159:1809-18.
5. Oyebode F. Clinical Errors and Medical Negligence, Advances in Psychiatric Treatment. 2006;2:22-27.
6. Gautum S, Avasthi A. Forensic Psychiatry, Clinical Practice Guidelines for Psychiatrists in India, published by Indian Psychiatric Society.
7. Gutheil TG. Paranoia and progress notes: A guide to forensically informed psychiatric record keeping. Hosp Community Psychiatry, 1980;31:479-482s.

8. Hand Book of Psychiatry, Bhugra D (ed.), Year 2005.
9. Hippocrates, the 5-4 Century, BC.
10. Journal of Behavioural Sciences. 1992;2(1):3-10.
11. Mathiharan K, Tiphagne H. Resource Materials for doctors and psychiatrits, National Project on Preventing torture in India 2006, published by People's Watch—Tamil Nadu.
12. Medilaw. A Newsletter on Medical Law and Ethics, Year 2002-2, Issue 2.
13. Nagaraja J. Mental Health Limits. Priorities and psychoethics. Presidential Address. Indian J Psychiat, 1983;25(1):3-6.
14. Nambi S. Legal Aspects of Psychiatry—Indian Perspective, 2009, Manashanthi Mental Health Care Publications, 2008.
15. Nambi S. Negligence in Medical Practice, Tanpsycon 97, Indian Psychiatric Society, Tamil Nadu Branch, 12th Annual Conference, 12th and 13th July, 1997.
16. Neki JS. Confidentiality, Secrecy and Privacy in Psychotherapy: Sociodynamic Considerations, Indian Journal. Psychiatry. 1992;34(3):171-73.
17. Rastogi CK. Role of Ethics in Indian Psychiatry, Presidential Address, Indian.
18. Slovenko R. On the need for record-keeping in the practice of psychiatry. J Psychiatry Law, 197;7:399-440.
19. Slovenko R. Psychotherapy and Confidentiality. Springfield, IL: Charles C Thomas 1998.
20. Tharyan P. Ethics committees and clinical trials registration in India: Opportunities, obligations, challenges and solutions. Indian J Med Ethics 2007;4:1689.
21. The Journal of the American Academy of Psychiatry and the Law, 2007;53:3.
22. Thomas G Gutheil, Paul S Applebaum PS. Clinical Handbook of Psychiatry and Law. Lippincott Williams & Wilkins Publications, New Delhi, 2007.
23. Warner JP, King M, Blizard R, et al. Patient-held shared case records for individuals with mental illness. Brit J Psychiatry, 2000;177:319-24.

4 Chapter

Mental Health Legislation in India

EVOLUTION AND EVALUATION OF THE VARIOUS ACTS

Almost every aspect of life in the modern days is regulated or affected in some way by law. All civilizations in the world have enacted laws to regulate human behaviour so that the weakest can live freely and enjoy all his human rights. Legislation forms an important component in the implementation of mental health care. There is a dynamic relationship between the concept of mental illness, the treatment of the mentally ill and the law. "Forensic psychiatry is a poorly defined speciality, with little organised training in most countries."—(WHO Working Group, 1975). A working knowledge of the Mental Health Act, 1987 is essential for all psychiatrists in India.

In the Indian Context, many acts are directly related to mental health. Among them, the Mental Health Act, 1987 is a Major legislation and it has become operational in 1994 in all States of the Indian Union. The Act replaces the Indian Lunacy Act, 1912.

The various enactments controlling the care and treatment of the mentally ill of the British India could be enumerated as follows:

1. The Lunacy (Supreme Courts) Act, 1858 (Act XXXIV of 1858)
2. The Lunacy (District Courts) Act, 1858 (Act XXXV of 1858)
3. The Indian Lunatic Asylums Act, 1858 (Act XXXVI of 1858)
4. The Military Lunatics Act, 1877 (Act XI of 1877)
5. The Indian Lunatic Asylums (Amendment) Act, 1886 (Act XVIII of 1886)
6. The Indian Lunatic Asylums (Amendment) Act, 1889 (Act XX of 1889)
7. Chapter XXXIV of the Code of Criminal Procedure, 1898
8. Section 30 of the Prisoner's Act, 1900.

The first three Acts were enacted immediately after Queen Victoria's proclamation and India came under the rule of the British Crown. In her proclamation, she promised, amongst other things, "By the blessing of providence internal tranquility, it is our earnest desire to stimulate the peaceful industry of India to promote the works of public utility and improvement and to administer the government for the benefit of all subjects." (I presume she had the interests of the mentally ill in India in her mind!)

A short review of the following three Acts including the Mental Health Care Act Draft, 2012 is to be discussed:

1. Indian Lunacy Act, 1912.
2. Mental Health Act, 1987.
3. Mental Health Care Act Draft, 2012.

THE INDIAN LUNACY ACT, 1912

With this British background, the curtain rises in the Viceregal Lodge of Shimla on Monday the 18th September 1911 with Baron Harding of Penshurst presiding over the Council of the Governor-General of India. The honorable Mr Jenkins moved to introduce a bill to consolidate and amend the law relating to Lunacy. He observed, "We propose to consolidate these enactments and to introduce certain amendments and especially to bring the Law in certain important particulars into line with the Modern English Act." The Lunacy Act, 1890 as amended by the Lunacy Act, 1891. The Legislative Department of the Council was complimented for its painstaking labor. He considered that it is more fit for careful examination with regard to all details in the Select Committee, than for general discussions in the Council. The Council met on Wednesday the 10th January 1912, under the presidentship of the hon'ble Sir Guy Fleetwood Wilson and referred the Indian Lunacy Bill to the Select Committee.

EARLY MENTAL HOSPITALS

During the middle ages, a few monasteries harboured lunatics, but it appears that the first asylums for their care were built by the *Moslems*, whose ideas on the treatment of mental patients were derived from Eastern physicians. In Europe, the Bethlem Royal Hospital (the original Bedlam) was first used as an asylum in 1247, the second was opened in 1448 at Valencia in Spain. Further asylums were established in Europe during the following century. In America, the first hospital for insane was opened in Virginia in 1773 (WHO, 1955; Bluglass, 1984). Although, hospitals in India were popular since the time of Ashoka the Great (274–235 BC), the first mental hospital was probably established by Mahmood Khilji (1436–1469) at Dhar near Mandu in Madhya Pradesh and the second one was built in Calcutta in 1787 (Verma, 1953). The first unaided private mental hospital in India was established in Calcutta in 1935 by Kaviraj Atul Behari Dutt.

HIGHLIGHTS OF THE INDIAN LUNACY ACT, 1912

Repealed	The Indian Lunacy Act, 1977 (Jammu and Kashmir Act)
Policy	Not based on any mental health policy or program.
Main objectives	1. Protection of society from the presence of mentally ill persons who have become or might become a danger or nuisance to others.
	2. Protection of the citizens from being detained in psychiatric facilities without sufficient cause.
Mental retardation	Excluded from the purview of the Act (The expression mentally ill person means person suffering from any mental disorder excluding mental retardation).
Psychiatric nursing home and residential home	Included
Board/Authority	Mental Health Authority without any fund established.
Appointment of visitors	Old provision retained and extended to psychiatric nursing home.
Voluntary admission	Formal
Services of magistrates for involuntary admission	Retained except for admission under special circumstances for a period not exceeding 90 days.
Mental health review tribunal	No provision
Rules	Rules u/s 91 (mandatory legal aid to mentally ill persons in Court) not made in any state. Principles of rule of construction not followed.
Forms	No provision for use of forms for orders. All forms mentioned in the Act have not been prescribed, some are inconsistent with the Act.

THE EVOLUTION OF MENTAL HEALTH ACT, 1987

The enactment of Mental Health Act, 1987 is a landmark in the history of care of mentally ill in India. This Act is not simply a cosmetic improvement over the outdated Indian Lunacy Act, 1912, but represents the conclusion of Lengthy persuasion by Indian Psychiatric Society to Government of India.

Establishment of Lunatic asylums was primarily a British concept. The rule and laws relating to mentally ill were much influenced by European ideas and concepts at that time. The British enacted the first Indian Lunacy Act in 1858 in India, which was modified in 1883 the objective was simple.

Insane persons are troublesome and dangerous to the community. Thus asylums were considered as simple places of detention and not for treatment. In early 20th century, there was adverse publicity about the condition of Mental Institutions in India as well as abroad. Due to this awareness, British brought out the Indian Lunacy Act in 1912, (ILA). In early 20th Century, the names of all lunatic asylums were changed to mental hospitals.

Before the Independence of India, "Bhore Committee" was asked to survey mental hospitals in India. The committee recommended that ILA 1912 was outdated and outlived its usefulness. As a follow-up, the Indian Psychiatric Society appointed a three member adhoc committee, consisting eminent psychiatrists of yester years like Dr Roy of Nagpur, Dr RB Davis, and Dr Hasib of Ranchi.

This committee prepared a draft: Indian Mental Health Act. Later repeated attempts were made by IPS to enact new Mental Health Act. The Ministry of Health introduced Mental Health Bill first in 1980 and later in 1981. The Bill was referred to the joint committee of parliament members in 1982. The committee held 22 meetings in various places and submitted its recommendations. But the Lok Sabha was dissolved in 1984. Later, a joint committee was formed in 1985. This suggested some amendments to the original Bill. Finally, the two houses of parliament passed the Bill in 1986. The present Mental Health Act was enacted in May 1987. The Central Government passed orders that this Act would come in force with effect from April 1, 1993 in all the States. The Central and State Mental Health Authority rules were framed in 1990. Thus, such a long and tiresome process was involved in the enactment and implementation of the MHA, 1987.

Definition of Mental Health Act, 1987

"An Act to consolidate and amend the law relating to the treatment and care of mentally ill persons, to make better provision with respect to their property and affairs and for matters connected therewith."

The Objectives of The Mental Health Act, 1987

1. To regulate admission to psychiatric hospital of psychiatric nursing homes, of mentally ill persons who do not have sufficient understanding to seek treatment on a voluntary basis, and to protect the rights of such persons while being detained.
2. To protect society from the presence of mentally ill persons, who has become a danger or nuisance to others.
3. To protect citizens from being detained in psychiatric hospitals or psychiatric nursing homes without sufficient cause.
4. To regulate responsibility for maintenance charges of mentally ill persons who are admitted to psychiatric hospitals or psychiatric nursing homes.
5. To provide facilities for establishing guardianship or custody of mentally ill persons who are incapable of managing their own affairs.
6. To provide for the establishment of Central Authority and State Authority for mental health services.
7. To regulate the powers of the Government for establishing, licensing and controlling psychiatric hospitals and psychiatric nursing homes for mentally ill persons.
8. To provide legal aid to mentally ill persons at State expense in certain cases, Government of India has constituted a Central Mental Health Authority.

Before implementing Mental Health Act in the States, the States have to take action regarding the following:

- Establishment of State Mental Health Authority.
- Spell out guidelines for establishment of private psychiatric hospitals and Nursing Homes.
- Formation of Board of Visitors.

Salient Features of Mental Health Act, 1987

The Mental Health Act, 1987 has 10 chapters in total:

1. *Definitions*: The Mental Health Act, MHA 1987 brings out number of changes based on newer concepts and knowledge in mental health field. It modified certain terms and definitions. The Act uses the term,

ILA	MHA
• Lunatic	Mentally ill person.
• Criminal lunatic	Mentally ill prisoner.
• Asylum	Psychiatric Hospital.

2. *Mental health authorities*: A provision of establishing Mental Health Authorities at centre and state levels have been made for the first time. This will facilitate better implementation and monitoring of various aspects of Mental Health Act, such authorities may also advise the Government on matter related to mental health activities in the country.
3. *Establishment and Maintenance of Psychiatric Hospital and Psychiatric Nursing Homes:* MHA lays down guidelines for establishment and maintenance of psychiatric hospitals and nursing homes. Also, there is a provision for a Licensing Authority, who will process application for licenses. No private Psychiatric hospital or nursing home will be allowed to function without a valid licence, which has to be renewed every 5 years. There is a provision for an Inspecting Officer who will inspect these institutions to prevent irregularities. Mention has been made about the establishment of separate psychiatric hospitals for children, addicts, and psychopaths.
4. *Admission Procedures*: Admission procedures are simplified and more progressive concepts have been incorporated. Medical officer in charge of psychiatric hospitals are given more powers and the powers of judiciary and visiting committee members relating to admission are minimized. The admission procedures are:
   a. Admission on voluntary basis.
      - By the patient
      - By the guardian (for minor)—A new provision.

   b. Admission under special circumstances: (A new provision). Admission of a mentally ill person who does not or is unable to express his willingness for admission may be admitted and kept for maximum 90 days. Admission can be made at the request of a relative or friend of the mentally ill person.

c. Admission through reception orders—
   - Reception order or application:
     – Application can be made by a medical officer or a relative along with medical certificates, on production of mentally ill person before magistrate, a reception order may be issued for admission.
   - Reception order on production of mentally ill person before magistrate. (Admission of a dangerous wandering mentally ill person)

     On production of a wandering mentally ill by the police before the magistrate, a reception order for admission may be made.
   - Further provision regarding admission and detention of mentally ill persons:
     – Admission as inpatient after inquisition
     – Admission of mentally ill prisoners:
       - Convicts (Under section 30 of the Prisoners Act, 1900 (3 of 1900)
       - Undertrial prisoners (Under section 330 of code of criminal procedure, 1973 (2 of 1974)
       - Guilty, but mentally ill (Under section 335 of code of criminal procedure, 1973 (2 of 1974)
   - Admission of military persons:
     — Under Section 144 of Air Force Act, 1950
     — Under Section 145 of Army Act, 1950
     — Under Section 143 and 144 of Navy Act, 1957.

d. Inspection, discharge, leave of absence and removal of mentally ill person: This chapter deals with the formation and functioning of visitors to the psychiatric hospital or nursing home. This chapter deals with procedures for discharge of mentally ill persons admitted in the psychiatric hospital. There is a provision for Leave of Absence for patients admitted under reception orders. The maximum duration of leave of absence is 60 days. The application may be made by the relative or through magistrate.

5. *Judicial Inquisition and Appointment of Guardian and Manager:* Inquisition is an investigation or examination whether the person who is alleged to be mentally ill and incapable of managing his affairs. An application for judicial inquisition may be made by his relatives, public curator (prosecutor), Advocate General of the State or by the District Collector.

   Guardian to be appointed by the court for a mentally ill person who cannot look after himself and his properties. Manager to be appointed for a person who can take care of himself, but unable to manage his properties.

6. *Maintenance of Mentally Ill Persons in a Psychiatric Hospital or Psychiatric Nursing Home:* Chapter VII of MHA, 1987 deals with the liability to meet the cost of maintenance of mentally ill persons detained in hospital or nursing homes by the relatives or by the government.

7. *Protection of Human Rights of Mentally Ill Persons:*
   a. This is a humanitarian approach of MHA, 1987 towards the unfortunate, underprivileged mentally ill persons.
   b. No mentally ill person shall be subjected to any indignity (whether physical or mental) or cruelty during treatment.
   c. No mentally ill person, under treatment, shall be used for the purpose of research unless.
      - Such research is of direct benefit to him
      - A consent has been obtained in writing from the person (if a voluntary patient) or from the guardian/relative (if admitted involuntarily).
   d. No letters or communications sent by or to a mentally ill person shall be intercepted, detained or destroyed.
8. *Penalties and Procedures:* In chapter IX MHA, 1987 deals with penalties and procedures for establishment or maintenance of psychiatric hospital or nursing homes in contravention of the Act.
9. *Miscellaneous:* Here the Act deals with matters not covered in other chapters, like keeping medical report about the patients, etc.

The Positive Qualities of the Mental Health Act, 1987

Mental Health Act, 1987 represents a pleasant departure by incorporating the latest scientific knowledge and social concepts. A modest attempt has also been made to bring mental illnesses at par with physical illnesses thus reducing the stigma attached with the mental illnesses (Sharma, 1991).

1. The definitions in this Act are in a progressive way, e.g. mentally ill persons is one who is in need of treatment by reason of any mental disorder other than mental retardation. Hence, "treatability" is considered as a major criterion. Hence, the Act does not apply to untreatable conditions like mental retardation and dementia.
2. The Act does not apply to general hospitals or general nursing homes which also may provide psychiatric services.
3. The formation of mental health authorities in the centre and state level provides opportunities for monitoring and suggesting improvements in the mental health care of patients.
4. Out patient services should be available at every psychiatric hospital or nursing home—A welcome approach.
5. Admission procedures are simplified and made more convenient to the relatives. A voluntary patient can be admitted or discharged merely on request. Minors can be admitted by the guardians. A relative or a friend can admit a mentally ill person who does not or who is unable to express his willingness under special circumstances. The two medical certificates required can be made by the doctors working in the psychiatric hospital or nursing home. Any private person can report to the magistrate if a mentally ill person is not under proper care. Inclusion of such a provision brings out the role of community for the welfare of the mentally ill.

6. Discharge procedures are made easier. A person admitted through reception order need not be discharged by the visiting committee; on the recommendation of two medical officers the patient may be discharged.
7. Provisions have been made for establishing separate hospitals for those under 16 years, addicts and psychopaths.
8. Due to growing global human right concerns, efforts have been made to safeguard the human rights of the mentally ill person, stringent punishment has also been provided for those who subjects the mentally ill to physical and mental indignity.

Criticism Against Mental Health Act, 1987

1. The notion of a care in the community has not been addressed to in the current legislation. No effort has been made to provide after-care services for the discharged patients. There seem to be no thinking over the alternative to the hospital care. No mention is made about rehabilitation.
2. Psychiatrists running private psychiatric nursing home are facing too many medicolegal problems, difficulties and interference in the administration with regard to:
   a. Getting and renewing licence.
   b. Board of visitor's control over their nursing home.
   c. Consulting a medical board for their day-to-day hospital procedure like issuing certificates for admission, discharge, and leave of absence, etc.
   d. Inspecting officer can unnecessarily intervene the functioning of the hospital.
3. Patients examined by psychiatrists and admitted in a psychiatric nursing home should not be compelled to undergo further examination by medical and/or non-medical visitors. It goes against the fundamental rights of a citizen or his family and such a exposure of any responsible citizen or his family and disclosure of his psychiatric illness to the knowledge of the public may amount to indignity and cruelty.
4. In the Mental Health Act, 1987, the matter of consent and competence has not been adequately addressed to.
5. Does an involuntary admission (For example, Admission through reception order) necessarily imply incompetence? Can drugs and ECT be given without any informed consent? What is the statuary criteria for competence? Who will judge the competence, doctors or the judges? These questions are to be answered.
6. The Act presumes that there are sufficient hospital beds for all the psychiatrically ill. Reality do not substantiate this presumption. There are hardly 20,000 hospital beds for a population of 900 million people. The need for more provisions for long-stay patients is not taken care of. The Act mostly talks about patients in hospitals. Thus keeping the realities of the Indian situation in mind, one is forced to say that the Mental Health Act, 1987 should be more appropriately called the Mental Hospitals Act.

7. For the patients admitted under special circumstances, no provisions has been made for continuation of his treatment beyond the period of ninety days. The only way left to the relative is to make an application before a Magistrate for a reception order, severe penalty may be imposed upon the Medical Officer in-charge for improper detention beyond a period of 90 days.

MENTAL HEALTH ACT: A REITERATION OF INSTITUTIONALIZATION

Involuntary commitment to mental hospitals is presently regulated by the Indian Lunacy Act of 1912. The Indian Lunacy Act antedates both current human rights thinking and therapeutic developments in the realm of mental health. In tune with times in which it was enacted, the ILA views mental illness as a "Law and Order" problem. Therefore, the procedure of involuntary commitment is required to be activated in order to protect society from the disruptive and dangerous manifestations of mental illness. Mental hospitals are in the main, required to function as custodial houses and not treatment centres (Dhanda, 1985).

This predominantly custodial policy of the ILA is obviously at odds with the NMHP. This legislation, however, is the prevailing law only as long as the Mental Health Act of 1987 is not brought into force. As the MHA is the incoming law, any strategy of coordination has to be dealt with in the context of this statute.

The MHA alters the predominantly custodial functions allocated by the ILA to mental hospitals and requires involuntary commitment for therapeutic considerations. However, despite several studies on the harmful effects of institutionalization and long-term stay in mental hospitals the MHA addresses the issue of compulsory care and treatment only in the context of "Psychiatric Hospitals" (Dhanda, 1985; 1986).

There is no provision which requires that commitments to a psychiatric hospital should be ordered only if less restrictive alternatives are inappropriate. Though Central and State Mental Health Authorities are to be established to regulate and superintend all mental health services in the country, there are no provisions whereby an inter-referral system is set up between these various services.

Section 5 of the MHA empowers the government to set up institutions such as halfway houses after-care homes, but there are no provisions spelling out the inter-relationship of these institutions and "psychiatric hospitals", in order to lessen the institutionalizing rigour of psychiatric hospitals.

Along with deinstitutionalism, the NMHP also advocates deprofessionalised delivery of mental health care. On this aspect, a curious position is adopted in the MHA. General practioners of *Allopathy*, *Ayurveda*, *Unani*, and *Homeopathy* systems of medicine have been empowered to issue medical certificates to a "mentally ill person". For purposes of seeking admission in a psychiatric hospital the responsibility for providing mental health treatment has been exclusively accorded to psychiatrists. The role of other mental health professionals such as clinical psychologists, psychiatric social workers, and psychiatric nurses has been accorded no recognition either for certification or for care and treatment.

CONSEQUENCES OF LACK OF COORDINATION

The consequence of the non-recognition of the deinstitutionalization programs of the NMHP in the MHA is that the poor and vagrant, mentally ill persons, who is routed to the mental health system from the criminal justice system is deprived of access to the less restrictive services. Authorities empowered to make compulsory commitment decisions are not authorized to refer them to the less restrictive services even if appropriate (Dhanda, 1988). Since compulsory admission to mental hospitals is controlled, legislatively any change in the functional role of these institutions cannot be achieved without amending the statutory regime.

Studies on mental hospitals (Gupta, et al. 1968; K Bhaskaran, 1970; Gupta, et al. 1980; Sharma, 1990), show that the inmate population can be broadly divided into three categories;

- Persons, who need active treatment
- Chronically ill persons, who need no active treatment but require custodial care
- Psychiatrically fit persons, who need after care and rehabilitation.

Mental hospitals can acquire their NMHP designated status of "active treatment centers" only if services are established for fulfillment of the other needs, and distinct grounds and procedures for the use of those services are articulated. In order to remodel mental hospitals as active treatment centres, it is essential that the other functions fulfilled by these institutions are reallocated both in law and in policy.

Due to the amalgamated role of "therapist cum custodian" being performed by mental hospitals, a number of these institutions have come to function as dumping houses for the rejects of society (Kalbag, 1982; Sagar, 1983; Singh, 1984; Bonnerjee, 1985; Munshi, 1987; Hindustan Times, 1988; Philips, 1988; Times of India, 1990). Commitment to such an institution deprives a mentally ill person of his life and personal liberty without any attendant benefits of treatment or care.

Through delivery of mental health care is not exclusively provided by mental hospitals, they are the most visible caretakers of the mentally ill. Hence the abysmal conditions prevalent in these state-administered and funded institutions becomes a major indicator of societal attitudes towards the mentally ill. For promotion of community care of the mentally ill, it is essential that stigma-promoting or perpetuating agents should be deactivated. The continuance of mental hospitals as custodial houses both strengthens the stigma of mental illness and obstructs social reintegration of the mentally ill. In order to protect the constitutional rights of the mentally ill and to promote their social acceptance, the restructuring of these institutions needs to be accorded high priority.

THE ADVANTAGES OF CONSONANCE

The NMHP adopts the policy of deinstitutionalization and deprofessionalization on an "inadequate resources logic". The policy of deinstitutionalization cannot be supported only because the country does not possess adequate resources to deliver mental health services through specialist institutions and personnel. This rationale can be criticized as being discriminatory to the poor sections of the populace, who are being provided substandard care without any safeguards against misuse.

This criticism could have been obviated if the program makers had adopted the logic of constitutional rights as the basis of the program. This logic would require the program to state that the policy of deinstitutionalization was being advocated because institutionalism entails a deprivation of life and personal liberty of the mentally ill persons. As the process harms the personality of the mentally ill person and obstructs his reintegration into society. Article 21 of the constitution requires that the denial should not be greater than is required for fulfilling objectives of either therapy or custody. The constitutional principle of "least restrictive alternative", could have been the reason for constructing the inter-referral system of the program.

If the NMHP has been based on a "constitutional rights logic" the program makers would have clearly made the point that the policies of the program are motivated by the best interests of the mentally ill and not a compromise with an inadequate resources position. A constitutional basis to the program would have increased its implementational priority. Also a statutory incorporation of some of the policy thrusts of the program would have been greatly facilitated.

A statutory incorporation of the policy preferences of the program should increase its implementation momentum, such a statute could introduce mechanisms to monitor the quality of mental health care and thus obviate one of the major criticisms against the NMHP.

It may be feared that if the "least restrictive alternative" principle is inducted in legislation, an integration of all mental health services will result. Such integration whether it benefits the institutionalized patient or not, can stigmatize the remaining mental health services and the legal restrictions which at present operate for treatment in mental hospitals could extend to all other services.

It cannot be denied that till date, legislation in our country has emanated from a coercive model and constructed a negative image of the mentally ill. Whilst it has provided procedures for making treatment inaccessible, it has provided procedures for making treatment inaccessible, it has offered little or no protection against wrongful confinement. However, such use of the legislative instrument does not have to continue. A facilitative legislation promotive of the treatable nature of mental illness can also be made. The need for such legislation is underscored by the above analysis which shows that lack of coordination between law and policy makes the law insular and lessens the efficacy of the policy.

RECOMMENDATIONS OF THE INDIAN PSYCHIATRIC SOCIETY ON MENTAL HEALTH LEGISLATION

1. The professional Bodies are given importance in other countries. Likewise, Indian Psychiatric Society, the National Organization of Psychiatrists in India, should be consulted in the matters related to Mental Health Policy and Mental Health Legislation by the Government.
2. Since the Mental Health Act, 1987 is not based on any Mental Health Policy and plan of the Government of India is urged upon to declare its Mental Health Policy and the plan and program based on the said policy. The policy should be drafted in consultation with the Indian Psychiatric Society.
3. The Mental Health Act, 1987, be repealed by a mental health legislation based on:
   a. Mental health policy of the Government.
   b. Modern concepts of psychiatry.
   c. Basic statutory structure of Mental Health Legislation as laid in the guiding principles and alternative approaches recommended by the WHO in 1978.
   d. Recommendations of the British Royal Commision of Law relating to Mental Deficiency based on which the English Mental Health Act, 1959 was framed.
   e. Principles, guidelines and guarantees for the protection of persons detained on grounds of mental ill health or suffering from mental disorder adopted by the UN in 1991.
   f. Changes made in the English Mental Health Act, 1959 (repealed by Mental Health Act, 1983), especially regarding dispensing with the services of the magistrate in matters relating to admission of mentally ill patient to any medical facilities, dispensing with the services of the visitors and formation of Mental Health Tribunals.
   g. Memorandum of the Indian Psychiatric Society on the Mental Health Bill, 1981 suggesting large number of specific amendments (Annexure B).
4. Among others the following changes should be made:
   a. Inconsistencies between the provisions made in different sections and subsections of the Act must be corrected and the rules made under the Act must be consistent with the provisions of the Act and all the rules (including rules regarding aid to mentally ill persons) must be framed before the Act is given effect to.
   b. The expression "mentally ill persons" should be redefined as suggested by the WHO Expert Committee on Mental Health, 1955. A single Mental Health Act covering both mentally ill and mentally retarded persons is the most useful form of legislation. Minimum qualifications of all Mental Health Personnel mentioned in the Act and rules should be clearly stated in the definition.

c. Mental Health Authority should function in an advisory capacity and licensing Authority should function in the administrative capacity. Members of the Mental Health Authority should be qualified Mental Health Professionals with special knowledge in Mental Health Legislation and Mental Health Services. The functions of the Mental Health Authority under a separate Mental Health Unit or Directorate or Division in the Ministry of Health should include—
   - Promoting mental health program
   - Compiling educational materials
   - Coordinating with other bodies to increase human resource in the field of mental health.

d. Adequate funds should be provided for proper functioning of any forum or authority constituted under the mental health legislation and for execution of all provisions made under the said legislation.

e. All "Mental Health Services" including residential establishments for the mentally retarded should be required to obtain licence under the Mental Health Act and consideration be given to the need to provide effective management policy and quality control standards for all Mental Health facilities, regardless of whether these facilities are publicly or privately owned.

f. Voluntary admission to any medical facility should be made informal as in English Mental Health Act, 1993.

g. Changes of status from voluntary and vice-versa should be done by the medical officer in charge of the psychiatric facility.

h. The minimum structure required for a 10-beded psychiatric facility should be amended and must be considered with the availability of qualified Mental Health Personnel and financial resources of the psychiatric facility and/or the financial status of the community it serves.

i. Forms should be prescribed for all orders passed under the Act and its use should be mandatory.

j. Violation of the human rights of the mentally ill persons at any place or by any person or authority should invite action by the Mental Health Commission.

Although amendments of clauses would take lesser time than replacing the Act by a new one, the Indian Psychiatric Society feels not only large number of amendments is necessary in almost every section of the Act and every clause of policy, as recommended above, would call for further changes in the Act and the rules. Drafting of a new bill would be much easier than large scale amendments of the existing Act as would be found by the large number of specific amendments suggested by the Indian Psychiatric Society in the Memorandum on the Mental Health Bill, 1981.

SUGGESTIONS FOR AMENDMENT

As it is believed that the law should be in consonance with policy; it is suggested that in this period of suspended animation, the MHA should be amended as follows:

1. The functions of therapy and custody should be separated and the principle of least restrictive alternative adopted.
   - Two separate institutions to fulfill functions of therapy and custody to be established.
     – Institutionalization for active treatment and
     – Community based programs for long-term care and rehabilitation.
   - Institutionalization for custody should be ordered when a mentally ill person is dangerous and unable to look after himself and cannot be managed in the community.
   - Mentally ill persons institutionalized for treatment or custody should later be transferred to less restrictive facility after improvement.
2. Professional management of institutions.
3. Safeguard against wrongful commitments.
4. Adoption of principle of right to treatment.
5. Quality of care guidelines.
6. Civil status matter of separate judicial determination.

SUGGESTIONS TO IMPROVE MHA, 1987

- A National Mental Health Policy should be formed before Mental Health Act.
- Need not have a blanket requirement for licence.
- Same standard should be prescribed for both Government and private psychiatric facilities.
- The inspecting team should include a medical person.
- Provision should be made available for special group like elderly, destitute women, etc.
- For 10–30 bedded psychiatric facility, one psychiatrist is enough.
- The format for various certificates should be made available.
- There should be provisions to open the daycare centres, rehabilitation centres, halfway homes, long-stay facilities for chronic patients outside the hospitals. In the Community Mental Health Centres, there should be a mention about "Community Care", "Rehabilitation", "Informed consent", etc.
- Both Central and State Mental Health Authorities should be made more effectively functioning. There should be periodical review of existing legislation, plan amendments and bring in new legislation from time to time.
- Law does not ensure implementation, it needs support and involvement from public and professionals, above all, blessings from the governments.
- There are lacunae in mental health legislations even in developed countries.

- There was a period of Euphoria when the bill was submitted. They thought that MHA would be "*Sarva Roha Nivarani*" for all their problems alas! Many were disappointed when the Act really came into force.
- To achieve quality mental health care a cross-sectional interdisciplinary work is essential.
- Any new rule of Act is found to face criticism and comments in initial stages: only after implementation of the Act the exact problems can be assessed. Even though the Central Mental Health Authority is formed, the State Authorities have not been established in some states, even where they are established they are non-functional due to various reasons.
- There is no point in having a law unless it can be implemented and this country is full of laws, which have not been implemented. With all our positive efforts, we can make this country as diligent in its treatment of the mentally ill as we are in the treatment of any other major health problem.

MENTAL HEALTH CARE ACT, 2012—DRAFT

- Ministry of Health and Family Welfare
- Government of India
- New Delhi

Overview and Comments

The government of India Ministry of Health and Family Welfare has brought out a draft of the Mental Health Care Act 2012 based on the inputs from the five regional consultations and those provided by the professional bodies and other stakeholders.

Mental Health Care in India is gaining a momentum in the recent past. Almost every aspect of life in the modern days is regulated or affected in some way by law. Most of the civilization in the world has enacted laws to regulate human behavior, so that, the weakest can live freely and enjoy all his human rights. There is a dynamic relationship between the concept of mental illness, the treatment of the mentally ill, and the law.

In the Indian context, many acts are directly or indirectly related to mental health. Currently, the Mental Health Act, 1987, (MHA 1987) is a major legislation and it has become supposed to be operational in 1994 in all States of the Indian Union, but, only after the Erwadi tragedy in 2004 many States started implementing, as per the order of the Supreme Court. This Act replaces the Indian Lunacy Act, 1912.

Even though, lot of new developments and modifications have been included in the MHA 87, many of the mental health professionals, NGOs, and other stake holders felt there are lot of lacunae and deficiencies in this Act. Hence, in the last 15 years, many organizations including Indian Psychiatric Society consumers started demanding a new Act which can fulfill the aspirations and improve the quality of care of the mentally ill. Based on this, the Government of India,

Ministry of Health has taken steps to bring about a new Act, Mental Health Care Act 2012. (MHCA, 2012) and after wide consultations released the draft on December 6, 2010. This draft will take a final shape after suggestions and some more recommendations, which will then be circulated to the Law Ministry and later the Bill will be introduced in both the Houses of Parliament. The bill should be passed in both the houses and it will be enacted after getting the President of India's approval.

The basic requirements of a new Mental Health Act:

- A comprehensive mental health policy of the government drafted in consultation with professional bodies.
- Incorporation of modern concept of psychiatry.
- Basic statutory structure of mental health legislation as laid down in the guiding principles and alternative approaches recommended by the WHO.
- Apart from the care of the mentally ill and their rights the act should comprise facilities to promote mental health program.
- Should take into account the care of the common (minor) mental disorders.
- The new MHA should focus on community psychiatry and rehabilitation programs.
- Should coordinate with other agencies/institution to increase human resources in the field of mental health.
- Same standard should be prescribed for both government and private psychiatric facilities.
- Provisions should be made available for special groups like elderly, destitute women, etc.
- There should be provisions to monitor effective functioning of the central and State Mental Health Authorities.

The draft of the Mental Health Care Act, 2012, consists of 9 Chapters and 67 Sections. The proposed Act is more comprehensive, specific, and consumer oriented. This Act resembles some of the advanced countries legislations in that sense, that very great importance is given to the rights of persons with mental illness. The Act's concern to give a quality mental health care and to treat the persons with mental illness with humanity and dignity is evidenced by Chapter II, wherein the various rights of persons with mental illness has been detailed. They are:

- Right to access mental health care.
- Right to community living.
- Right to protection from cruel inhuman and degrading treatment.
- Right to equality and non-discrimination.
- Right to information.
- Right to confidentiality.
- Access to medical records.
- Right to personal contacts and communication.
- Right to legal aid.
- Right to make complaints about deficiencies in provision of services.

In the title description of Mental Health Care Act 2012, it is described as an Act to provide access to mental health care for persons with mental illness and to protect and promote the rights of persons with mental illness during the delivery of mental health care. Hence, it is understood that the two important objectives of this MHCA 2012 are access to mental health care and protection and promotion of rights of persons with mental illness. Unlike the MHA, the present Act talks about rehabilitation also as a part of the care.

In the Chapter I, where the definitions are prescribed lot of new concepts have been included like caregiver, informed consent, Least Restrictive Alternative or Less restrictive Option, mental health facility, mental health professional, mental health review commission, and district panel of the mental health review commission have all been included.

The definition of mental illness is more specific and comprehensive compared to MHA, 1987. This Act defines mental illness as "a disorder of mood, thought, perception, orientation or memory which causes significant distress to a person or impairs a person behavior, judgment, and ability to recognize reality or impairs the person's ability to meet the demands of normal life and includes mental conditions associated with the abuse of alcohol and drugs, but excludes mental retardation."

In Section 4 of Chapter I, the concept of competence or competent to make a decision has been very clearly put forth. In Section 5, a new concept of Advance directive has been specified. Every person has a right to make an advance directive in writing, specifying any or all of the following:

- The Way the Person Wishes to be cared for and treated for a mental illness and/or
- The way the person wishes not to be so cared for and treated for a mental illness and/or
- The individual or individuals shall appoint a nominated representative.

The concept of advance directive and Nominated Representative are all going in hands with the modern concept of mental health care delivery. There are different terms like relative, caregiver, guardian, and nominated representative have been mentioned. Even though, they seem to be synonyms each one has a different meaning and purpose in this act. The nominated representative has to be appointed by the district panel of the Mental Health Review Commission and he is responsible for all the legal and health care protection of the person with mentally ill. This term has almost replaced the concept of guardian. In minors, below 18 years, the legal guardian need not always be the nominated representative of the child.

The very positive note in using terminology in this new Act is evidenced by using the phrase "Person with mental illness" rather than using the term "Mentally ill person", in accordance with the WHO guidelines.

In Chapter III, the duties of government in promoting mental health program and creating awareness about mental health problems and to improve the human resources are mentioned.

The Chapter IV deals with Mental Health Review Commission (MHRC), this mental health review commission would replace the Central Mental Health Authority of MHA, 1987. The Central Government shall constitute MHRC within three months of the Act coming into force. This will have the jurisdiction all over the country.

The MHRC consists of:

- A President (High Court Judge)—to be appointed by the President of India.
- One Member—a psychiatrist with 15 years experience.
- One Member—a representative of persons with mental illness or families or caregivers or NGOs.

Members to be appointed by the Central Government.

Section 22 of Chapter IV describes the constitution of district panels of the mental health review commission (District Panel of MHRC). The MHRC shall appoint and function through the District Panels in the districts. The District Panels functions as per the guidance of MHRC. Each District Panel of the commission shall consist of:

a. Chairperson—a District Judge.
b. Two Members—Mental health professionals of which one shall be a Psychiatrist and other a mental health professional.
c. Two Members from the stakeholders—either the persons with mental illness or caregivers or representatives of NGOs.

The President of the MHRC shall constitute a committee for each state to appoint members of the District Panel. The state committee consists of—

- The President or one of the members of the MHRC—he is the Chairperson.
- Chief Justice of the State or his nominee.
- Secretary, Ministry of Law of the State Government or his nominee.
- Secretary, Ministry of Health of Family Welfare of the State or his nominee.
- Secretary, Ministry of Social Welfare of the State or his nominee.

Any person with mental illness whose rights are violated or his nominated representative or an NGO may make an application to the District Panel for redressal.

Section 28 of Chapter IV describes the functions of MHRC and District Panel of the MHRC.

The Functions of the MHRC

- Appoint and remove members of District Panel.
- Guidance to District Panel.
- Periodic review of the use of advance directives.
- Advise Central Government on matters relating to the promotion and protection of rights of persons with mental illness.

The Functions of District Panels of MHRC

- To review, alter, modify and advance directive.
- To appoint a nominated representative.

- To decide applications from persons with mental illness or caregivers.
- To decide applications regarding nondisclosure of information.
- To decide complaints regarding deficiencies in the care and services.
- To visit prison or jails and question the responsible medical officer taking care of mentally ill.

From the Draft, it looks as if the MHRC is replacing the existing Central Mental Health Authority, even though, it is not specifically mentioned in the Draft.

Chapter V describes about the formation and functions of the State Mental Health Authority (SMHA). The State Government shall constitute the SMHA within three months of the Act coming into force. The SMHA has totally 13 members. They are:

a. Ex-Officio members:
    - Secretary, State Department of Health.
    - Representative of State Department of Health, who is responsible for mental health.
    - Head of the Mental Hospital.
b. Other members:
    - A Prominent Psychiatrist from the State, who is not in government service.
    - A Psychiatric Social Worker.
    - A Clinical Psychologist.
    - A Mental Health Nurse.
    - Two Persons representing who have or have had mental illness.
    - Two Persons representing caregivers.
    - Two Persons representing NGOs working in the field of Mental Health.
    - The term duration for each member is three years.

Section 34 talks about the Executive Officer of SMHA (EO of SMHA). The Chairperson (Health Secretary) shall appoint an EO to the authority. The EO shall be a full-time employee of the authority. He controls and monitors the functioning of SMHA.

The functions of SMHA are almost like what has been detailed in MHA 1987.

Chapter VI deals with mental health facilities. The existing term of psychiatric hospital has been removed, instead, the organization or institution taking care of the mentally ill is now known as the Mental Health Facility. The Mental Health Facilities are categorized and minimum standard of care is provided. The Mental Health Facility is defined (as per Chapter I, Section 2 (h)) as "all facilities either wholly or partly, meant for the care of the persons with mental illness, establish or maintained by the govt or any other person or organization, where persons with mental illness are admitted or reside at, or kept in, for care, treatment, convalescence, and/or rehabilitation, either temporarily or otherwise; and includes any general hospital or general nursing home established or maintained by the govt or any other person or organization; and excludes a family residential place if a person with mental illness resides with his or her own family."

The Mental Health Facility should obtain registration from the State Mental Health Authority. Hence, the SMHA functions as the licensing as well as inspecting authority unlike in MHA, 1987. After the State Government fix the standards and categories of Mental Health Facilities and officially notified, the Mental Health Facilities should get their permanent registration within a period of six months.

Chapter VII deals with admission, treatment, and discharge. Following are the different types of admissions as per Mental Health Care Act, 2012.

- Independent (without support) admission and treatment—at the request of the individual himself.
- Admission of a minor—at the request of the nominated representative.
- Admission and treatment of persons with mental illness, with high support needs, in a Mental Health Facility, up to 30 days (supported admission).
  - Admission and treatment of persons with mental illness with high support needs, in a Mental Health Facility beyond 30 days (supported admission beyond 30 days).
  - Admission of wandering mentally ill or a person at risk to himself or to others due to mental illness or a person with mental illness, who is ill-treated or neglected.

It is the duty of the police officer to take these mentally ill persons into protection and produce them before the magistrate for authorizing the admission of the person with mental illness in a Mental Health Facility for such period not exceeding 10 days for assessment and planning of the treatment.

Section 59: Deals with admission of prisoners with mental illness. Section 60 deals with admission of person with mental illness for judicial process.

Section 51: Deals with prohibited treatments, where it is mentioned that ECT without muscle relaxant and anesthesia should not be given for minors and during emergency treatment. Sterilization of men and women shall not be performed when such sterilization is intended as a treatment for mental illness and persons with mental illness shall not be chained.

Section 52: Gives the consent and the procedure for psychosurgery for persons with mental illness.

Section 53: Deals with guidelines for restraints and seclusions for unmanageable or risky mentally ill persons.

Chapter IX deals with the penalties and miscellaneous provisions.

Section 61: Deals with penalties for establishing and maintaining a Mental Health Facility in contravention of this act.

Section 63: Deals with special relaxation applicable for the states of North East Council. There is a provision of MHCA, 2012 for emergency treatment for a maximum period of 72 hours by any medical practioner to prevent death or irreversible harm to the health of the person or the person inflicting serious harm to himself or to others or the person causing serious damage to the property belonging to him or others.

COMMENTS

Even though, the modern concept of Mental Health Care has been formed as the basis for this Act, it is better for our Nation to have a comprehensive Mental Health Policy to be framed before any Mental Health Legislation or program to be charted out. There are a lot of positive thinking in defining many terms in Mental Health Care including the mental illness.

The qualification of psychiatric social worker and the clinical psychologist should be more specified like "the psychiatric social worker means any person holding MA in Social Work/MSW/MPhil in Social Work, who have obtained their Masters Degree in Medical and Psychiatric Social Work in a recognized institution."

The term Clinical Psychologists means after Post Graduation, a recognized qualification in Clinical Psychology in a recognized institution or an institution attached to a hospital. The term "psychiatric hospital" has been replaced by a comprehensive term "Mental Health Facility". The Mental Health Review Commission to monitor the countries Mental Health Care delivery and the district level panel of this commission will facilitate the smooth functioning of the Mental Health Care Delivery. The term "Licence" instead, the term "Registration" has come in. The term licensing authority and the inspecting authority have gone. The admission procedures have been modified for betterment. The emphasis of the New Act is mainly given for Protection of Human Rights and delivering dignified quality Mental Health Care to the persons suffering from mental illness.

Mental illness should not be viewed as either a "medical" or "legal" conditions alone, but a sociological dimension has to be incorporated. Exclusive judicial preoccupation with the medical concept of mental illness is not preferable. Each case has to be considered on its own merits. (Justice Venkatachalliah, 1988).

Since Law is the King of Kings, nothing can be mighter than the law by whose aid; even the unfortunate mentally ill may have the rights to have equal opportunity, rights to have protection of legal rights and rights to have full participation in the affairs of life on par with those who are non-disabled.

SUGGESTED READING

1. Agarwal AK. The Mental Health and the Law (editorial), Indian Journal of Psychiatry, 1992;34(2).
2. Desai NG. National Seminar on Mental Health Legislation, WHO, Delhi, 8th and 9th May, 1999.
3. Dhanda A. Legal Order and Mental Disorder, Sage Publication, New Delhi 2000.
4. Dutt AB. The Long March of Mental Health Legislation in Independent India, LP Shah Oration at the Western Zonal Conference, Indian Psychiatric Society, Goa 2001.
5. Mental Health Care Act 2010. Ministry of Health and Family Welfare, Government of India, New Delhi.
6. Nambi S. Legal Aspects of Psychiatry—Indian Perspective, 2009. Manashanthi Mental Health Care Publications, 2008.
7. Nambi S. Mental Health Care Act 2012, Draft-Overview and Comments—Guest Lecture at the CME—Indian Psychiatric Society, Tamil Nadu Branch, Trichy 2010.

8. Sethi BB. Mental Health Bill, 1981. A Ray of Hope (editorial). Indian Journal of Psychiatry;1982;24(4).
9. Somasundaram O. Presidential address Indian Lunacy Act, 1912. Paper presented at the Indian Psychiatric Society, Tamil Nadu Branch, Trichy, 2012.
10. The Mental Health Act, 1987 (Bare Act, 2003), Delhi Law House with Mental Health Authority Rules, 1990 along with State Mental Health Rules, 1990.
11. Trivedi JK. Satellite workshop on MHA under auspices of IPS at Lucknow, 1.5.99;1999.
12. Trivedi JK. The Mental Health Legislation: An ongoing debate, Indian Journal of Psychiatry, vol. 44(2)s.

5 Chapter

Mental Illness, Disability, Rehabilitation and the Recent Legislations

Rehabilitation in psychiatry is the process which attempts to benefit a mentally ill person back, as near as possible, to his original state. It is the process designed to help the handicapped individuals to make maximum use of their residual capacities and to enable them to lead a beneficial and meaningful life in the community. Rehabilitation of the mentally ill is an essential component of any therapeutic programme that proposes to tackle effectively the maladies of mental illness.

Rehabilitation is the restoration of the handicapped to the maximum possible physical, mental, social, vocational, and economic usefulness of which they are capable. Psychiatric rehabilitation differs from its medical counterpart in a number of respects. The poor insights associated with major mental disorder hampers rehabilitation process in psychiatry. Rehabilitation necessitates a long term commitment to the patient. Rehabilitation facilities and services are a link between the hospital and community and between the productive, and sociable person. According to WHO estimates, approximately, two-fifths of all disability, the world-over, is related to psychiatric conditions. The magnitude of the problem can be imagined as the prevalence of psychiatric problem in developing countries is approximately the same proportion as in the developed countries (WHO, 1975).

At the outset, it is essential to understand the definitions of related terminologies, the concepts were clarified and unified by International Classification of Impairment, Disability and Handicap—ICIDH.

Illness: Physical, mental states or processes, which are perceived as deviations from normal state of health, involves some lesions or physiological dysfunction and described as symptoms and signs.

Impairment: Any loss or abnormality of psychological, physiological or anatomical structure or function.

Disability: Any restriction or lack of ability to perform an activity in the manner or within the range considered normal for a human being.

Handicap: This is the disadvantage resulting from impairment or disability that limits or prevents the fulfilling of a role that is normal for the individual.

The Disability Assessment Schedule: WHO/DAS defines social disability as "any temporary or persistent restriction resulting from mental disorder or impairment of the individuals" capacity to perform the social roles that are considered normal for someone.

There are three recent Acts in India in relation to the mental illness, the disability and the rehabilitation. They are:

- The Mental Health Act, 1987 (MHA).
- The Persons with Disability (Equal Opportunity, Protection of Rights and Full Participation) Act, 1995 (PDA).
- The Rehabilitation Council of Indian Act, 1992.

The Mental Health Act insists the need to get a valid license for the treatment and care of the mentally ill persons and include a convalescent home. It also mentions about the provision for rehabilitation activities in psychiatric hospitals. Apart from these, MHA is not much bothered about rehabilitation programme or community care of the mentally ill.

The Persons with Disability Act which came into effect from February 7, 1996, is a step towards accelerating this process in India. Legislation of this kind provides a much needed legitimacy. The concern for the disabled in India is a recent origin. PDA is a major milestone in the protection of rights and providing equal opportunities for mentally disabled. The inclusion of mental illness in PDA is a positive gain.

The purpose of PDA (Gazette No. 1 of 1996) is to fix responsibilities on the Central and State government to ensure that disabilities do not prevent individual citizens of this country living a full life and making full contribution each in accordance with his/her ability. Mental illness and Mental Retardation are the two types out of the seven disabilities specified in PDA. It defines mental illness as any mental disorder other than mental retardation. It defines mental retardation as the condition of arrested or incomplete development of the mind.

A person with mental disability has to be certified by a medical authority that he/she is suffering from not less than 40% of the disability.

The PDA provides better care, job opportunities, and other concessions to the mentally ill and mentally retarded persons. There are some lacunae in PDA concerned with mental illness. First of all, the definition is not clear and specific. It says "any mental disorder" will come under PDA, stress related disorders, and psychoactive substance abuse disorder can be treated on par with major mental disorders (psychoses). This needs clarification and more specification.

The next important issue is the assessment of disability. It may not be easy to assess the disability of a mental illness like other disabilities at the clinician's routine assessment. The disability assessment scales available now may be research oriented and may not be used in day-to-day practice. The disability assessments in relation to mental illnesses need to include some specific criteria like the diagnosis, severity and duration. Some uniform and practically simple assessment schedule to assess the disability is essential before we implement the PDA. There is also a need to understand the magnitude of the problem, nature of rehabilitation programmes required, and available mental health professional. There is a need to create awareness and train the Mental Health Professionals in this regard.

The third recent legislation in relation to the rehabilitation Council of Indian Act (RCIA) 1992, which came into force from July 31, 1993. The RCIA is an Act to provide for the constitution of the Rehabilitation Council of India for regulating the training of rehabilitation professionals and the maintenance of a central Rehabilitation Register. The RCIA is concerned about the "handicapped" persons. It includes persons suffering from mental retardation apart from visual and hearing impairment and persons suffering from locomotor disability.

The RCIA defines mental retardation as a condition of arrested or incomplete development of mind of a person, which is specially characterized by subnormality of intelligence. The RCIA gives recognition to the persons/professionals taking care of mentally retarded persons. It conducts orientation course for these persons know as Bridge course in the field of mental retardation and associated disabilities. Selected centres are giving training to these personnel in the areas of mental retardation.

The RCIA includes only the mental retardation as the "handicapped" but not mentioning anything about the other mental illnesses, whereas, the PDA includes both "mental illness" and "mental retardation" as "disabilities".

There are positive and negative impacts about these legislation's in relation to the rehabilitation of the mentally disabled persons. Mental Health Professionals, who wants to start rehabilitation centres for mentally ill will now be governed by all these three legislation's. Regulation by these authorities may interfere with the very idea of service to the mentally ill and psychiatrists in future may hesitate to start such centres, which defeat the very purpose of caring for the mentally ill.

The positive features about these acts is that the Government of India, now recognizing mentally ill as a disabled category. With careful planning and after removing the deficiencies of these Acts, more effective rehabilitation programmes can be carried out on a long-term basis for the mentally disabled persons.

DISABILITIES ACT, 1995

This is an Act to give effect to the proclamation of the full participation and equality of the peoples disabilities in the Asian and Pacific region. The Act was enacted by parliament in the 46th year of the Republic of India. The Act extends to the whole of the India except the state of Jammu and Kashmir.

The Persons with Disabilities Act (PDA), which came into effect from February 7, 1996, is a step towards accelerating rehabilitation programs for the mentally ill in India. Legislation of this kind provides a much needed legitimacy. The concern for the disabled in India is of recent origin. PDA a major milestone in the protection of rights and providing equal opportunities for mentally disabled.

The purpose of PDA (Gazette No. 1 of 1996) is to fix responsibilities on the central and state government to ensure that disabilities do not prevent individual citizens of this country from living a full life and making full contribution each in accordance with his/her ability. Mental illness and mental retardation are two types out of the seven disabilities specified in the PDA. It defines mental illness as any mental disorder other than mental retardation. It defines mental retardation as the condition of arrested or incomplete development of the mind provision. A person with disability has to be certified by a Medical Authority that he/she is suffering from not less than 40% of the disability.

The PDA has 14 chapters. In the first chapter, legal definition of the terms used in the Act are given. Disability means blindness, low vision, leprosy-cured, hearing impairment, locomotor disability, mental retardation and mental illness. The other chapters of the PDA describes the formation and functions of the Central and State coordination committees, prevention and early detention of disability, free education upto 18 years, the integration of normal and special schools, and vocational training facilities. The PDA mentions in detail about the employment of the disabled, their identification, reservation, formation of special employment exchange and the incentives. It also insists on the non-discrimination of disabled in transport and government employment. The disabled should not be reduced in a rank or denied promotion. Care is taken to encourage research and manpower development. The PDA specifies the needs and ways to recognize institutions for persons with disability. The Act mentions about appointment of the Chief Commissioners for persons with disabilities. The PDA mentions various social security systems in the rehabilitation of the disabled, which include insurance scheme and unemployment allowance.

The advantages of PDA in relation to Mental Health Care are many fold. The PDA provides better care, job, opportunities, and other concessions to the mentally ill and mentally retarded persons. It is a major milestone in the protection of rights and providing equal opportunities for the mentally disabled. The inclusion of mental illness as a disability is a positive gain. It removes the barriers to full participation. In future, we can anticipate that the Mental Health Care Programmes will get greater support. There are some issues to be clarified in PDA with regard to mental illness. First of all, the definition of mental illness is not clear and specific. The Act says that any mental disorders will come under it's purview. This needs modification. Only major mental disorder, which exists for some considerable period, which in turn disturbs and disables the persons and which cannot be totally cured even after a specific period of continuous treatment should be taken into account.

The next important issue is the assessment of disability. It may not be easy to assess the disability of a mental illness like other disabilities during the clinician's routine assessment. The disability assessment scales that are available now are research oriented and may not be suitable in day-to-day practice. The disability assessment in relation to mental illness needs to include some specific criteria like the diagnosis, severity and duration. Some uniform and practically simple assessment schedule to assess the disability is essential before we implement the PDA. There is also a need to understand the magnitude of the problem, nature of rehabilitation programmes required, and available mental health professionals. There is a need to create awareness and train the mental health professionals in this regard.

Some advocacy group fighting for the rights of mentally ill insists that the mental illness should be considered on par with any other physical illness and there should not be any separate stigma attached to mental illness alone. The feel that mental illness cannot be considered on par with physical disability. Mental illness can be cured and there is a wide spectrum of mental disorders and including them in the disability category will dilute the very objective of this Act.

The positive feature about this Act is that the government of India is now recognizing mentally ill as a disabled category. With careful planning, lobbying, and rectifying the defects, we hope that this Act can form a basis for better and effective mental health care program in future. The need of the hour is "Disability Solidarity" rather than "Disability Politics", to get things done in the right perspective.

SUGGESTED READING

1. Banerjee A, Sengupt P. Mental Illness and Disabilities Act, 1995—An Overview, Official Publication of IPS, Bengal Journal of Psychiatry, December 2000(10)1.
2. Nambi S. The Persons with Disabilities Act, Overview and Comments, 1985. Souvenir released at the IPS, Tamil Nadu state conference. The Rehabilitation Council of India Act, 1992.
3. Sethi BB. Mental Health Bill, 1981. A Ray of Hope (editorial). Indian Journal of Psychiatry; 1982;24 (4).
4. The Persons with Disabilities Act, 1995, Bare Act.

6 Chapter

Crime and Mental Illness

The widespread concern over the apparently increasing crime rate needs no documentation. The role of psychiatry in understanding and modifying this extensive and costly criminal behavior is not clear and is a subject of controversy.

Traditionally, criminality has been associated with mental illness, though there is no definite evidence. The studies of the relationship between dangerous behavior and mental disorders reveal that "There did seem to be a greater than chance association between mental disorder and crime." (Monahan and Steadman, 1985)

The frequency of the association between crime and mental illness depends on the sample being studied, which could be mental illness among criminal offenders, the history of criminal offences in psychiatric patients and correlation in community samples.

While some studies suggest a weak association, if any, between crime and mental illness (Rapoport, et al. 1965, Hafner and Borker, 1982) assessment of frequency of a history of crime among psychiatrically ill has shown a consistent association at least in several of the offences. (Cohen, 1980; Sosowsky, 1980).

An analysis done by (Walker and McCabe, 1973) of hospital order cases, showed that 41% of the count could be diagnosed as having schizophrenia, 35% mental subnormality, 12% psychopathic disorder and 8% affective disorder (Gunn, 1977). It is to be understood that crime may not always be directly related to current psychopathology, other factors such as the personality structure and the social setting may be equally important.

The pattern of crime is severely mentally disturbed offenders is the same for the general population. Mentally ill persons also commit the offences.

a. As a result of delusion and hallucination.
b. Due to the problems arising from the stress produced within the family and due to personality structure and the problems they fear in the social setting. Mental illness and crime are common phenomena and as a result, it is no wonder that some people with mental illness commit crime and that some offenders are mentally ill in the question. Most often asked in forensic psychiatry research is whether there is a specific link between crime and mental illness. This is often colored by the Public Perception and that patients with mental illness are dangerous. (AN Chowdhury, et al.)

While it is common knowledge that many mentally ill persons end up in prison there is a death of comprehensive surveys of psychiatry morbidity in prisons in South Asia. Regarding, the association of psychiatric disorder and criminal behavior. The results of studies are mixed by the emerging consensus that major mental illness does increase the chances of having a criminal conviction. There may be a link between specific psychiatric disorders and criminal behavior. Criminality has been associated with mental illness for a long time. There did seem to be a greater than chance association between mental disorder and crime. (Monahan and Steadman 1985). The frequency of the association between crime and mental illness depends on the sample being studied which could be mental illness among criminal offenders, the history of criminal offences in psychiatric patients and correlation in community samples. While some studies suggest a weak association, if any between crime and mental illness, (Rapopert, et al. 1965, Hafner and Borker, 1982). Mental illness assessment of frequency of a history of crime among psychiatrically ill has shown a consistent association at least in several of the offences. An analysis done by (Walker and McCabe, 1973) of hospital order cases showed that 41% of the court could be diagnosed of having schizophrenia, 35% mental subnormality, 12% psychopathic disorder, and 8% affective disorder.

(Gunn, 1977), it is to be understood that crime may not always be directly related to current psychopathology, other factors, such as the personality structure and the social setting may be equally important.

CRIME AND SCHIZOPHRENIA

Research provides limited answers to some important questions:

- Does, having schizophrenia led to a greater risk of offending.
- What sort of offending might this be and what stage of illness might it occur?
- What clinical features are important and what steps can be taken to prevent or at least diminish the risk of similar behavior in the future?

The relationship found between schizophrenia and offending depends on the nature of the sample under study. People with schizophrenia show a similar rate of offending in general as the rest of the population (Lind Qrist and Alleybeck, 1990). Although, they are more likely to commit the crime of violence this will usually be minor in degree. They are more likely than other offenders to be detected and arrested. In prison remand populations, a person with schizophrenia is six times more likely than other prisoners to be facing a charge for violence. (Taylor and Gunn, 1984)

HOMICIDE

A homicide is an appalling tragedy for all directly concerned, but single cases however, shocking and publicized, do not constitute the evidence for failure of a national system of care nor for far reaching changes in legislation and service delivery.

People with mental illness account for a minute amount of risk to the general public; their contribution has been falling over the years of major service change.

The Risk of Violence by People with Schizophrenia

Patients with schizophrenia who offend fall into two broad categories:

1. The acutely ill patients with positive symptoms.
2. Mostly they act in respond to delusions or to deal with a perceived threat. Patients with paranoid schizophrenia, in particular, may commit occasional, but often well-planned and serious violence.
3. Patients with more negative symptoms: These people are mostly chronic and disabled individuals. The offence is committed inadvertently or neglectfully only when confronted or threatened. In chronic patients, when there is acute exacerbations, the offending occurs.

Schizophrenia

In India, some studies of mentally ill criminals show schizophrenia to be the commonest diagnosis (Soma, 1960; Varma and Jha, 1966; Nambi, 1992). Schizophrenia was the commonest (74% diagnosis among 58 Broadmood patients, who killed their relatives. Taylor, 1982; reviewing schizophrenia and violence came into the following conclusions:

- That schizophrenia disposes the patients to violence though the overall numbers are small.
- That paranoid and catatonic excitement are the subgroups most likely to be assisted with violence.
- That the violence is more common as a late accompaniment of the illness.
- That the violence is more common in those patients who have recurrent exacerbations rather than those who are continuously ill.
- That at the time of the offence, the offender is generally psychotic and without insight.
- Minor offences are more common than serious offences.
- People with schizophrenia over representative among violent offenders and violent inpatients.
- Violence may occur in acute or chronic phases of illness.
- Acting on delusions is common in schizophrenia.
- Individuals phenomenology, situational factors, and features of the victim may also contribute to violence.
- Substance misuse is commonly a contributory factor.

Epilepsy and Crime

The association of offending and epilepsy is summarized by (Gunn, 1969).

- The offence may occur in a disturbed state induced directly by a fit. This appears to be rare.
- The offence and the fit may be coincidental.
- The brain damage which caused the epilepsy may have led to personality problems resulting in antisocial behavior.
- The subject may have developed strong antisocial attitudes as a result of the difficulties he has experienced in life as a consequence of his illness.

- An early deprived childhood environment may have both, engenerated antisocial attitudes and exposed the subject to epileptogenic features.
- Antisocial subjects may expose themselves to dangerous situations and sustain more head injuries than normal which may cause epilepsy.

Epilepsy crimes are of historical importance from the forensic psychiatric point of view for it was in a case of an epileptic murder in Scotland that the plea of diminished responsibility was accepted by the Law there (Whitlock, 1963). In a Chennai study of crimes committed by persons with epilepsy, out of 115 criminally mentally ill, 15 were found to be suffering from epilepsy, i.e. 13% (Somasundaram, 1972).

The various abnormal mental states associated with epilepsy, like confusion, stupor, depression, or excitement could be raised in the Court of Law, but automatism is a comparatively simple defence raised in many cases.

Epilepsy poses a problem to the psychiatrist especially in relation to crime, but in many cases, this could be untangled by careful history taking, observation, and EEG findings.

PERSONALITY DISORDER AND CRIME

There are close associations between crime and personality disorder, particularly antisocial personality disorder. Gunn, 1977; diagnosed abnormal personality in 20% of prisoners in prisons in South East England. Bluglass found psychopathic personality disorder in 40% of newly convicted prisoners in a Scottish prison; and Guze, 1976; described 70% of prisoners discharged from American Prisons as "sociopathic"; Guze, 1976; recommended that psychiatrists should use the word "psychopathic disorder" in current legal proceedings. It is widely held that the legal concept of psychopathy is unsatisfactory. The legal definition is difficult to apply in practice.

Close association exists between crime and personality disorder especially ASPD. 20% of prisoners in South England had abnormal personality (Gunn, 1977). 40% of newly convicted prisoners in Scotland are persons with psychopathic personality disorder (Bluglass, 1990). 70% of prisoners discharged from American prisons were "sociopathic" (Guze, 1976). The legal concept of psychopathic is unsatisfactory. The legal definition is difficult to apply in practice.

Antisocial Personality Disorder and Offending

- The term "psychopathic disorder" should only be used as a legal category.
- Personality disorders in forensic psychiatry are usually mixed in type.
- Diagnosis should be based upon longitudinal assessment and information from other sources. A wide range of abnormal personality traits contribute to offending behavior.
- Substance misuse is a commonly associated finding.
- There is an increased likelihood of other psychiatric symptoms and disorders.
- Features of borderline personality disorder are common in female offenders in secure settings.

Affective Disorders and Offending

Offending is less common than in other functional psychoses. Violent offending in depressive disorder is rare but may be serious in severe depression, enquiry should be made about homicidal ideation.

A family member is the usual victim in altruistic homicides, shop lifting, particularly in middle-aged offenders, may be associated with depressive disorder. Offending is more common in mania and hypomania than in depression, and may be serious.

Rapid-cycling bipolar disorder may be missed in offender patients.

MENTAL RETARDATION

- Offending is more likely in mild and moderate than in severe mental retardation.
- Offending is more likely in association with family, social, and environmental disadvantage.
- Offences are broadly similar to those of offenders without mental retardation.
- Some evidence exists for increased rates of sex offending and fire-raising in the mentally retarded.
- Learning disability together with antisocial personality features carries a high risk for offending.
- There has been a recent fall in the use of compulsory admission for people with mental retardation.
- Earlier there was a belief that most criminals are of low intelligent, now it is disproved.
- MR people may commit offence because:
  - They do not understand the implication of their behavior or
  - Because they are susceptible to exploitation by their people.

Common Offences by MR People

- Sexual offences (pimp, prostitution)
- Arson
- Drug peddling.

Alcohol, Drug Addiction, and Crime

After a long controversy about the relationship between crime and addiction, recent research has unequivocally demonstrated that criminality is an integral part of established addiction. In the USA, it is estimated that narcotic addicts commit over 50 million crimes per year. Much of the crime relates to the need to purchase drugs. There is strong evidence suggesting a high incidence of criminal record in established drug users. In an American Study of 354 narcotic addicts (Shoffer, et al. 1984) delinquency was committed by every addict in the sample. Offences committed by the addicts are of two types.

- Drug related
- Non-drug related.

With the implication that drug related offence (Possession, supply, and larceny) are an inevitable aspect of the lifestyle of the street addict. An FBI analysis in 1966 indicated that 26% of heroin addicts had a conviction of violence and 74% were convicted for larceny.

In a study of 243 Baltimore narcotic addicts. (Ball, et al. 1983) the main offence behavior emerged as theft (38%), followed by 27%, pimping and gambling (26%), confidence games and forgery (8%), and violence (2%).

The link between cannabis used and offending are complex. Abuse itself may give rise to offences, apart from crimes related to illegal trafficking. It is widely believed that cannabis takers are much less delinquent than other drug abusers, such as users of heroin, cocaine and morphine.

Crime and Dementia

Only 6 person of the sample of 533 mentally abnormal offenders had dementia (Hafner and Borker, 1973).

It is likely that dementing patients with all but the most serious antisocial behavior can be contained within the Health Care System. Roth, 1968; outlined the likely associations between senility and offending, in particular, the link between disinhibition of behavior and sexual offending.

Deutsch, et al. (1991) described physical aggression in nearly one-third of patients with Alzheimer's disease attending a research clinic in the USA (Johns Hopkins).

Neurosis and Crime

The incidence is unknown. In a study of shop-lifters, 10% were found to be neurotic but there was no control study. Gunn, 1978; gave a primary diagnosis of neurosis to 9% of a prison population; but it is difficult to know how this would compare with the general population. There is one particular syndrome, the Ganser Syndrome, which has been described as a reaction to imprisonment. Ganser was certain that the condition was not malingering but a genuine illness which he believed was hysterical in nature.

CHARACTERISTICS OF INSANE IN MURDER

Persons with mental illness at times commit major crimes like murder, persons suffering from schizophrenia especially paranoid and catatonic type, epilepsy, organic mental disorder like, Huntington chorea, mental retardation, etc. are notable to commit this type of crime. There are some unique features of the murder committed by mentally ill.

- The victim maybe very closely related or totally unknown person.
- More than necessary force could have been used.
- The accused mostly do not try to escape from the scene of crime.

- Usually they do not conceal or destroy the material evidence of the crime.
- Often they immediately accept that they have done the act.
- Most of the cases, a past history of severe mental illness might be available.

Criminal Responsibility: Mentally ill offenders usually stand trial in their same way as their offender, but when sentence is passed, consideration is given to their mental state and to the responsibility of psychiatric treatment. In determining whether or not a person is guilty it is necessary to consider his mental state at the time of the Act.

Before anyone can be convicted of a crime, the prosecution must prove.

- That he carried out an unlawful Act (Actus reus) (Intent).
- That he had a certain guilty state of mind at that time, namely mens rea (Guilty mind).

When a person is charged with an offence, the defence can be made that he is not a capable because he did not have a sufficient degree of men's rea. This defence can be raised in several ways.

- Not guilty by reason of insanity (under the McNaughton Rules).
- Diminished responsibility (not guilty of murder, but guilty of manslaughter, which requires a lesser degree of criminal intent).
- Incapacity to form an intent because of an automation.

For example, if mother kills her child in the first year of its life, she is not usually held legally responsible for murder but only for the less serious crime of infanticide.

Can a person commit a crime and plead "unsound mind" as a defence for escaping punishment?

Yes, if he could prove that he was of unsound mind at the time of committing the crime.

The Indian Penal Code, The IPC in short is a general enactment providing for punishment for every Act or omission contrary to its provisions. However, in chapter titled "General Exceptions", certain categories are excluded from punishments for committing offence. One such category is a person of unsound mind.

According to IPC, Section 84, any offence done by a person who is incapable of knowing ione, is not an offence in the Eye of Law. A person therefore shall be deemed to be of unsound mind if he is incapable of knowing:

1. The Nature of his Act.
2. That the Act is wrong.
3. That the Act is contrary to law.

Of one cuts the throat of a sleeping person, without being capable of knowing that he is causing the death, then that person is of unsound mind. If a person causes the death of another, without being capable of knowing that it is wrong or contrary to the law, then that person is of the nature of his Act and that is wrong, but is not capable of knowing that it is contrary to law, then, that person is not of unsound mind. If a person commits an offence knowing the nature of his Act and also that is contrary to law, but is incapable of knowing that it is wrong, then that person is not of unsound mind.

Therefore for a person to plead unsound mind as defence he is to establish that either he is incapable of knowing the nature of the Act or he is incapable of knowing it is wrong or contrary to law.

A person cannot plead that he did not know that having sexual relationship with a minor girl with her consent is contrary to law for availing the defence of unsound mind. Ignorance of law is no excuse. The only criteria for the defence of unsound mind is the lack of perception of the incapability of knowing that such an Act is contrary to law. At what time the state of unsound mind existed is very relevant—the state of unsound mind should have been present at the time of committing the offence.

A person of sound mind can avoid punishment if he can establish that he was of unsound mind at the time of committing the offence. A person of unsound mind can be punished if it can be established that he was of sound mind at the time of committing the offence. The law has recognised four broad types of unsoundness of mind:

1. Idiot
2. Unsoundness due to illness
3. Lunatic or mad man
4. One who is drunk.

Medical insanity differs from legal insanity. Legal insanity is based on the accused person's consciousness of the bearing of his Act on those affected by it. Mere abnormality of mind, partial delusion, irresistible impulse, are all cases of medical insanity but are not held to be legal insanity. For example, a poojari sacrificing a child to appease the goddess is held to be NOT a legal insanity.

Inspite of the vigorous criticism from so many knowledgeable quarters, the McNaughton Rules have found a secure place in the Indian Statute Book from the time when Queen Victoria took over the control of the colonial Indian Empire-Indian Penal Code: Section 84- Nothing is an offence which is done by a person, who at the time of doing it is incapable of knowing the nature of the act or that he is doing what is either wrong or contrary to law.

We can now look at some of the Indian Cases in which the above sections have been applied. It is evident from the study of these cases that many of the difficulties inherent in the interpretation of the rules are plain. The Following cases from the pre-independence era were taken from (Ratan, 1949).

In CJ Joseph's case: The accused was charged with having committed criminal breach of trust in respect of fines received by him in his capacity as head clerk in the sub magistrate court Kulitalai. The defence was that the petitioner was insane during the period in question and that he was generally subject to fits of insanity during the summer months. It was held that the petitioner did not come within the terms of Section 84 of the code and was convicted.

Emperor vs Bheleka Aham: The accused killed the deceased a young boy without motive. The accused was addicted to opium and for some days before and after the killing of the boy, he was irresponsible for his actions. It was held that the accused came with section 84 through the incapacity was caused by voluntary drunkenness and was of a temporary nature.

Queen Empress vs Venkatasami: The accused was charged with having committed the murder of a child. No motive could be assigned. The medical evidence showed that the act was committed under a sudden attack of homicidal mania. He confessed the crime to the village magistrate and denied the same to the sessions judge. It was held that it was not proved that the accused was incapable of knowing the nature of the act or that he was doing what was wrong or contrary to law and that he was guilty of murder.

In Vodde Subbigadu's case: There was no evidence of insanity except the motiveless act of the accused. The court held that it was one of the instance of the act being done by an insane impulse.

Karam Urang vs Emperor: The accused cut off his father's head picked it up, wrapped it and was proceeding along the road, when the matter was reported to the police. He was overtaken, and at the request of the Policeman accompanied him to the thana, he stated that the kali appeared to him in a dream and told him that he would have cut his father's head or his father would kill him and that unless he killed his father he would die. He wanted to dedicate his father's head to *Kali*. The judge acquitted him of the crime.

The following post-independence era cases were taken from the law journals:

Mohinder Singh vs State of Punjab (1983): Supreme Court Judgment; The appealant had been convicted under Section 302—IPC and sentenced to imprisonment for life. After going through the evidence of the two Doctors it was clear that the accused was suffering from schizophrenia. From the evidence, it was clear that he was talking in a very unusual manner saying things to the effect that he had seen *Lord Shiva* in front of him and alike. In view of the circumstances we are in a position to take a different view particularly when the appealant was suffering from Schizophrenia. The appeals are accordingly dismissed.

In Vemban's case (1988), Madras High Court: Vemban the appellant was charged for murdering his wife, by pushing her out from a taxi in which they were travelling along with her brother and when the vehicle was stopped by its driver, he got down and wriggled out of the hold of his wife's brother, took the water bottle and dealt a blow on her head and then he pushed her into the field into the slushy mud and he lay flat on the deceased. The trail court came to the conclusion that the appellant was responsible for the death of the deceased.

From the evidence, it was inferred that the appellant suffered from unsoundness of mind both at the time of occurance, as well as subsequent to the occurance. Taking all these factors into consideration, the court concluded that the act of violence was done while he was in an unsound state of mind and as such, he was incapable of knowing the nature of the act and he would not have been aware that the act done by him was wrong or contrary to law. The court held that the appellant is entitled to have benefits of the provisions of Section 84 of the IPC which will in turn give him the benefit of acquittal.

LEGAL INSANITY vs MEDICAL INSANITY

The word insanity has no technical meaning in law or in medicine. Insanity comprises a degree of mental disturbance, so menacing and so disabling, that the person may be considered to be legally immune from certain responsibilities. Insanity is a defence because, not knowing what he is doing or not knowing the moral nature of his Act. The insane person is incapable of forming the intentions that are required for unlawful killing. He has not the "Mens Rea" (guilty mind) for any offence. An insane person is an innocent person, who has nothing to answer for.

Medical insanity would cover abnormality of mind, delusion and cases of irrestibility, all of which warrant diminished responsibility. Legal insanity as such envisages that the unsoundness of mind of the subject must be such as to make the offender incapable of knowing the nature of the Act, or not knowing that what he is doing is wrong or contrary to the law.

THE McNAUGHTON RULES

Daniel McNaughton was a 29 year old, son of Glasgow wood-turner, a man of gloomy and reserved social habits, which included membership of religious groups and the Tory Party. He decided to murder Sir Robert Peel, the Prime Minister. He made elaborate plans and traveled to London, but in fact mistakenly shot and killed Edward Druminod, Peel's private secretary, in daylight in front of numerous witnesses on January 20, 1843. During the trial, McNaughton himself admitted that "they have accused me of crimes of which I am not guilty, they do everything to harass and prosecute me, in fact, and they wish to murder me. I was driven to desperation by persecution." McNaughton knew what he was doing and was aware that he was committing a criminal Act but felt compelled to do so, an Act he performed with cool deliberation.

Psychiatrists were called and it was expected:

- That his delusions were real.
- That the Act was committed under a delusion.

McNaughton was found "not guilty on the grounds of insanity".

McNaughton himself was sent to Bethlehem and later Boadmoor asylum, where he died in 1865.

In McNaughton's case, the Lord Chancellor put to a panel of his Majesty's judges five questions designed to clarify the legal position. Their replies given on June 19, 1843, constitute the so-called "McNaughton rules".

The following contain the main points of the McNaughton's rules:

- Every man is to be presumed to be sane, until the contrary be proved.
- An insane person is punishable, if he knew at the time of committing such a crime that he was acting contrary to law.
- To establish a defence on the ground of insanity, it must be clearly proved that at the time of the committing of the Act, the accused was suffering under such defect of reason, from disease of the mind, as not to know the nature and

quality of the Act he was doing, or if he did know it, that he did not know he was doing what was wrong.

- Finally, it is the jury's role to decide whether the defendant was insane.

The rules stressed the importance of—

1. The defendant's notion of understandability of right and wrong.
2. A causal relationship between the content of delusions and the crime.
3. The status of the offence is the contents of the delusion were true.

No reference was made to lack of control, irresistible drives or impulses.

There are three components of the mind, one controlling cognition, another controlling emotion and the third controlling will. This rule exempts only those whose cognitive faculties are affected, hence, the rule has been regarded as too narrow, more stringent and retrogressive. It makes no provision for cases where one's emotions and the will are so affected. Every type of insanity recognized by medical man is not legal insanity unless the cognitive faculty of mind is lost as a result of unsoundness of mind. The irony invested in the McNaughton rule is that if the right-wrong test has been applied at the time of McNaughton was tried, he could not have been found guilty on the ground of insanity.

In day-to-day practice, psychiatrists come across several cases where it is pleaded that criminal responsibility of the accused may be exempted and in several cases courts have done so for the accused suffering from unsoundness of mind, but in many cases, where it was not established that at the time of committing the crime, the person was of unsound mind, accused have been convicted also.

It is a crucial question for the psychiatrist to establish whether or not at the time of commencement of the criminal Act the person was suffering from unsoundness of mind. Invariably, in the present day procedure, the individual is brought for psychiatric evaluation after a gap of months, or even years, following the event. On psychiatric evaluation and observation, it is possible to comment on the present mental state of the individual but a comment in retrospect is possible based on reliable history of illness, which is quite likely to be distorted.

DURHAM RULE (1954)

"An accused person is not criminally responsible, if his unlawful Act is the product of mental disease or mental defect." In this, the casual connection between the mental abnormality and the alleged crime should be established. This rule is also known as "Product Rule".

AMERICAN LAW INSTITUTE (ALI) TEST

A person is not responsible for criminal conduct if at the time of such conduct, as a result of mental disease or defect, he lacks adequate capacity either to appreciate the criminality of his conduct or to confirm his conduct to the requirements of the Law.

The ALI Test is similar to the combination of the McNaughton and the Irresistible Impulse Test. This rule excludes psychopaths. This popular test is now used by all courts in the USA.

FITNESS TO STAND TRIAL

If the crime accused is probably suffering from mental illness and not fit to stand trial, the court can order a psychiatrist to observe, treat, and give an opinion regarding his fitness to stand trial. The dependent must be in à fit condition to defend himself. The issue may be raised by the defence, the prosecution or the judge. If the accused is found unfit to plead, an order is made for admission to a Psychiatric Hospital, where he will be detained and discharged later for trial after he is found fit for trial.

In ascertaining fitness to plead; it is necessary to determine whether the person:

- Is oriented to place, person and time.
- Understands the questions asked.
- Understands the nature of the charge.
- Understands the difference between guilty and not guilty.
- Is able to instruct his advocate.
- Is able to follow the evidence presented in the court
- Is able to challenge the selection of jurors.

A Person may be Suffering from Severe Mental Disorder, But Still be Fit to Stand Trial

Lucid Interval

Lucid interval is that space of time between two attacks and episodes of insanity during which a person is completely restored to the perfect enjoyment of reason upon every subject upon which the mind was previously cognizant.

A lucid interval is a period of relative mental clarity between periods of irrationality. It is commonly noted after head injury and in organic mental disorders such as delirium and dementia. The total remission period between two episodes of bipolar disorder can also be considered as a lucid interval especially in rapid cycling disorder.

The lucid interval has:

- A period of remission of symptoms in a psychosis.
- A brief return to consciousness after loss of consciousness in head injury.

  The concept of lucid interval is based on the notion that Author Name: individual with a major mental disorder may have an interval of remission of symptoms and during such an interval may have the mental abilities regulated by law to fulfill the criteria for testamentary capacity and Lucid Interval may be found in individuals who abuse alcohol and illicit drugs unless the substance abuse has led to some chronic significant mental deterioration. At times, the lucid interval doctrine has been extended to the individual who is lucid for a few minutes. However, those few minutes are usually insufficient for the individual to assess and comprehend the factors involved in the distribution of assets. In addition, the individual may be especially susceptible to undue influence during these few minutes of lucidity.

- Some neuropsychiatric disorder observes a law of periodicity, which is not uncommon.

Effect of this curious law consists in an intermission of the outward manifestations of the disease, so, complete as to bare the appearance of a perfect cure and in the present state of our knowledge, is all that we can with certainty say of it. Bipolar disorder is one of the diseases that is subject in some aspects to this law of periodicity, is universally admitted; but to what extent the law operates is a point on which there is much diversity of opinion:

- In the early periods of English Law, the Doctrine of Lucid interval was universally admitted and they seem to have been considered not a rare but a very common phenomenon of mental derangement. The principle law which holds the civil responsibilities of the insane to be impaired during the lucid interval, we are willing to admit, is generally correct, it should be the duty of courts, however, and view their acts done at such times.
- In emergency medicine, a Lucid Interval is a temporary improvement in a patient's condition after a traumatic brain injury, after which the condition deteriorates.
- In a typical case of extradural hematoma, there is history of injury which starts the bleeding and will usually cause temporary unconsciousness. This is followed by a period of normal consciousness, a lucid interval of few hours to a week. Lucid interval is seen only in 30 TO 40% of head injuries.

SUGGESTED READING

1. Chiswick D, Cope R. Seminars in Practical Forensic Psychiatry, 1995.
2. Devar BV. Mental health from a gender perspective. Sage Publications, New Delhi 2001.
3. Dhanda A. Insanity and Criminal Responsibility—Legal Order and Mental Disorder, New Delhi, Sage Publications, New Delhi 2000;79–180.
4. Foundoulakis, KN, et al. Personality disorders and violence. Current opinion in psychiatry 2008;21,1:84–92.
5. James Higgns, et al. Crime and Mental Disorder, Practical Forensic Psychiatry Seminars on The Royal College of Psychiatrists 1995;52–86.
6. Nambi S. Legal aspects of psychiatry—Indian perspective, 2009. Manashanthi mental health care publications, 2008.
7. Rangaswami K, Arunagiri S, et al. Personality dimensions of criminals and mentally ill criminals. Indian Journal of Psychiatry, 1982;24(1):88–91.
8. Rath NM, Dash B, et al. A study on insanity related homicide, Indian Journal of Psychiatry, 1990;32(1):69–71.
9. Somasundaram O. Criminal responsibility—An overview; Indian journal of psychological medicine, 2001;24(1) Indian psychiatric society, South Zone.

7 Chapter

Civil Issues (Responsibilities) in Psychiatry

All citizens have many civil rights, e.g. writing a valid will, entering into legal contract, to vote and right to get married, etc. All are considered to be sane; unless the contrary is proved. Mental illness can affect a person's legal capacity to make such decisions.

MENTAL CAPACITY

A "Normal" person must understand the nature of his act. Understand that what he is doing is right or wrong. Understand the consequences of his act. Psychiatrists may be involved in the assessment of the subjects. Mental state and his competence for the particular task in question.

TESTAMENTARY CAPACITY

The capacity to write a valid "Will". "A Will means a declaration of the intention of a testator with respect to his property which he desires to be carried into effect after his death." Will must be in writing, need not be registered. Section 59 of the Indian Succession Act (1925) states that every person of "sound mind", not being a minor may dispose of his property by Will.

A Will can be declared invalid if it is proved that at the time of making the Will, the testator:

- Was of unsound mind
- Did not have the mental capacity to understand the consequences of the act. In other words, any person of unsound mind cannot make a valid Will.

It is essential that at the time of making a Will, the person should possess sound and disposing mind.

- Should have an understanding of the nature of the Will.
- Should have knowledge of the property to be disposed off.
- Should have an ability to recognize those who may have justifiable claims on property.

When a psychiatrist is called upon to examine a testator as to his witness to make a valid Will, the above points must be kept in mind.

CONTRACT

A "contract" is a written or spoken agreement between two parties consisting of an offer and its acceptance. The person should understand the nature and effect of the contract.

Agreement may be oral or in writing; may be registered. The proposal (agreement) is revoked by the death or insanity of the proposer, Section 12 of the Indian Contract Act (1872).

A person is said to be of sound mind for the purpose of making a contract, if at that time, when he is capable of understanding it and forming a rational judgment as it affects upon its interest. Person during lucid interval may make a contract.

MARRIAGE

Marriage is a contract between an adult male and female of sound mind (Tables 7.1 and 7.2). Under the Hindu Marriage Act of 1955, a marriage with a person who was an idiot or lunatic at the time of marriage can be declared as null and void on application. If one of the marital partner has been suffering from an incurable unsoundness of mind or has been suffering continuously or intermittently from mental disorder of at least three years and the petitioner cannot reasonably expected to live with the other (respondent), as per Section 15 of Hindu Marriage Act, a divorce can be decreed.

Table 7.1: A unsoundness of mind as affecting the capacity to marry

Hindu Marriage Act, 1955 (HMA)

- A Hindu Marriage is voidable if either party is incapable of giving a valid consent as a consequence of unsoundness of mind, or
- Though capable of giving a valid consent as a consequence of unsoundness of mind, or
- Though capable of giving a valid consent has been suffering from mental disorder of such a kind or to such an extent as to be unfit for marriage and the procreation of children
- Has been subject to recurrent attacks of insanity.

The Special Marriage Act, 1954 (SMA)

Applicable to persons from any religion undergoing a civil marriage. Has provisions similar to the HMA except that a marriage under the SMA is void.

Indian Divorce Act, 1869

A Christian marriage is voidable if either party was a lunatic or idiot.

Parsi Marriage and Divorce Act, 1936

Unsoundness of mind is not ground for annulment.

Muslim Law

A person of unsound mind cannot contract a marriage and such a marriage if contracted is void. However, if the guardian of the person of unsound mind considers such marriage to be in his interest and in the interest of society and is willing to take up all the monetary obligations of the marriage then such a marriage can be performed.

Table 7.2: Unsoundness of mind as a ground for divorce

Hindu Marriage Act, Special Marriage Act and Parsi Marriage and Divorce Act Respondent has been incurably of sound mind or has been suffering continuous or intermittently from mental disorder of such a kind and to such an extent that the petitioner cannot reasonably be expected to live with him.
Dissolution of Muslim Marriage Act, 1939 A muslim woman can seek divorce on the ground that her husband has been insane for period of two years.
Indian Divorce Act, 1869 Amendment, 2001 (For Christians) Unsoundness of mind is a ground of divorce on two conditions that is it must be incurable and it must be at least for two years immediately before the filing of the petition.

Judicial Inquisition

Judicial Inquisition regarding alleged mentally ill persons possessing property, (Section 50 of Mental Health Act), where an alleged mentally ill person is possessed of property an application for holding an inquisition into the mental condition of such person may be made by the following persons.

- Any of his relative or
- Public Curator appointed under the Indian Succession Act (1925) or
- The Advocate General of the State or
- By the District Collector.

GUARDIANSHIP/MANAGER

Mental Health Act (1987) (Section 52) has the provision for appointing guardian or manager for mentally ill person. If the alleged mentally ill person is incapable of taking care of himself and also incapable of managing his property, the court can appoint a guardian (Section 53). If the mentally ill person is capable of taking care of himself, but is incapable of managing his property alone, the court can appoint a manager for him (Section 54). Just because a person is a legal heir of a mentally ill person, he cannot be assumed as the guardian or manager. The court should decide that. At times the District Collector can also appoint a Guardian or Manager.

ADOPTION: THE HINDU ADOPTION AND MAINTENANCE ACT, 1956

As per this Act, a father or mother of unsound mind cannot validly adopt a child. Likewise, a father or mother of unsound mind cannot validly give their child for adoption. Adoption is not legally recognized among Christians, Parsis, and Muslims; but based on custom and some court judgment, the same is permitted.

TORT

A "TORT" is a civil wrong (a non-criminal) committed by an individual or an entity (defendant) who has caused injury to a second individual (plaintiff).
Some of the varieties of Tort include:

- Bodily injury or death, injury to reputation, injury to domestic relation, injury to economic/business relation, abuse of legal process, nuisance and breach of duty.
- Mental illness is a good defense against Tort.
- Since the mentally ill does not know the degree and nature of the act and not knowing what he has done was wrong.
- Mere presence of mental illness is not a defense in Tort. It must be proved that individual was legally insane at the time of Tort being committed.

CONSUMER PROTECTION ACT, 1986

Medical profession has come under the purview of the Consumer Protection Act as per the Supreme Court judgment in 1995, which has created an anxiety among medical professionals. The law is trying to protect the interest of the consumers (patients and/or caregivers) and providing them means to get quick justice. The service rendered to a patient by a doctor would fall within the "Ambit of Service", only when a fee is charged for the service. If there is no fee, the Consumer Protection Act (1986) is not applicable.

Objectives of Consumer Protection Act

- The rights of the consumer to seek redressal against unscrupulous exploitation.
- Right to consumer education and others.

The second objective is very relevant to the practice of psychiatry, which includes the informed consent. The three levels of implementing Consumer Protection Act:

- District forum with jurisdiction up to 5 Lakhs claim
- State forum with jurisdiction upto 20 Lakhs claim and
- National forum far beyond 20 Lakhs.

Even though psychiatrists have a fear whether any of their patients turn out to be a litigant and go to the consumer forum, most of the time, it is not happening so. The incidents of claim against psychiatrists still remain much lower than that of claims against other medical specialists (Less than 3%).

Steps for prevention—

- A good doctor-patient relationship
- Psychoeducation
- Proper record keeping
- Obtaining informed consents wherever necessary.

Above all—A good ethical psychiatric practice.

WITNESS

Under the Evidence Act, 1872, (Section 118) a lunatic is incompetent to give evidence in the Court of Law, if he is unable to understand the questions asked or to give rational answers to them by "Virtue of Lunacy".

RIGHT TO VOTE AND RIGHT TO STAND FOR ELECTION

Under Article 326 of the Constitution of India, no person declared to be of unsound mind could vote. Under Article 102 of Constitution of India, a person is disqualified from being chosen as or for being a member of either House of Parliament, if he is of unsound mind and stands so declared by the competent court.

This is true for practically all official and responsible positions.

DRIVING

Anyone applying for a "Driving License" or who holds the license must declare whether he has suffered from any mental disorder. A person who is suffering from severe mental disorder, which includes severe learning disability, dementia, etc. are not entitled to have a valid driving license as per the Road Traffic Act and Driving license Act of India.

MEDICAL TERMINATION OF PREGNANCY (MTP)

The MTP act (1971) was passed in parliament in 1971 and came into the implementation from April 1972. The act liberalized the abortion laws as a family welfare and health measure to ensure better health and prevent risks to the liver of women from the hazards of criminal abortion.

Mental Health Aspects of MTP

- Insanity of parents is considered as an indication for termination of pregnancy. A written consent of the guardian is necessary for performing abortion in women who is suffering from severe mental illness irrespective of whether their age, above or below 18.
- This fact of severe mental illness should be certified by a qualified psychiatrist.

ORGAN TRANSPLANT AND MENTALLY ILL

Transplantation of Human Organs Act (2009) permits the transplantation of human organs. For the mentally ill recipient, the consent must be given by the Guardian. Whether, a mentally ill person (both related and unrelated) can donate his/her organ is a difficult problem; the guardians cannot give consent because it is impossible to assess whether donation is in the interest of the patient. Occasionally, the Courts may give permission; but it is prudent not to seek donation from mentally ill persons, who is incapable of taking decisions about their affairs. It is a routine to have potential donors examined by qualified psychiatrists to assess their mental status; to ascertain whether he can give valid consent and rule out any mental disorder. It is better to certify fitness with more than single Interview and Assessment.

MEDICAL INSANITY vs LEGAL INSANITY

When civil issues related to the mentally ill come to the Court of Law, the concept of mental illness viewed in the court is different from medical concept. In the Court of Law, a person is considered to be insane or of unsound mind, he is determined by the following facts:

- A person is incapable of knowing the nature of the act he is doing
- Not knowing what he is doing is wrong or contrary to Law
- Not knowing the consequences of the act, hence, only those who suffer from severe mental illness with the above criteria fulfilled and also, the presence of the illness at the time of carrying out the act is considered as mentally ill.

CONCLUSION

A working knowledge of the law that regulates the practice of Psychiatry, assist clinicians to provide good care and their patients and avoid unnecessary and counter-productive defensive practices. Psychiatrists cannot be expected to be as knowledgeable of the Law as Lawyers, but they do need to understand how the law and psychiatry interact in various common clinical situations. Good psychiatry and law are complementary.

SUGGESTED READING

1. Njenga FG, Acuda W, Patel V, et al. Essentials of clinical psychiatry for Sub-Saharan Africa; Masson, 2005.
2. Park K. Park textbook of preventive and social medicine, 2nd edition, 2009.
3. Ray I. Medical jurisprudence of insanity, classics in psychiatry; New York, Arno Press 1976.
4. Reddy KNS. The essentials of forensic medicine and toxicology 2008.
5. Rosner R. Principles of practice of forensic psychiatry; Arnold Publications, 2003.

8 Chapter

Forensic Aspects of Sexual Offences

INTRODUCTION

Sexual violence in general terms is often misunderstood even amongst forensic psychiatrists. This means that other mental health professionals probably also struggle with the concept. The reasons for this are complex, however, it is a field that is clinically challenging and often does not receive the interests it deserves from the various professional fields in psychiatry, psychology, and other mental health professions. It is clearly a very important area ideally suited for biological, psychological and psychosocial research.

SEXUAL VIOLENCE AND SEXUAL SADISM

Various studies have shown that sexual sadism is associated with brain damage most commonly in the anterior temporal lobe region of the brain. How underlying cerebral damage manifests in criminal and sexually violent behavior is still.

Theories of sexual offence have been well reviewed by Lanyon (1991). He pointed out that theorist have concerned themselves with global explanations for sexual derivation.

1. Freud (1905), for example, regarded them as representing a single type of psychopathology and highly resistant to change. His explanations involve oedipal conflicts and castration anxiety.
2. The behaviorist seem to believe that there is no particular character do present in the sexual deviant, the behavior itself is the disorder.
3. FLor-Henry (1987) suggested that sexual derivations are overwhelmingly a consequence of the male pattern of cerebral organization.
4. Biological factors may have important influences on types of human and sexual aggression. Biological here seems to mean physiological either a genetic factor or a neurochemical factor underlies some forms of deviants. Temporal lobe pathology has been found unduly prevalent among transsexuals. Higher serum level of testosterone were found to be associated with a higher likelihood of sexual violence.

An ethological explanation by Welsn (1987) suggested that the sexual derivation or aggression results from the males struggle for access to young healthy females and that the difficulty stem from the problems which unsuccessful males have in managing their sexual drive some sexual derivations are inevitable and should be tolerated rather than treated.

6. Holmstrom's and Burgess (1980) suggested four meanings for sexually aggressive behavior.
   a. The assertion of power and control.
   b. The expression of anger and hatred.
   c. Camaraderie in a group of rape.
   d. Sexual experience per second (John Gunn/Pamela J Taylor).

PARAPHILIAS

Arousal from	
Interaction with persons of the same sex	Homosexuality
Interaction with children	Pedophilia
Genital exposure to strangers in public places	Exhibitionism
Handling, possessing or wearing certain articles, e.g. underwear, rubber	Fetishism
Inflicting pain or humiliation	Sadism
Receiving pain or humiliation	Masochism
Spying on naked persons or sex acts	Voyeurism
Spraying urine ("water sports")	Uralagina
Rubbing against strangers in crowded places	Frottage
Cross dressing	Transvestism
Contact with corpses	Necrophilia
Making obscene telephone calls	Scatologia
Sexual activity from non-human mammals	Bestality

SEXUAL ASSAULT/SEXUAL OFFENCES

Sexual assault has taken place since earliest times. The women's moment, changes in the social role of women, their relationship to men, and publications by mental health professionals interested in the effect of the commonly occurring private violation of sexual assault upon women initiated a more human attitude towards women who has been sexually assaulted. One of the most challenging and important tasks for the Mental Health Professional is the appropriate application of theory; investigates skills and therapeutic expertise to relevant social problems. Undeniably, undoubtedly, rape is one social problem which requires such attention with rape recognized as most rapidly increasing reported violent crime, greater attention is being focused upon the victims.

The sexual crimes are as old as mankind. Many sexual acts, irregularities and sexual crimes are as a result of deviation from the normal sexual activity when the Law intervenes to regularize to curb such activities.

Sexual Offences, Indian Law Recognizes Three Types of Sexual Offences

1. Rape.
2. Unnatural offences.
3. Obscene acts.

The rape, the rape victim and her experience and the forensic aspects of rape: Day-in and day-out, women irrespective of their age are subjected to rape. Rape is considered to be an age long psychosocial and a medicolegal problem. Because of the social stigma attached to the victim of rape, several cases go unreported.

Definition

According to IPC Section 375, A man is said to commit rape, if he has sexual intercourse with the women under circumstances falling under any of the following descriptions:

- Against her will.
- Without her consent.
- With her consent, whether the consent has been obtained by putting her to fear of death or any person in who he is interested in fear of death or hurt.
- With her consent, when the man knows that he is not her husband and that her consent is given because she believes that he is another man to whom she is or believes herself to be lawfully married.
- With her consent when at the time of giving such consent by reason of unsoundness of mind or intoxication, or the administration by him personally are thought another of stupefying or unwholesome substance, unable to understand the nature and consequence of that which she gives consent.
- With or without consent, when she is below the age of 16 years,
- The explanation to this Section says that penetration is sufficient to constitute the sexual intercourse necessary to the offence of rape. Therefore, mere partial penetration would attract this provision and total and complete penetration is not required to constitute the offence of rape.

Section 375 of IPC provides for punishment which varies from one situation to the other, from imprisonment of not less than seven years which may extend to either ten years or even life imprisonment. The offence of rape is cognizable, bailable, non-compundable and triable by the Court of Sessions.

Some drastic changes have been brought into the area of punishment for the offence of rape, through the Criminal Law (Amendment) Act, 1983 in Section 376. This amendment, in addition, has also introduced some new provisions like Section 376 A to 376 D. Section 376 A provides for sexual intercourse by the husband with his own wife without her consent who is living separately from him under a decree of separation or under custom or usage, shall be punished with imprisonment to an extent of two years and also be liable to fine.

Section 376 B, 376 C, and 376 D deal with the offence of custodial rape committed by public servants, jail, and remand home authorities and management staff of a hospital, taking advantage of official position are punishable with imprisonment to an extent of five years and also be liable to fine. The offence given in these sections is cognizable, bailable, noncompundable and triable by the Court of Sessions, but no arrest shall be made without a warrant or without an order of a Magistrate. The punishment for custodial rape or rape on a girl under 12 years of age or a rape on a pregnant women or gang rape; Section 376 (2) prescribes rigorous imprisonment for a term not less than ten years but which may be for life along with fine. In rape cases, the onus is always on the prosecution to prove affirmatively each ingredient of the offence it seeks to establish and such onus never shifts. They have been taken note of as a much more serious crime than an ordinary rape and therefore deterrent punishment needs to be imposed to the accused in such cases. Similarly, the Supreme Court has also observed that "a sentence of only six months rigorous imprisonment on an accused who raped a six year old girl makes mockery of justice and because of the beastliness of the crime it deserved to be increased much more. In State vs Sunderlal, the Supreme Court observed that the victim of rape, a thirteen year old girl, could not have forgotten the face of the man who had committed ghastly crime on her, and the identity of the accused could be said to be amply established by her evidence and hence, his conviction on that basis was proper, where a prostitute who was in police custody was forcefully raped by the Sub Inspector of police, the contention of the accused, that the victim was a prostitute and offence of rape cannot be attributed, was not accepted by the trial court and he was convicted. The High Court reversed the judgment of the trial court. On appeal, the Supreme Court; while confirming the punishment on the accused, observed that the "unchastely of a woman could not make her open to any and every person to violate her person as and when she wishes". She is entitled to the protection of law. Therefore, merely because she is a woman of easy virtue her evidence cannot be thrown overboard. The accused being a police officer should abide the law and should protect the helpless. Here the accused violated the duties entrusted to him. Where the accused raped a handicapped helpless young girl, taking advantage of her blindness was convicted for the offence of rape. The court, held, in such cases, her passive submission cannot be treated as consent but it was due to her physical impairment.

In another case, where the victim of rape, due to shame and humiliation committed suicide, before the trial started. The Supreme Court by taking medical report and circumstantial evidence into consideration, reversed the High Court decision of acquittal, convicted the accused.

There is an alarming and shocking increase of sexual offences committed on children due to the reason that they are ignorant of the act of rape and they are unable to resist and become easy prey for lusty male who lure the children by their deceitful and insidious Act. While lamenting on this alarming situation the Supreme Court observed that "such offenders who are menace to the civilized society should be mercilessly and inexorably punished in the severest terms. Judges who bear the sword of Justice should into hesitate to use the swords with the utmost severity, to the full and to the end of the gravity of the offences so demand."

The relationship between mental illness and violence has stimulated much debate among both researchers and the public alike. There is undoubtedly considerable tension between public perception of the mentally ill person representing a high risk of violence and the reality of statistics that demonstrate relatively low levels of violence among this group. Given the steady increase in the proportion of sex offenders relative to the total offender population in recent years (Motiuk & Belcourt, 1996), it is perhaps not surprising that current public opinion is that individuals with a mental illness are primarily responsible for sexual offences, particularly those perpetrated against children. (Murray, et al. 1992). Given that the majority of those who commit sexual offences are not in fact suffering from a mental disorder (Chiswick, 1983), such fears are largely unfounded. Nonetheless, a small number of sex offenders are present in criminal mental health services who are suffering from a mental illness and who pose considerable challenges to forensic practitioners in relation to risk assessment and future planning.

The particular difficulties associated with working with this group of offenders will be highlighted by outlining briefly some of the work which has been carried out on the links between mental disorder and violence. This leads into a review of the small body of literature addressed specifically at sexual violence and psychosis. Discussion of a particular case illustrates the need for broad-based assessments which do not focus exclusively on psychopathology but also include consideration of relevant criminogenic factors.

Mental Disorder and Violence

Their work highlighted the fact that the strongest predictor of adult offender recidivism in mentally disordered offenders was criminal history, a finding consistent with earlier work carried out by Monaghan (1993). Similarly, variables including juvenile delinquency, family problems, poor living arrangements and substance misuse were also shown to play an important role in respect of risk prediction. This is identified by the authors as providing substantial support for adopting a sociopsychological approach to understand the anti-social conduct of mentally disordered offenders. Interestingly, the clinical variables which were included in the meta-analysis yielded little in relation to predictive validity. Indeed, the more severe mental disorders such as psychosis and schizophrenia were in fact inversely related to both general and violent recidivism, a finding that is in contrast to work by other authors in the field such as (Robins and Regier, 1991 and Swanson, 1994). The author note that one explanation for the variability across some of the studies may be due to the way mental disorder is defined in the country where the research is being carried out.

Research to date, which has looked at particular psychotic symptoms and their relative contribution to future violence, has yielded some interesting findings. Recent research has certainly indicated that the presence of specific symptoms may increase the likelihood of violence taking place. For example, organised delusions (Nestor, et al. 1995, Taylor, 1993) thought disorder (Gardner, et al. 1996) and command hallucinations (Bartels, et al. 1991).

The apparent lack of consensus regarding the role and relative influence of psychotic symptoms in relation to violent behavior may in part be attributable to the paucity of literature which looks at specific categories of violence, thus failing to account for relevant criminogenic factors. This poses particular challenges for the forensic practioner who is faced with the task of carrying out individual risk assessments on mentally disordered offenders. According to Bonta, et al. (1998), theories which have been identified as providing explanation for the behavior of so called rational offenders are likely to have significance for understanding mentally disordered offenders. What appears to be central to this field is clarification regarding which specific symptoms may, in conjunction with other risk factors result in an increase in the likelihood of violent behavior or, specifically, sexual violence occurring. The behavior of mentally ill sex offenders might, therefore, be better understood in the context of criminological theory in addition to psychopathological frameworks.

Sexual Offending and Psychosis

Chiswick (1983), in his review of psychiatric aspects of serious sexual offences, concludes that only a small number of sex offenders are suffering from mental illness. Research on adolescent sex offenders also indicates that conduct disorder is more commonly diagnosed in this group than mental illness (Kavoussi, et al. 1988). Chiswick (1983) goes on to suggest that understanding of offences in this group requires a comprehensive understanding of the offender, the victim and the environment, warning against adhering to rigid psychiatric nosology. Given the small numbers of sex offenders, who have a mental illness, together with some of the methodological and conceptual complexities briefly alluded to, it is perhaps not surprising that research in this area has been sparse and has tended to report on surveys (Henn, et al. 1976, Gibbens & Robertson, 1983, Murray, et al. 1992) or case studies (Craissati & Hodes, 1992, Huckle & Jones, 1993, Meloy & Gacono, 1992).

Surveys in this area have generally comprised mentally ill sex offenders as a sub-sample. Henn, et al. (1976) examined records of 239 individuals charged with sexual offences and found that major mental illness was very rare among both those who had been charged with rape and those who had offended against children. The subjects in Gibbson & Robertson (1983) survey of all men receiving hospital orders in the UK in the year 1963–64, excluding those given restriction orders were followed up over 15 years with regard to subsequent offences and convictions and hospital admissions. The authors noted that out of a sample of 378 patients with a mental illness, 17 had committed a sexual assault, of which five were described as 'serious assaulters' defined as having three or four convictions.

In what is the largest published review of sex offenders in the Special Hospital System, Murray et al. (1992) identified 32 patients with a mental illness out of a group of 106 sex offenders, with five subjects being excluded from the study because of a dual diagnosis of psychopathic disorder and mental illness. Of interest, here are the apparent similarities and differences between this age group and the other social hospital sex offenders. Significantly, choice of victim was noted to be different among the mentally ill group with only 6% targeting victims under 11 years of age, compared to 28% and 33% in a psychopathic disordered group and mentally handicapped group respectively. Further 94% of the mentally ill group had offended against females compared with 72% and 43% in the other groups. Interestingly, the range of sexual offences committed by the three groups was consistent with a high percentage of subjects engaging in at least one offence in the "sexual touching", 'exhibitionism' and other including 'sexual threats' categories. The authors concluded that in light of their findings overall, there may be a case for including mentally ill sex offenders. Such an assertion would indicate that factors other than those associated with the offenders' illness may also be an important target for treatment.

In addition to Special Hospitals, sex offenders with a mental illness are also located in medium secure provision. Craissati & Hodes (1992) described a sample of 11 male sex offenders suffering from a psychotic illness resident in a medium secure unit with 10 of the patients reported to have a diagnosis of schizophrenia. Interviews with nine of the patients revealed that the offences involved minimal violence, leading the authors to conclude that sociopathic traits were not a feature of this group. This work provides an interesting contrast with Kalichman's (1990) findings, which suggest that rapists have traits in common with other offenders in general. These include poor impulse control and significantly sociopathic traits. Somewhat surprisingly, in light of work described above, Craissati & Hodes also reported that a history of delinquency or family history of criminality was not a feature of this group. Rather, they concluded that the primary casual factor in their offending was sexual disinhibition. While phallometric assessment was not employed in this particular study, it might be useful for future research to delineate further the nature of this sexual disinhibition.

Huckles & Jones (1993) provided a commentary on the above study suggesting that there may be an alternative explanation for the mentally ill sex offenders' behavior. They stress the importance of carrying out a full mental state examination as soon as possible after the commission of the offence to ensure that the practioner does not miss the presence of command hallucinations at the material time. However, they suggest that patients may actively hide their symptoms at the time of the assessment. In an attempt to provide some empirical support for their position, Jones, et al. (1992) explored the possible links between the role of command hallucinations and sexually assaultive behavior by examining four case studies in which the two were reported to co-exist. It is reported that there is a possible link between the role of command hallucinations and sexually assaultive behavior.

Assessment of Sexual Offending

Sexually offending can be assessed by using the following rating scales:

1. The Minnesota Multiphasic Personality Inventory-2 (MMPI-2) (Hathaway & McKinley, 1989). This is a broad band test comprising 567 items which asseses a number of the major patterns of personality and emotional disorders.
2. The Rust Inventory of Schizotypal Cognitions (RISC): This is a 26-item, self-report scale for assessing the Schizotypal cognitions associated with the positive symptoms of schizophrenia and schizotypal personality.

3. The Multiphasic Sex Inventory (MSI) (Nicholls & Molinder, 1984): This is a 300-item, self report questionarrie comprising 20 scales which assess sexual deviance, treatment attitudes, social sexual desirability, sexual obsessions, lie scale, cognitive distortions, immaturity, justifications, paraphilias, sexual dysfunction, sexual knowledge and beliefs and sexual history.
4. The Hypermasculinity Scale (HIS) (Mosher & Sirkin, 1984): This is a 30-item, forced choice questionnaire which measures macho personality constellation consisting of three components; violence as manly, danger as exciting, and callous sexual attitudes towards women.
5. The Rape Myth Acceptance Scale (RMAS) (Burt, 1980): This is a 19-item, self-report questionnaire, which measures adherence to common myths about rape.
6. Attitudes to Women Scale (AWS) (Spence, et al. 1973): This is a 45-item, self-report scale which measures stereotyped and traditional attitudes to male/female roles.

This list is not meant to be definitive for this type of assessment, but merely serves to illustrate some of the available measures appropriate for this area.

Adolescent Sex Offenders

Sex offences committed by adolescents are a rising problem according for 20 to 30% of rapes and 30 to 60% of child molestation cases. Half of all adult offenders began their aberrant pattern of sex offending while juveniles. It is of vital importance to identify the type of offending pattern in juvenile sex offenders as outcome research has shown an excellent response to specialized treatment and supervision in this population of offenders. We illustrate the spectrum of juvenile sex offenders with two brief vignettes. Research on this population shows that although each case adjudicated must be individually scrutinized the vast majority are best left in the juvenile justice system.

The following are some of the facts regarding adolescent sexual offenders:

- Their offending behaviors are not simply attempts to learn about sex.
- Not all offenders are male (see Mathews et al. 1997).
- They derive from all races, socio-economic classes and levels of intellect.
- The victims are often known to the perpetrator.
- Adolescent sexually deviant conduct will not go away with simply maturity.
- The label of sex offender will not predispose the youth to re-offend.
- Sexual assaults are not primarily sexually motivated behaviors.
- Sexual offences are largely planned actions.
- The trauma to victims does not vary with the age of the offender.
- Adolescent offenders typically have committed more than one offence when apprehended.
- Adolescent sex offenders require sex offender specific treatment.
- Not all adolescent sex offenders have been victims of sexual abuse.

Psychological reactions of rape

- Anxiety and fear
- Post traumatic stress disorder
- Depression
- Sexual dysfunction
- Rumination
- Refused to cooperate.

Long-Term Consequences of Rape

It is difficult to predict all the long-term needs of the rape victim, because individual response patterns and circumstances differ so much. A few of the reactions that do appear clinically, often at a later date, are as follows:

1. Mistrust of men with consequent avoidance or hesitation to form relationships.
2. A variety of sexual disturbances, often presenting as sexual dysfunctions and marital conflicts.
3. Persistent phobic reactions.
4. Anxiety and depression, which may be precipitated by seemingly unrelated events that in some way bring back the original trauma.
5. Persistent anxiety and avoidance of gynecologic examinations or procedures.
6. Suicide and suicide attempts. Preliminary studies of female suicide attempters suggest the possibility of a relationship between an earlier rape experience and suicide attempts.

There are two potential problems related to rape victims.

1. Only minority of the victims seek medical and psychological help probably due to the stigma attached to the rape.
2. Even though during the acute critical phase, they come for medical help for the long-term assessment and management, most of them are reluctant to come for followup. Apart from this, there is resistance from the community, hospital authorities, and women voluntary organizations to recognize rape as a health issue requiring medical and psychological intervention. Even now, the participation by psychiatrists in the management of rape victim is very scarce. Hence, there is an urgent need to educate the women organizations, community-health workers, social workers, and hospital professionals and women organizations are to be sensitized about the importance of utilizing the psychiatric services.

Long-term follow-up data on the effects of rape as well as research on the effects of therapeutic intervention with rape related problem is needed. The research on the sociological and psychological reactions aftermath of rape to be dealt with.

The Mythology of Rape

The mythology which surrounds rape has been developed, perpetuated and reinforced by a number of attitudes and values which are reflected in both the medical and legal systems.

A few of these myths are discussed below:

1. Women can't be raped unless they want to be. A corollary of this might be that women enjoy rape. Or that they at least unconsciously want it, therefore, there is no such thing as rape.
2. The rapist is a sexually unfilled and/or disturbed man carried away by a sudden, uncontrollable rage.
3. Rapists are always strangers to victims.
4. Rape occurs primarily on the street, and as a long as a woman stays home, she is safe.
5. Most rapes involve black men raping white women.
6. Women are raped because they ask for it by dressing seductively and walking provocatively; thus only "bad" women are raped.

The first of these myths represents a serious misperception of the situation, as well as of the concept of the unconscious. The prevalence of conscious or unconscious rape fantasies hardly make every woman a willing victim and every man a rapist. The fantasy does not remotely capture the actual violence or degradation of the experience. Although fantasies in which rape plays a part are frequent, the rape victim in a real situation knows that she is submitting because there is no choice without real danger to her person or to her life.

Although definitive data are lacking, there are studies that shed light on a few of the other myths involving rape. In 1971, Amir published data that encompassed all cases of rape, not including incest or statutory rape, listed by the police in 1958 and 1960 in the city of Philadelphia. The data included 646 victims and 1291 offenders. Three-quarters of the rapes involved one or two assailants (single rape, 57 percent, pair rape, 16 percent) group rape (three or more assailants) was the pattern in 27%. Of the total number of incidents 71 percent were planned in advance, and only 16 percent could be considered as resulting from an uncontrollable impulse. Group rapes were planned in 90 percent of cases, and single and two-assailant rapes in 58% of cases. Thus the "uncontrollable urge" theory of rape is challenged.

The myth that staying at home is safe fails to recognize that 56% of rapes in the Amir study occurred in the victim's residence, and the remainder was divided among automobiles, outdoors, and other indoor places. Moreover, in only half of the cases was the rapist a stranger to the victim, the remainder included casual acquaintances, neighbors, boyfriends, family friends, and relatives. Indeed, a recent study concluded that the number of victims who know their assailants is probably higher than 50 percent. Husbands were not included in these statistics because, until quite recently, a sexual act between husband and wife was not considered rape under American Law.

Hayman and Lanza report on 1223 cases in which the age of the victim ranged from 15 months to 82 years. Twelve percent were victims under 12, 25 percent were between 13 and 17, and 32 percent were between 18 and 24, and 30 percent were over 25. The rapists were almost all less than 30 years of age. The majority of reported rapes involved rapists and victims of the same race. Earlier studies suggested a high proportion of black rape, but the significance of this is unclear. It is possible that black rapists are most likely to be reported and apprehended and that white rape may be grossly underreported or less aggressively pursued when reported. A Denver *Study 12* is an exception in that 71 percent white, 15 percent black, and 11 percent chicano.

More recent studies lend support to the view that rape is a crime of opportunity. Rape is largely an intraracial event and is ecologically bound, occurring as it does between members of the same race, economic class, and geographic neighborhood. Rape is most likely to occur in areas with higher unemployment rates and lower median incomes and in areas where there are higher number of unemployed youths between the ages of 14 and 21 years.

In Amir's study, physical force was present in 86 percent of cases, the remainder involved various degrees of nonphysical force such as coercion or intimidation with or without weapons. Amir characterizes physical force in the following way:

- Roughness (holding, pushing around) 29 percent
- Nonbrutal beating (slapping) 25 percent
- Brutal beating 20 percent
- Choking and gagging 12 percent

These statistics do not include rape that ends in death. This group is reported in the homicide statistics rather than in rape statistics. Thus, in one third of the cases, in which physical force occurred, extreme brutality was used.

In group rape, there is evidently a higher frequency of both alcohol intake and prior criminal records, especially of sexual offenses. The assault is usually planned and is more brutal in terms of beatings and subjecting the victim to sexually humiliating practices in addition to the rape.

Victim behavior is described by Amir as submissive in 55% with some degree of resistance in the remainder. At the time of assault, the victim must decide whether she has a greater fear of the rape or of physical injury. Her actions will reflect her decision, usually without opportunity for thought. A dilemma is presented in that resistance increases the victim's chance of escape, but also increases the likelihood of violence towards her should she not escape.

Rape occurs in a context of violence rather than of passion; "Rape is a deviant Act, not because of the sexual Act per se, but rather in the mode of the Act, which implies aggression, whereby the sexual factor supplies the motive." Mythology has it that most rapists are sexually perverted, but Amir suggest that rapists are a danger to the community not because they are necessarily sexually perverted but because of their violence and aggression. They often may appear to be "normal" but they tend to have criminal records of offences committed with brutality and violence.

Medico Legal Aspects of Rape

The law relating to rape has undergone a tremendous change after amendment of the Section 375 and 376 and the insertion of new sections 376A, 376B, 376C, and 376 D of IPC. Section 228 A of IPC has been incorporated to protect the victim of rape, a girl or woman, from embarrassment due to the glare or damaging publicity.Section 228 A reads as follows:

1. Whoever prints or publishes the name or any matter which may make known the identity of any person, against whom an offence under sections 376, 376 A to D, is alleged or found to have been committed, shall be punished with imprisonment of either description for a term which may extend to two years and shall also be liable to fine.
2. Under section 327 of the CrPC, similar protection is extended to a rape victim to the effect that the enquiry should be conducted "In Camera". Section 114A of the Indian Evidence Act provides that where the sexual intercourse by the accused is proved and she alleges that she has been raped the court shall presume, she did not consent for the same.

Unnatural Offences

The following are considered to be unnatural sexual acts and offences are listed as follows:

a. Homosexuality/lesbianism
b. Bestiality
c. Sodomy
d. Sadism
e. Masochism
f. Frotteurism
g. Voyeurism
h. Exhibitionism
i. Necrophilia
j. Pygmaliomism.

INTERNET, SEXUAL PREDATORS AND FORENSIC PSYCHIATRY

Forensic psychiatrist involved in the evaluation of stalkers, pedophiles, and other sexual predators requires at least a basic understanding of the internet, its uses and misuses,

The forensic psychiatrists benefit from specific knowledge of how offenders use the internet. This knowledge will help in gaining an understanding the offenders' temptations, choices, and potential online behavior.

Whether online support encourages sexual predators to act on impulses that would have otherwise remain dormant?

Whether the internet is leading to an increase in stranger stalking?

PORNOGRAPHY AND SEXUAL OFFENDING

- There is a relationship between pornography and sexual crime.
- Sexual offenders are known to be heavy users of dornography (Blackburn, 1993).

- Commercially produced pornography, marketed as entertainment promotes sexual objectification.
- Generally and features specific themes of control and domination.
- Pornography contributes to a climate of institutional sexism, exploitation and intimidation.

INDECENT ASSAULT

- Sec. 354 of IPC deals with this offence.
- A man who behaves indecently with a woman commits an assault.
- This shall be punishable with two years imprisonment with or without fine.
- Indecent assault means outraging the modesty of a women.
- The Indian Law has taken all the care about the potention of the women from the sexual assaults on them, but had taken for granted that the Indian women always speak the truth.

HOMOSEXUALITY

- Viewed as illegal in India.
- No longer illegal in many Western countries.
- Now, considered as sexual orientation disturbance sexual offences.

Homosexual Offences

- Buggery
- Acts of gross indecency
- Attempts and assaults
- Prostitution
- Homosexual rape
- Homosexual as victims.

Miscellaneous Anomalous Sexual Behaviors

- Indecent exposure (Exhibitionism).
- Obscene telephone calls (Scatologia).
- These offenders mostly have other associated sexual deviations. It is an offence under telecommunication Act.
- Sexual asphyxia—induction of sexual pleasure by anoxia; a form autoeroticism—confined to males.
- Necrophilia—sexual arousal with dead bodies.

Incest

- The sexual relation between family members forbidden by taboos, social norms and the law.
- Incest is a specific offence in many countries.
- The incest laws were passed in the hope of deterring the behavior, this has not happened.
- Vast majority of the cases do not come to the surface at all due to areas reasons.

In India, the impact and influence of the pseudowestern culture and the communication media will increase the risk of sex related crimes. When human beings deviate from the very biological aspect of the sex and abuse, there would always be a danger. The stringent law alone cannot change the sexual deviations and sex related crimes. It is healthy sex which pleasures, propagates and protects the human race.

CONCLUSION

Significant research in sexual sadism, serious sexual violence and biological causes is in progress. Internet sexual offending is the new frontier for study of child and adolescent sexual offenders. Ongoing research into the characteristics of offenders and the process of treatment continued to be important in reducing sexual violence.

Assessment of sexual violence is gaining greater importance. Cognitive distortions are fundamental to the assessment and treatment of pedophilia. The Sexual Offenders Assessment Package (SOAP). Which measures social functioning, personality profile, and a measure of obsessive compulsiveness in sexual deviants.

SUGGESTED READING

1. Bhujang, PM. Mentally ill and the law. Universal publishing corporation, Mumbai, 2003.
2. Blueglass R, Bowden P. Principles and practice of forensic psychiatry, 1990.
3. Chiswick D, Cope R. Practical forensic psychiatry, Royal college of psychiatry, 1995.
4. Gunn J, Taylor P. Clinical, legal and ethical issues in forensic psychiatry 1993.
5. Nambi S. Legal aspects of psychiatry—Indian perspective, 2009. Manashanthi Mental Health Care Publications, 2008.

9 Chapter

Forensic Psychiatric Services—A Feasible Model for Developing Countries

FORENSIC PSYCHIATRY

Forensic psychiatry is a subspecialty of psychiatry in which scientific and clinical expertise is applied to legal issues in legal contexts embracing civil, criminal, correctional, or legislative matters. The treatment of mentally disordered offenders (or even potential offenders) as a primary function.

Law Relating to Psychiatry

1. The Care and Treatment Legislation (Mental Health Legislations).
2. Criminal Responsibility Formulation (Criminal Laws).
3. Civil Status Provisions (Civil Laws).

THE RIGHTS OF THE MENTALLY ILL

Right to:

- The same fundamental rights as their fellow citizens, including the right to a decent life, as normal and full as possible.
- Legal safeguards against abuse appeal.
- Necessary treatment in the least restrictive setup and as far as possible to treatment and care in the community.
- Rehabilitation.
  - Personal autonomy, privacy, freedom of communication
  - Education
  - Training
  - Economic and social security
  - Family and community life employment
  - Protection against exploitation and discriminator.
- Abusive or degrading treatment.
- Assistance, including legal to protect their neglects.

FOUNDATIONS OF A MENTAL HEALTH SYSTEM

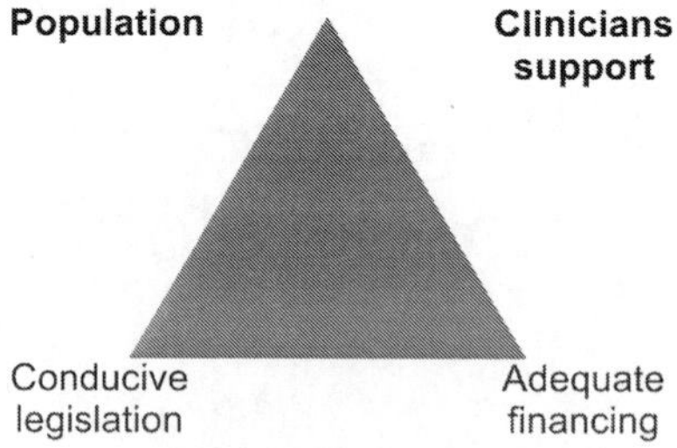

Epidemiological surveillance, data and evidence-based medicine.

DIFFERENT TIMES—DIFFERENT SYSTEMS

Custodial care (Asylums)
↓
Mental hospitals
↓
Mental health institutes (Psychiatric hospital)
Deinstitutionalization ↓
Community care

Admission and detention of mentally ill prisoner in psychiatric hospital in India.
1. Undertrial prisoners
2. Not guilty by reason of insanity
3. Convicts.
(Those who are undergoing imprisonment)

Characteristics of Mentally Ill Criminals in India

- Male out number female—95%:5% majority of them are undertrial prisoners (nearly 80%)
- Majority of them suffer from psychotic disorders, especially schizophrenia
- Most of the patients referred committed major crime (Murder)
- A significant proportion of patients were abusing alcohol and other drugs.

Crime and Psychiatric Disorders

- Criminality has been associated with mental illness for a long time
- There did seem to be greater than chance association between mental disorder and crime
- The current psychopathology need not be always the cause for the crime. Other factors like personality structure and the social setting may be equally important
- Management of forensic psychiatric patients:
  - Psychiatrists provide treatment to criminal offenders is often in conflict concerning the selection of patients and the purposes of therapy.

  - The selection of patients should always constitute and independent judgment by the therapist based on clinical diagnosis, need for treatment and the effectiveness treatment.
- Clinical forensic services are a liaison function, not an independent therapeutic practice.

THE ROLE OF MEDICATION

- Medication is only one aspect of patient management and is complementary to psychological and social interventions.
- Treatment should be aimed at the underling mental disorder rather than aggression perse.
- Parenteral use of Haloperidol and Benzodiazepines like Lorazepam preferred.

MANAGEMENT OF FORENSIC PSYCHIATRIC PATIENTS

Security: Maximum security is provided by the staff by keeping the mentally ill prisoners in a ward made of high walls like prison.

Seclusion: A widely practiced procedure. Seclusion is defined as the supervised confinement of a patient specifically a space alone in a loft room for a period for the protection of the patient, staff or others from series harm.

Physical restraint: Can be used very rarely without injuring the patients.

MANAGEMENT IN FORENSIC PSYCHIATRY

- In Forensic Mental Health practice, an environment with compulsion and coercion play greater a role.
- The institutionalized (prison or forensic hospital) management is often less than optimal for therapeutic activities and often inimical .
- Dual mandate for forensic mental health professionals—containing and controlling at the same time as treating and caring .
- The outcome in terms of social goals such as the prevention of recidivism as well as health goals such as reduced symptoms and improved function.

THE PLIGHT OF THE MENTALLY DISORDERED OFFENDERS

The insane criminal has nowhere to go no go age or nation has provided a place for him. He is everywhere unwelcome and objectionable. The prisons thrust him out, the hospitals are unwilling to receive him. The law will not let him stay in his house, the public will not let him go to the community, and yet humanity and justice, the sense of common danger, and a tender regard for a deeply degraded man all agree that something should be done for him. The mentally ill criminal offenders have double disqualification being considered both 'mad' and 'bad' (Halleck, 1986).

The Guiding Principles for the Care of Mentally Disordered Offenders (Reed Report)

- By Health and Social Services.
- With regard to the quality of care and proper attention to the needs of the individual.
- As far as possible in the community, rather than in institutional settings.
- Under conditions of security no greater than is justified by the degree of danger they present to themselves or others.
- In such a way as to maximize rehabilitation and their chances of sustaining an independent life.
- As near as possible to their own homes or families, if they have them.

Where they Want to be?

- Psychiatrists, in prison, in forensic unit of a psychiatric hospital, or a visiting psychiatrist to prison.
- Mentally ill prisoners—in Prison or in psychiatric hospital.
- What the human rights activists think?

Maximum Secure Hospitals–the Clinical Issues

- Mental Disorder is probably more commonly associated with dangerous actions, than would be expected by chance.
- Minority of these mentally disordered people need treatment is a maximum security hospital.
- Good Treatment is not incompatible with security, indeed, it is essential to it.

A Balance between Treatment and Security

Factors to ensure the balance:

- Replacement or upgrading of old buildings with modern facilities
- The discarding of prison style uniforms
- Emphasis on individual based treatment program
- Efforts to decrease the institutionalization.

FORENSIC PSYCHIATRIC SERVICES

1. Prison
2. Exclusive Forensic Psychiatric Hospitals (special hospitals)
3. Forensic Psychiatric Unit in Psychiatric (mental) hospitals
4. Correctional settings for juveniles.

PSYCHIATRIC DISORDERS IN PRISONERS

- Psychiatric symptoms are common in the first two months of imprisonment.
- Between a third and a half may have ICD-10 classifiable psychiatric disorder.
- Personality disorder and substance abuse are the most common diagnoses.

- High rates of psychotic disorder exist in prisoners remanded for psychiatric reports.
- In sentenced prisoners the prevalence of psychotic disorder is similar to that in the general population.

MENTALLY ILL OFFENDERS

- From prison to psychiatric hospital
- Whom to be transferred? (Forced Treatment)—Violent, unmanageable:
  - Potentially dangerous to himself or to other inmates
  - Whose psychiatric illness showing irreversible deterioration
  - Very disturbed patient who refused to take treatment.

FORENSIC PSYCHIATRIC SERVICES IN PRISON SETTINGS

- Exclusive for mentally ill offenders and for psychopaths
- Mental health professionals constantly station at prison or
- Service by visiting Mental Health Professional.

FORENSIC PSYCHIATRIC HOSPITALS (SPECIAL HOSPITALS)

- An exclusive treatment center for persons involved with legal implications
- High security hospital with emphasis more on containment and coercion along with treatment and care of the mentally ill offenders
- A centre in between psychiatric hospital and prison.

THE MEANING OF SPECIAL HOSPITAL CARE

- Physical security
- Prisons although, unlike
- Security by staff numbers
- Security by training
- Security by selection
- Political and administrative security
- Psychiatric treatment as security.

FORENSIC PSYCHIATRIC SERVICES IN PSYCHIATRIC HOSPITALS

- A highly secured separate ward for mentally ill prisoners (mentally ill offenders)
- Services for involuntary admissions of dangerous, unmanageable and uncooperative patients
- Services for persons admitted for judicial inquisition.

FORENSIC PSYCHIATRIC SERVICES FOR CHILDREN AND ADOLESCENTS

- Children and adolescents need special care and attention.
- Juvenile delinquents have immunity against punishment.
- The crime committed by children is usually not considered as an offence.
- For treatment, care and protection they need to have special correctional settings.

FORENSIC PSYCHIATRIC SERVICES

System that is:
1. Patient focused
2. Respectful of rights of patients
3. Aimed at recovery from illness
   - Least restrictive alternative respects of autonomy empowering
   - Normalization including expectation of quid pro quo (duties and obligations)
4. Responsive to local needs
5. Information based and accountable.

FORENSIC PSYCHIATRIC SERVICES—A FEASIBLE MODEL FOR DEVELOPING COUNTRIES

- The most feasible model is the forensic psychiatric unit/ward in a psychiatric hospital with high security and constant care by mental health professionals.
- A separate, special, forensic psychiatric hospital has its own disadvantages like cost, human resource and double stigma.

PSYCHIATRIC HOSPITALS—NOT PRISONS

- The emphasis should be on therapy and rehabilitation rather than control and containment.
- High security forensic units will again oppress the mental health services.
- Risk of detaining non-criminal mentally ill is high in prison setup.

10 Chapter

Prediction of Dangerousness and Management of Violent Behavior

In the day-to-day practice of psychiatry, especially, those who practice psychiatry in hospitals do come across mentally ill persons who are dangerous and indulge in violent behavior. Hence, it is essential for the practicing psychiatrists to have knowledge and skills in predicting dangerousness and if possible preventing, otherwise, treating the violent behavior. Very often, the dangerous offender is equated with the violent offender. One definition of dangerousness is "A propensity to cause serious physical injury or bringing psychological harm to others" (Butler 1975). According to Law Dictionary, the word "dangerous" means "exposing to" or "involving danger", able or likely to inflict injury. From medicolegal point of view, dangerousness may be classified as follows (AB Dutt, 1997).

Dangerous persons maybe either:

1. Patients or
2. Accused.

A and B mentally unsound are the mentally ill more dangerous than the non-mentally ill? The most obvious problems concern the definition of terms such as "mentally ill", "dangerous", and "violent". We can consider the following three questions:

1. Does the psychiatric disorder contribute significantly to dangerousness?
2. What happens to dangerous patients after discharge?
3. Are there any factors associated with dangerousness?

It is proved beyond doubt that persons suffering from severe mental illness exhibit more dangerousness and violent behavior. This is more than a chance

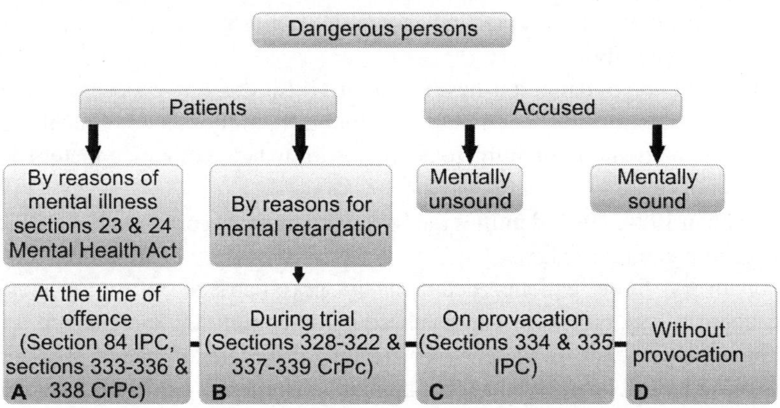

Mentally ill and dangerousness in—Indian legal view

coincidence. Lindquist and Alleybeck 1990 found the risks of serious violence in schizophrenia to be four times that of normal control. Similarly, Wessely, et al 1994 found that violent offence in men with schizophrenia was 3.8 times more likely than with other mental disorders. Apart from schizophrenia, other psychotic disorders like acute psychosis, postpartum psychosis, substance-induced psychosis, bipolar disorder—Mania and organic psychotic conditions are more vulnerable for violent behavior.

RISK FACTORS ASSOCIATED WITH DANGEROUSNESS

The factors which need to be taken into account in assessing dangerousness can be summarized as follows:

1. Being a male.
2. Being young.
3. Coming from an economically deprived sub-group.
4. Substance abuse.
5. Lacking social supports.
6. Having an established pattern of violent behavior.
7. Having a personality structure given to conflict, lacking impulse control and marked by a paucity of feelings for others.
8. Having shown conduct disorder as a child delinquent behavior as an adolescent.
9. The previous offence or offences taking particular note of:
   - The context
   - The predispositions revealed
   - The state of mind at the time
   - The behavior of the victim
   - The intentions of the perpetrator
   - The outcome for the victim and the subsequent behavior of the attacker.
10. Mental disorder, having regard to:
    - Its type and likely natural history
    - The associated disturbances of mental state
    - Its relationship, if any, to previous offences
    - Its likely effect on social and economic supports
    - Its manageability.

The prediction of dangerousness is dubious business, but on occasion, it is our business. In situations of uncertainty and doubt, the only help is clinical method applied with meticulous attention to detail and knowledge of which factors do and which do not relate to violent behavior.

Monahan 1984, 1993 identifies the following three important factors to predict violence in mental disorders.

1. For every three patients detained by psychiatrists on the grounds of dangerousness, only two would subsequently commit the violent Act.
2. The basic predictors of violence for mentally disordered offenders are the same as those for offenders, who are not mentally disordered, e.g. previous violence.
3. Diagnosis, severity of disorder, and personality traits are the poorest predictors.

THE MACARTHUR VIOLENCE, RISK AND ASSSESSMENT STUDIES

The MacArthur study is the largest study to examine risk factors for violence in patients in the community. It consists of a descriptive, a 12-month-follow-up of 1136 patients discharged from general psychiatry hospital in three US Cities.

Baseline Research Diagnosis in the MacArthur Violence Risk Assessment Study (%, N = 1136)

Depression/dysthymia	40.3
Alcohol or drug abuse/dependence	23.9
Schizophrenia/schizoaffective disorder	17.2
Bipolar disorder	13.3
Other psychiatric disorder	3.5s
Personality disorder only	1.8

The main findings of MacArthur are:

1. Violence is common in mental health population.
2. Substance misuse is more important than mental illness as a cause of violence.
3. Psychopathy is a riskful predictor of violence in general mental health population.
4. Violence in mental health population is related to many of the same factors as in the general population.

MANAGEMENT OF VIOLENCE

A three-stage model at risk management is essential in assessing and managing the risk of violence.

The components are:

1. What is the nature and extent of risk?
2. To what extent can the risk be reduced by treatment?
3. Is the residual risk acceptable?

Monahan, 1993 Suggested the following principles of risk containment.

1. Risk assessment
2. Risk management
3. Documentation
4. Policy and
5. Damage control.

Appleby, et al. (2001) enumerated 12 point to a safer service in violent management.

1. Staff should receive training in the management of risk every three years.
2. All patients with severe mental illness and a history of self-harm or violence should receive the most intense level of care.
3. Individual care plans should specify action to be taken if the patient fails to attend or to comply with treatment.

4. There should be prompt access to services for patients in crisis and for their families.
5. Assertive outreach teams should be used to prevent loss of contact with vulnerable and high-risk patients.
6. Atypical antipsychotic medication should be available to all patients with severe mental illness, who are non-compliant with "typical" drugs because of side-effects.
7. There should be strategy for dual diagnosis patients covering training on the management of substance misuse, joint working with substance misuse services, and staff with specific responsibility to develop the local service.
8. In-patient wards should remove or cover all likely ligature points.
9. There should be follow-up within seven days of discharge from hospital for everyone with severe mental illness or a history of self-harm in the previous three months.
10. Patients with a history of self-harm in the last three months should receive supplies of medication covering no more than two weeks.
11. There should be local arrangements for sharing information with criminal justice agencies.
12. There should be a policy of post-incident multidisciplinary case review and the information should be given to families of involved patients.

Hence, Mental Health Professionals working with persons suffering from severe mental illness should be sensitized to understand, assess, predict the dangerousness, so that, not only they can minimize the violent behavior of the patient, but also to prevent the harm to the caregivers and other members of the community.

The first law of forensic psychiatry should be "always protect your back."

SUGGESTED READING

1. Kapur RL. Oration DLN Murthy Rao. Violence in India. A psychological perspective. IJP, 1994;36(4):163–9.
2. Sethi BB. Indian Journal of Psychiatry, 1984;26 (4).
3. Sharma S. Violence among psychiatric patients and criminals. IJP, 1988;30 (4):409-13.

11 Chapter

Admission and Discharge Procedures of Persons with Mental Illnesses

ADMISSION INSIDE A PSYCHIATRIC HOSPITAL/NURSING HOME AS PER MENTAL HEALTH ACT, 1987 (MHA)

It includes the following:
- Admission without reception order
- Admission with reception order
- Admission with detention order.

Admission without Reception Order

Voluntary:
a. Informal (Psychiatric Unit of Government Hospital).
b. Formal 1 under/section 15-17 Mental Health Act, 1987.

Section 15

Request by Major for Admission as Voluntary Patient

Request by major for admission as a voluntary patient—Any person (not being a minor) who considers himself to be a mentally ill person and desires to be admitted to any psychiatric hospital or psychiatric nursing home for treatment, may request the medical officer in-charge for being admitted as a voluntary patient.

Section 16

Request by Guardian for Admission of a Ward

Where the guardian of a minor considers such minor to be a mentally ill person and desires to admit such minor in any psychiatric hospital or psychiatric nursing home for treatment, he may request the medical officer in charge for admitting such minor as a voluntary patient.

Section 17

Admission and Regulation with Respect to Voluntary Patients

On receipt of a request under section 15 or section 16, the medical officer in charge shall make such inquiry as he may deem fit within a period not exceeding 24 hours and if satisfied that the applicant or, as the case may be, the minor requires treatment as an inpatient in the psychiatric hospital or psychiatric nursing home, he may admit therein such applicant or, as the case may be, minor as a voluntary patient.

Every voluntary patient admitted to a psychiatric hospital or psychiatric nursing home shall be bound to abide by such regulations as may be made by the medical officer in charge or the licensee of the psychiatric hospital or psychiatric nursing home.

DISCHARGE OF VOLUNTARY PATIENT

If a voluntary patient/guardian request for discharge the medical officer, in charge shall discharge the patient within 24 hours (Section 18), and if a minor admitted turn to be a major during hospitalization within one month, he shall request for continuation; otherwise to be discharged. If the patient continues to be ill, the medical officer in opines that discharge is not desirable, within 72 hours constitute a board consisting of two medical officers. If the board also opines is continuation of stay is desirable, the medical officer shall not discharge the patient.

ADMISSION PROCEDURES OF MENTALLY ILL IN PSYCHIATRIC HOSPITALS AS PER MENTAL HEALTH ACT (1987)

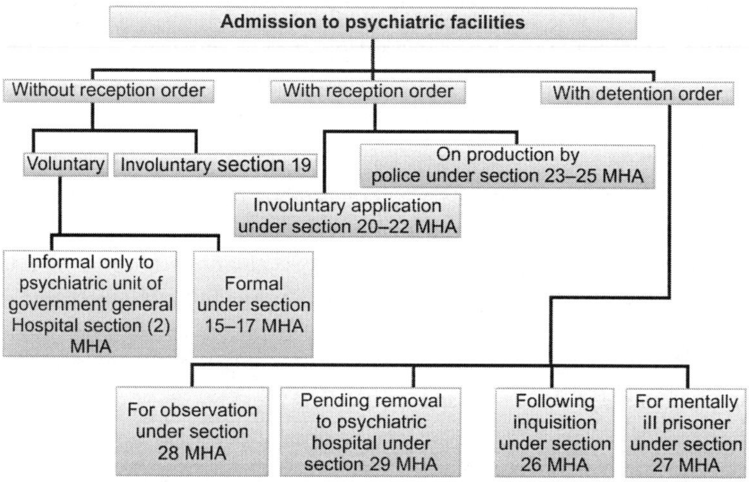

A welcome step to admit mentally ill, who does not, or is unable to express his willingness for admission, to be converted as voluntary basis, to get the reception order and the medical officer can request extension of the stay.

Dutt AB (2001), the long march of Mental Health Legislation in Independent India.

The patient or the relative can apply for discharge to the magistrate. If he is fit for discharge the magistrate shall pass the order, otherwise, dismiss to the application for discharge.

CRITERIA FOR PERSONS WHO CAN BE ADMITTED AS INVOLUNTARY IN THE TREATMENT

The criteria includes the following:

- Presence of mental illness.
- Immediate physical danger to himself and/or others because of his mental illness.
- Inability to engage in rational decision making, regarding the acceptance of mental illness.
- Absence of less restrictive alternative.
- Admission includes a therapeutic purpose.

VARIOUS TYPES OF INVOLUNTARY ADMISSIONS AS PER MHA—1987 INCLUDE

1. Admission under special circumstances—section 19
2. Admission through reception order:
   - Reception order on application—section 20, 21, 22.
   - Reception order in the case of wandering, dangerous mentally ill—Section 23 and 24.
   - Reception order in the case of mentally ill who are cruelly treated or not, under proper care—section 25.
3. Admission as in-patient after inquisition—under section 26.
4. Admission and detention of mentally ill prisoner under section 27.
5. For observation—under section 28.
6. Pending removal to psychiatric hospital—under section 29.

Admission Through Reception Orders (RO)

- Reception order on application section 20–22, MHA.
- Reception orders on production of mentally ill persons before magistrate Section 23–25, MHA.
- Further provisions regarding admission and detention of certain mentally ill persons Section 26–29.
- Miscellaneous provisions in relation to Order Section 30–36.

Admission and Detention of Mentally Ill Prisoner

WHO Expert Committee on Mental Health, in its fourth report (1955) suggested that should be cared in special establishments for criminals. If detained in mental hospital premises security by police to be provided in a specially created ward for mentally ill prisoners

However, National Human Rights Commission Orders states that the mentally ill persons should not be kept in prisons.

Admission and Detention of Mentally Ill Prisoner in Psychiatric Hospital in India

- Under trial prisoners—Section 330 of the code of criminal procedures, 1973.
- Not guilty by reason of insanity—Section 335 of the code of criminal procedures, 1973.
- Convicts—Section 30 of the Indian Prisoners Act, 1990.

DETENTION OF ALLEGED MENTALLY ILL PERSON PENDING REPORT BY MEDICAL OFFICER

When a person alleged to be mentally ill person appears or his brought before magistrate under section 23 or 25, the magistrate can order for detainment of this person in a Government Hospital/GHPU/Psy. Hospital/Nursing home for a period not exceeding 10 days for observation, assessment and issue a certificate (Maximum 30 days).

DISCHARGE OF PERSONS ADMITTED THROUGH RECEPTION ORDER (SECTION 40 TO 44)

Order of discharge by the medical officer—the medical officer on recommendation of two medical practioners (one to be a psychiatrist) may discharge any person other than voluntary patient or mentally ill prisoner. This to be informed to the admitting authority.

Discharge of mentally ill person on application—medical officer can discharge on an application made in that behalf. If dangerous or unfit, need not discharge (Section 42).

Persons admitted under section 22, 24, and 25—even if not improved, the relative, friend, may apply for discharge to the medical officer, he shall forward this to the admitting authority. By producing a bond and undertaking that the applicant is responsible to give care and the treatment to the patient, the admitting authority shall discharge the patient.

Discharge of Person on his Request (Section 43)

If a person feels that he is recovered, he may take an application to the magistrate for discharge. This application to be supported by the medical officer of the hospital. If patient is fit, the magistrate shall pass an order for discharge.

Discharge of Person Subsequently Found on Inquisition to be Sound Mind (Section 44)

If any person detained in the psychiatric hospital after inquisition, if he is of sound mind and can look after himself and/or his properties, the medical officers in charge shall discharge the person after certified by the District Court.

THE ROLE OF THE POLICE OFFICERS IN THE CARE OF THE MENTALLY ILL

- In case of the wandering, dangerous mentally ill—MHA Section 23
- In case of the mentally ill person cruelly treated or not under proper care and control – MHA, Section 25.
- Commissioner of police can function as magistrate—MHA, Section 38.
- Accompanying mentally ill prisoners formally to the prison and mental hospital.
- In the case of juvenile—mentally ill conflict with law Juvenile Justice Act, 2000, Section 10,13, and 32.
- In the case of attempted suicide—IPC Section 309.

Powers and Duties of Police Officers in Aspect of Wandering/ Dangerous Mentally Ill

- Every Officer in charge of police station shall take or cause to be taken into protection any person who is found wandering at large or dangerous by reason of mentally ill.
- The person or his relatives or friends has to be informed.
- The mentally ill person has to be produced before magistrate within 24 hours.
- Commissioner of police can function as Magistrate—Section 36 MHA, 1987.
- In any area, where a commissioner of police has been appointed, all the powers of the magistrate under section 23, 24, 25 and 28 may be exercised or discharged by the commissioner of police.

LEAVE OF ABSENCE (LOA)

Application for LOA can be made on behalf of any mentally ill person undergoing treatment as inpatient in psychiatric hospital/nursing home. Every application should be accompanied by a bond and undertaking to take care of the patient. Medical officer can grant LOA, for a period not exceeding 60 days (Section 45). If not returned in time, the matter to be informed to the magistrate/commissioner of Police. If a medical officer refuses LOA, the applicant may apply to magistrate. If he feels it is necessary, so, he may grant LOA after obtaining a bond.

Provisions on Admission and Treatment	
30. A person who presents himself or herself voluntarily to a mental health care facility for treatment or admission shall be entitled to receive appropriate care and treatment or to be referred to an appropriate mental health care facility.	Voluntary admission.
31. (1) No mental health care, treatment or admission shall be accorded to a person with mental illness without the person's informed consent or that of his or her representative.	Informed consent.

Contd...

(2) In order for consent to be valid under this section, it shall satisfy the following conditions— (a) The person with mental illness or his or her representative shall be competent to give the consent; (b) Consent shall be given freely without threats or improper inducements; (c) There shall be appropriate and adequate disclosure of all relevant information relating to treatment, including information on the kind, purpose, likely duration and expected benefits of the treatment; (d) Choices, where available, shall be given to the person with mental illness in accordance with prescribed clinical practice; (e) Consent shall be documented in the person's records.	
32. (1) A person may be admitted involuntarily to a mental health care facility as a person with mental illness, or, having been admitted voluntarily as a person with mental illness, be retained involuntarily as a person with mental illness in the mental health care facility, if a qualified mental health care medical practitioner determines, in accordance with this Act, that the person has a mental illness or disorder and considers that— (a) Because of mental illness or disorder, there is a serious likelihood of immediate or imminent harm to that person or to other persons; (b) In the case a person whose mental illness or disorder is severe and whose judgment is impaired, failure to admit or retain the person is likely to lead to a serious deterioration in his or her condition, or will prevent the giving of appropriate treatment that can only be given by admission to a mental health facility in accordance with the principle of the least restrictive alternative. (2) A mental health care facility may receive an involuntarily admitted person with mental illness, only if the facility has been designated to do so by law and only for the duration necessary to stabilize the person with mental illness, and provide mental health care services to him or her. (3) The following factors shall be considered in cases of involuntary admission— (a) There is evidence of a mental illness of a specified severity; (b) There is likelihood of immediate or imminent harm to the person with mental illness or others, and a deterioration of the person's condition if treatment or admission or both are not given; (c) The treatment can only be given by way of admission to the health facility.	Involuntary admission.
33. An emergency admission or treatment of a person with mental illness shall be administered where there is immediate and imminent danger to the health and safety of the person with mental illness or other people, and the nature of such immediate and imminent danger is such that there need to be urgent care and treatment to stabilize the person with mental illness.	Emergency admission and treatment.

34. (1) For any case to be considered an emergency, there shall first be shown that the time required to comply with substantive procedures would cause delay and lead to harm to the person with mental illness or to other people. (2) Where the requirements in subsection (1) have been satisfied, the person with mental illness may be admitted to the health facility or be given treatment based on the assessment carried out by a qualified medical practitioner or other accredited mental health practitioner.	Considerations for emergency cases.
35. (1) Emergency admission or treatment shall not be prolonged for duration longer than necessary to stabilize the person with mental illness and in any case, shall not be prolonged beyond a period of seventy-two hours, and shall be allowed only to the extent that it is necessary to treat the person with mental illness. (2) Emergency treatment shall not include— (a) Depot neuroleptics; (b) Electroconvulsive therapy; (c) Dterilization; (d) Psychosurgery or other irreversible treatment. (3) Procedures for emergency treatment or admission or both may be initiated immediately by a spouse, next of kin, partner, parent or guardian and authorized by a qualified medical practitioner if it is assessed that the person with mental illness is likely to require care beyond the stipulated time limit for emergency treatment. (4) The family of the person with mental illness or their representative shall be immediately informed of the emergency procedures undertaken. (5) A person with mental illness, his or her family or representative have the right to appeal against emergency admission or treatment to the Board. (6) The Cabinet Secretary may, on the recommendations of the Board, make regulations on emergency treatment and admission.	Duration of emergency treatment.
PART VI—Mentally Ill Offenders	
36. (1) Whenever a medical practitioner is of the opinion that a prisoner or a remandee is of unsound mind, the practitioner may, by order under his or her hand in the form prescribed, direct that such prisoner be removed to a mental health facility within the prison or outside the prison and be treated while under detention. (2) Where a prisoner or remandee transferred to a mental health facility pursuant to subsection (1) is, in the opinion of the person in charge of such mental health facility, no longer mentally ill, the person in charge of the mental health facility shall inform the officer in charge of the prison from which the prisoner was removed, and the prisoner shall then be delivered into the custody of the officer of that prison if still liable to be confined in prison, and if not so liable, shall be released. (3) The period during which the prisoner has been detained in the mental health facility under this section shall be recorded as part of the prisoner's term of imprisonment.	Facilities for mentally ill offenders.

(4) Mentally ill offenders shall be entitled to have their criminal cases expedited and given priority over other cases. (5) The Director of Public Prosecutions and other state officers shall expedite the process of granting mentally ill offenders within the criminal justice system the necessary authorizations and examinations and at no cost. (6) Mentally ill offenders shall be provided mental health care and treatment by the government. (7) There shall be special cells for mentally ill prisoners within which they shall be held separately from the rest of the prisoners or other persons with mental illness, and receive mental health care and treatment of the same quality and with the same frequency as other person with mental illness. (8) Mentally ill prisoners with severe mental illness may be transferred to a mental health care facility where they can receive appropriate treatment and care.	
Part VIII—Review, Appeals, Discharge and Transfer of Person with Mental Illness	
39. (1) The mental health status of a person with mental illness shall be reviewed periodically by a mental health care practitioner, and such review shall include a review of— (a) The nature of the illness; (b) The need for care and treatment; (c) The type of care and treatment provided; (d) The need for referral, transfer or discharge; and (e) Any other matters related to the mental health status of the person with mental illness. (2) The review of the mental health status of a person with mental illness may be initiated by— (a) The person with mental illness; (b) The mental health care practitioner in charge of managing the person with mental illness; (c) A representative of the person with mental illness; (d) The mental health care practitioner in charge of the facility; (e) Any other person upon proof of the nature of their interest; or (f) The Board. (3) The procedure for review shall be as prescribed under this Act.	
40. (1) Any decision made under review shall be subject to appeal in the first instance to the mental health care practitioner in charge of the facility, and further to the Board. (2) A person with mental illness or his or her representative who is not satisfied with the decision of the Board on appeal may appeal further to the High Court.	Appeals
41. A person with mental illness shall be discharged where— (a) The mental health care practitioner in charge of managing the person makes a decision to discharge the person as a result of a review; (b) The person can no longer receive any other or further treatment from a mental health care facility and appropriate efforts are being made towards re-integration of the person into the community, and for specialized and personalized after-care service.	Discharge of person with mental illness

42. (1) Where a mental health care practitioner is of the opinion that it would be for the benefit of a person with mental illness admitted in a mental health care facility, or that it is necessary for the purpose of obtaining special treatment for such person, the person may be transferred to another mental health care facility after obtaining consent from— (a) The person with mental illness; or (b) The representative of the person with mental illness; or (c) The other mental health care facility where the person with mental illness is being transferred to. (2) A person with mental illness in a health facility other than a mental health care facility may be transferred from the health facility to a mental health care facility.	Transfer of person with mental illness

CONCLUSION

The above new procedures of Admission and Discharge of mentally ill persons are as per the Mental Health Care Amendment Bill, 2012.

We have to wait and watch whether all these provisions are going to be enacted in the New Act. Till then, we are going to follow the admission and discharge procedures of Mental Health Act, 1987.

SUGGESTED READING

1. Dutt AB. "The Long March of Mental Health Legislation in Independent India".
2. Mental Health Care Bill 2012, Ministry of Health and Family Welfare, Government of India, New Delhi.
3. Nambi S. Legal Aspects of Psychiatry—Indian Perspective, 2009. Manashanthi Mental Health Care Publications, 2008.
4. Shah LP. Oration-2001. Indian Psychiatric Society, Western Zonal Conference, Goa.
5. The Mental Health Act, 1987 (Bare Act, 2003), Delhi Law House with Mental Health Authority Rules, 1990, along with State Mental Health Rules, 1990.

12 Chapter

Ethical and Legal Aspects of Electroconvulsive Therapy

ETHICAL AND LEGAL ISSUES WITH SPECIAL REFERENCE TO INDIA

Electroconvulsive therapy (ECT) is a time tested biological treatment method in Psychiatry. ECT has been considered as a life saving treatment for over five decades. It is a unique treatment in the field of psychiatry and powerful therapeutic force. The consumer protection movement is gaining momentum and the practice of psychiatry is no exception to this. Many Human Rights Activists have started fighting for the less privileged mentally ill persons. There is no antipsychiatry movement in India, which questions efficacy and desirability of ECT, except a few public interest litigation and adverse criticism by some media. In India, ECT is being used not only for its valued indications, but also for cost effectiveness of the treatment. In a developing country like India, when we plan treatment for mental disorders, some important issues are to be taken into account.

Some of them are:

Minimal duration of hospital stay, less cost of the treatment, try to achieve the earliest return to normal functioning, minimizing the family burden, etc.

In India, the practice of ECT has neither a legal regulation nor have any guidelines or code of conduct prescribed by any professional body. The new Mental Health Act, 1987 has no mention or regulation about this sensitive method. The scientific materials concerning ECT published in India only during the last decade including the National workshop on ECT at NIMHANS in 1990 and Bombay Psychiatric Society Guidelines, 2002. The psychiatrists in India can benefit from the international reports regarding the practice of ECT. The practicing psychiatrists should come to the conclusion upon whom he is going to administer the ECT based on his physical condition, history, symptomatology and other contraindications. He should be convinced himself that he has made every effort to minimize the risks and maximize the benefits.

A letter by a citizen to the Honorary Chief Justice and other of the High Court of Maharashtra considered by the High Court as a public interest litigation at the Central Institute of Mental Hygiene and Research, Yervada, Pune. The judgment incorporates a recommendation regarding ECT (PIL Shankari vs State of Maharashtra; Dated 10/11/1989. To quote "Hospital authorities should review the effects of the direct ECT on the patients and should decide whether the method should be continued in view of the fright taken by the patients, modified ECT is recommended."

It is always ideal to have modified ECT. In a country like India, considering the lack of infrastructure, anesthetists, practically, it may be difficult to strongly advocate that only modified ECT's should be given. If the psychiatrists have administered the ECT for his patient in the right place having the entire necessary infrastructure available and having selected, the patient on reasonable clinical judgment, usually the law cannot find fault on him. Universally, there is a decline in the use of ECT in the management of mental illness in the recent past. This applies to India also. The attitude towards ECT among the public and the practicing psychiatrists is so negative that the ECT administration has gone down drastically. The decline of ECT may be due to scientific and nonscientific reasons (Abhayankar, 1995). The scientific reasons are: Post ECT and lack of memory impairment, availability of safe and effective newer drugs, poor quality of research on ECT and lack of proper scientific and technical guidelines about the improved methods of ECT for practicing psychiatrists. Medicolegal problem, adverse publicity in the mass media, negative emotional and political factors are some nonscientific reasons for the decline in ECT.

It is not correct to judge that most of our people have negative attitude towards ECT often lack of information, explanation, and education may mislead the public to have negative attitude towards ECT. This will apply not only to the general public, mentally ill persons, but also to the non-psychiatric medical professionals. Hence, the very essential aspect to change this attitude is to disseminate the correct information and the efficacy regarding the ECT.

Few psychiatrists still use ECT excessively and indiscriminately to many patients, where it is not essentially needed, that is personality disorders, etc. a few mental hospitals in India in the recent past have come into the scrutiny of the courts. Misuse of ECT in these hospitals has been decried. The commission investigating Shahadra Mental Hospital observed that though most of the patients suffered from schizophrenia is highly doubtful (Supreme Court Enquiry Report 1984). The Commission also found that a fixed number of ECT's were being given without proper monitoring of the patient.

In India, all patients are administered ECT after getting the informed consent of the patient and also preferably of the relatives except those admitted by the Magistrate with reception order. Mental Health Act, 1987 is silent on administration of treatment to non-consenting certified. Even though, in the past, the Indian courts have taken some lenient attitude on some cases, it is extremely important that the informed consent is to be obtained from the patient and preferably from a relative also. Usually in our practice, the relatives often leave the decision making about ECT to the psychiatrists himself. A healthy, active doctor-patient relationship often helps to prevent medicolegal complications, but yet not always, because of the more and more awareness of consumerism. Administration of ECT against a patient's will is considered to be legal, but at the same time, it is highly unethical in not administering ECT to a deserving patient.

Informed consent is a basic requisite for administration of ECT. In some countries, it may even be considered a legal requirement. The basic issues involved in the informed consent are:

1. How much to be informed? How, to whom and by whom?
2. Is the person giving consent, competent to give consent?
3. Is the choice voluntary or involuntary?

Psychoses per se are not a contradiction to competence (Culvet, et al. 1980). The concepts of understandability comprehension), the reasonable outcomes of choice on rational reasons are important determinants. American Psychiatric Association Task Force of 1990 recommends a list of information to be provided in the consent document in which inclusive of very minor and sometimes delicate issue. Providing all such delicate issues may at times proved negative impact in our Indian patients. It is also essential to inform the positive aspects of the ECT like life saving methods, which relief in the symptoms and the most effective treatment if pharmotherapy fails. (AK Agarwal, 1997)

The legal, ethical, and social aspects of ECT can be classified and evaluated under a 4C. They are:

1. Conceptualization
2. Communication
3. Consent and
4. Carrying out of the treatment (GG Prabhu, 1990).

The informed consent is not a matter of getting a signature in the prescribed form. The information regarding the procedure should be explained. Once the patient denies giving consent, another chance may be given to reconsider his decision. Another important aspect is that just because the patient has refused to give consent for ECT, in simple language, (the language they understand). They should be informed about the consequences of not having the ECT.

It is better to avoid giving ECT if:

- The indication is likely to be legally questioned.
- Relationship of the consenting relative in not well defined.
- The observation period is, in your own opinion, inadequate.
- There is history of trauma or assault prior to a psychotic spell.
- The patient is recently released from jail/judicial custody.
- The infrastructure is inadequate, as per standard norms.
- There are multiple medicolegal complications.
- A patient with a proven psychiatric disorder, but without any accompanying relative, requesting an ECT.
- The patient is an defence personnel.
- The patient is a foreign national, and consent from the concerned consulate is not available.
- There is evidence of dispute about consent amongst the relatives.

PRACTICAL GUIDELINES FOR CLINICAL USE OF ELECTRO-CONVULSIVE THERAPY

Consensus Recommendations of Bombay Psychiatric Society, 2004

- There is a pressing need for the Indian Psychiatric Society to give guidelines and form a code of conduct—regulating the administration of ECT's by the Indian Psychiatrists. It is high time to have a self-evaluating introspection before the law brings out its regulation.
- It is strongly recommended peer review and medical audit of all treatments including ECT, from each will be because Psychiatrists have failed to supervise or monitor its use adequately (Lancet, 1981).
- *Consent*: The nature of psychiatric illness for which ECT is indicated prevents the patient from having an awareness and/or insight into the disease. Therefore, the psychiatrist takes the consent of the nearest concerned relative in good faith and administers the treatment. The illness tend to be relapsing and therefore disclosing the ECT treatment to the patient even after his recovery can be counter-productive for the treatment of future episodes whether and when to disclose the nature of treatment is at the discretion of the treating psychiatrist.

Information About ECT

To be imparted to relatives/guardians of patient who would give consent

Electroconvulsive therapy is used in many psychiatric conditions, like depressive disorders, schizophrenia, mania, other allied psychotic disorders, etc. In most cases, it hastens recovery and may work where drugs have failed. In some cases, it may be even safer than some drugs.

Generally, the patient is given anesthesia, though, sometimes it may be decided not to use it. Irrespective of whether anesthesia is used or not, the patient does not experience any pain whatsoever. A small electric current is passed across the head and this causes a mild "fit" in the brain. If a muscle relaxant has been used, there is little movement of the body due to such "fit".

On waking up, the patient may complain of headache and remain confused for about an hour or so. Occasionally, fall of loose tooth, tongue-bite and minor bleeding from lips and gums could occur.

Forgetfulness, lasting upto few weeks, is common, but there is no scientific evidence of permanent brain damage.

It is not possible to predict the exact number of sittings/ECTs required for the patient, in advance, but usually 6 to 12 ECTs were found to be effective in one course.

The treatment is usually given 2 to 3 times a week, but this may vary from patient to patient. Like in other medical and surgical treatment modalities, risk to life is not ruled out. Fractures are rare.

It is a scientific and effective form of treatment. Use of electroconvulsive therapy does not imply means that further treatment is not required. It is always necessary to continue medicines and report for a regular follow-up for a certain period of time.

Informed Consent for Electroconvulsive Therapy

I hereby consent to the administration of a course of electroconvulsive therapy to myself/my .... (Relation) .... (Name of the patient) by Dr........................ (Or any other suitably trained Doctor disputised by him).

I also consent to the use of an anesthetic and/or a relaxant or sedative for this purpose, at the discretion of the doctors.

I have been explained the nature and the purpose of the treatments, and I have opted for this treatment.

As regards possible side effects and complications, I understand that headache and confusion, immediately after treatment, are common, but short-lasting.

Memory deficit, lasting for a few weeks, is common but there is no scientific evidence of permanent brain damage.

I also understand that, like in other medical and surgical treatments despite all precautions, risk to life cannot be ruled out. Rarely, fractures may occur.

I authorize the doctors concerned to administer emergency treatment for all such complications, shift the patient to other hospital, and/or seek help of other specialists if necessary. I also undertake to bear the financial.

I confirm that I have explained to the patient/relative the nature, purpose, and likely effects of this treatment.

Shri/Smt ....was the nearest relation available.

Date/Time/Place **Signature of Doctor**

RELATIVE'S APPROVAL: (Wherever relevant)

I .... (Name) .... (The closest available relative) of .... (Patient's name) confirm that an explanation of the nature, purpose and likely effects of ECT has been given to me by Dr....................................... and that I approve of the treatment being given to the patient ....

Date/Time/Place **Signature of Relative**

SUGGESTED READING

1. Abhayankar R. ECT: Indications and medicolegal aspects, Archives of Indian Psychiatry, 1995;2 (1).
2. Agarwal AK, Andrade C. The practice of ECT in India. Issues relating to the administration of ECT. Indian Journal of Psychiatry, 1997;34:385–97.
3. American Psychiatric Association. Task Force Report on ECT. Washington DC, American Psychiatric Press 1990.
4. Andrade C, Gangadhar BN. Electrical Aspects of Electroconvulsive Therapy. A Review I Electrical Issues, Indian Journal of Psychological Medicine, 1989a;12(1): 53–60.
5. Batra L. Short textbook of psychiatry for undergraduate students, PeePee Publishers 2006.
6. Channabasavanna. Presidential Address at the 5th Annual Conference of the Indian Association of Social Psychiatry, New Delhi, 1989.
7. Gada M, Cholera R. Practical guidelines for clinical use of electroconvulsive therapy. Consenus Recommendations of Bombay Psychiatric Society.
8. Gangadhar BN. Proceedings of the National Workshop on ECT. Priorities for Research and Practice in India, Bangalore NIMHANS, 1992.
9. Lancet (editorial). ECT in Great Britain, A shameful state of affairs. Lancet, 1981;2: 1207–8.
10. Trivedi JK. Indian journal of psychiatry, No 2, April 1992;34:67-77.

13 Chapter

Prison Psychiatry

INTRODUCTION

Mental health services in India as they exist today mostly follow the British model. Naturally, the early institutions for the mentally ill in the Indian subcontinent were greatly influenced by the ideas and concepts as prevalent in England at that time. Primarily, mental asylums were built to protect the community from the violent behavior of the insane and not necessarily for treatment. Accordingly, these asylums were constructed away from the towns with high fences, in buildings, similar to military barracks. Their function was more custodial than curative.

The functioning of mental health care delivery in the early years of independence in India was based on the following parameters:

1. The then existing mental health care system was based on the British concept and no knowledge and understanding of cultural underpinnings of mental illness in the Indian context was taught or studied.
2. Significant shortage of trained personnel.
3. Non-pharmacological treatments of psychiatric disorders were limited.
4. The research literature focused mainly on the phenomenology of mental disorders and almost no valid epidemiological data was available.

India with its population of nearly 1.2 billion faces a variety of health problems. The sociodemographic changes, epidemiological transition and media revolution consequent to urbanization, industrialization, migration, and changing lifestyles of people, have brought the severe burden of communicable and non-communicable diseases to the forefront.

Worldwide, on an average 32% of all prisoners require psychological help. If one includes substance abuse, the figure goes beyond 60%. Hence, there is a need for focused attention on mental health. There is a need for early identification of mental illness among prisoners and for taking consequent steps. There is little documentation of the problems of psychiatrically ill prisoners, problem of referrals, discharge, follow-up and care while in custody. Arrangements are being made for periodic visits by psychiatrists (Section, 31 and 32 of the National Human Rights Commission recommendations on Mental Health Issues of Detentions, 2008).

Mentally ill prisoners of India share a common plight with most of their counterparts in the developing countries. There is no dignified or safe place for many of them. Mentally ill prisoners are unwanted and neglected everywhere; prisons try to move them elsewhere, but psychiatric hospitals are reluctant to admit them and relatives often refuse to let them stay in their house. Mentally ill prisoners suffer double stigma being considered both "mad" and "bad".

MENTAL HEALTH IN INDIA

Mental health problems have long been recognized in every society. Communities had their own mechanisms of handling these problems; many of which are gradually being replaced by modern science. A greater understanding of mind and behavior from all dimensions has revolutionized the efforts of managing these problems in today's society.

A more recent meta-analysis of 13 epidemiological studies in India comprising 33,572 individuals concluded that the prevalence estimate of mental disorders is 52.2 per 1000 population. Among the various problems, organic psychoses—0.4 per 1000, schizophrenia—2.7 per 1000, affective disorders—12.3 per 1000, mental retardation—6.9 per 1000, neurotic disorders—20 per 1000, and alcohol related disorders—6.9 per 1000 are the major problems encountered in the country. Mental disorders were found to be higher in urban areas, among women in the age group of 35-44 years and in individuals of lower socioeconomic status. The study concluded that nearly 1.5 million persons suffer from severe mental disorders and 5.7 million persons suffer from various common mental disorders requiring immediate help.

Forensic psychiatric services in India are poorly developed compared to the West. Persons suffering from mental illness, who are also offenders are now considered as "mentally ill prisoners". Earlier, they were known as "criminal lunatics" but this terminology is not commonly used anymore. There are 37 state-run mental hospitals in India with a total bed number of around 20,000. The majority of these mental hospitals have a separate ward for mentally ill prisoners.

GENERAL CHARACTERISTICS OF MENTALLY ILL PRISONERS IN INDIA

- Mentally ill prisoners form less than 2% of the total admissions in a state psychiatric hospital.
- The majority of them suffer from antisocial personality disorders and psychotic disorders especially, schizophrenia.
- Most of the mentally ill offender patients referred to psychiatric hospitals committed a major crime (mainly murder).
- A sizeable proportion of mentally ill prisoners are known to have abused alcohol and other drugs like cannabis.

PRISONS IN INDIA

According to the National Crime Record Bureau 2008, there are total number of 1140 jails in the country of which 107 are central jails, 208 are district jails and 678 are sub-jails (smaller jails situated in every taluk-county-headquarter where usually the remand prisoners are kept for a short-term before they are sentenced and sent to the central jails), 14 are for women only; other jails number 73. (In India the name, jail is synonymous with prisons). Sub-jail: Although, the total capacity of jails in India is only 233,543, the total number of prisoners is 326,519, thus overcrowding of jail is a fact of life in India. Men are 24 times as likely to be incarcerated as women. The various categories of the prisoners in India are as follows:

- Sentenced prisoners: 28.1%
- Remand prisoners: 66.7%

Among the nature of crime, murder alone accounts for 58.6%. There are 333 convicts, including women, awaiting execution in the country and there are 48,334 convicts serving life-imprisonment accounting for 52.7%.

CRIMINAL RESPONSIBILITY

Can a person commit a crime and plead "unsound mind" as a defense for escaping punishment? The answer is yes if the person can prove that he/she was of unsound mind at the time of committing the crime. A defense can be raised in several ways.

- Not guilty by reason of insanity
- Diminished responsibility
- Incapacity to form an intent because of automatism.

As per law, only this first category is applicable in Indian courts. The law for criminal responsibility in India is based on the McNaughton rule first established in England. Section 84 of the Indian Penal Code states "Nothing is an offence which is done by a person of unsound mind, incapable of knowing the nature of the act or that what he is doing is either wrong or contrary to law". Thus, the person is deemed to be of unsound mind if he is incapable of knowing;

- The nature of the act or
- That the act is wrong or
- That the act is contrary to law.

Indian Courts also differentiate legal insanity from medical insanity. Medical insanity covers abnormality of mind, delusions and other psychopathology. Legal insanity envisages that the unsoundness of mind of the subject must be such as to make the offender incapable of knowing the nature of the act, or knowing that what he is doing is wrong or contrary to the law. There are not many offenders in India claiming the insanity defense. These persons may be acquitted under Section 84 of Indian Penal Code, which is based on the McNaughton's rule. Even among those who claim only a few have been considered to be not responsible for their crime because of their unsoundness of mind.

In spite of the vigorous criticism from so many learned quarters, the McNaughton rule has found a secure place in the Indian law dating back to the time when Queen Victoria took over the control of the colonial Indian Empire.

INDIAN LAW AND MENTALLY ILL PRISONERS

Within Indian law some regulations are of particular relevance for mentally disordered offenders.

The Code of Criminal Procedure, 1973 (Sections 328 to 333)

It has ample provisions to safeguard a mentally ill prisoner in India. Some of these provisions are:

Section 328: Procedure in case of the accused being a lunatic.

Section 329: Procedure in case of a person of unsound mind tried before court.

Section 330:
a. Release of lunatic to relatives for treatment pending investigation or trial.
b. Transfer of a lunatic to a psychiatric hospital for treatment pending investigation or trial.

Section 331: Resumption of inquiry or trial.

Section 332 Procedure for an accused appearing before Magistrate or Court.

Section 333: Procedure if an accused appears to have been of unsound mind.

Section 334: Judgment of acquittal on ground of unsoundness of mind.

Section 335: Detention in safe custody of a person acquitted on grounds of unsoundness of mind.

Section 336: Power of the State Government to empower an officer in charge to discharge.

Section 337: Procedure by which a lunatic prisoner is reported capable of making his defense.

Section 338: Procedure by which a lunatic detained is declared fit to be released.

Section 339: Delivery of lunatic to care of relative or friend.

Section 84 of Indian Penal Code

Based on the McNaughton rules it is stated that "Nothing is an offence, which is done by a person of unsound mind who is incapable of knowing the nature of the act or that what he is doing is either wrong or contrary to law."

Prisoners Act

The Indian Prisoners Act 1900 (Act III) has provision to transfer mental ill prisoners sentenced to a custodial sentence to a forensic ward of the psychiatric hospital for treatment.

MENTALLY ILL PRISONERS IN INDIA

There are three groups of mentally ill prisoners in forensic units of psychiatric hospitals and in secluded wards inside prisons in India.

1. Prisoners under-trial: Mentally ill prisoners who were mentally ill at the time of committing a crime and are unfit to stand trial.
2. Sentenced prisoners: Convicted prisoners who develop a mental illness during the course of imprisonment.
3. Guilty but insane: mentally ill prisoners who are acquitted at trial. Since no social support systems exist to provide for their care and treatment in the community, these prisoners continue to stay in the forensic units of psychiatric hospitals as per Section 27 of the Indian Mental Health Act, 1987.

There has been a serious concern about the inadequate medical and psychiatric care for all the above mentioned three groups of mentally ill prisoners.

For many decades, many mentally ill, both those with criminal record and those with no criminal record, have been admitted to jails, especially so in the Eastern part of India. Following a public interest litigation, the Supreme Court of India on July 18, 1993, passed a landmark judgment ruling that "The admission of non-criminal mentally ill persons to jails is illegal and unconstitutional". As a result, the admission of mentally ill persons to prisons has almost ended all over the country.

Some of the (unpublished) studies of psychopathology of prisoners in Indian prisons reveal that there are nearly 60 to 80% of prisoners who have one or more diagnosable psychiatric conditions. The majority of male prisoners suffer from antisocial personality disorder and alcohol and drug addiction. Among women, most suffer from neurotic disorders. Nearly 95% of mentally ill prisoners are men.

Among the mentally ill-prisoners in forensic units of psychiatric hospitals, the majority are under-trial prisoners (nearly 80%); many of them suffer from psychotic disorders, especially schizophrenia, followed by antisocial personality disorder and substance use disorders. Most of the mentally ill in the forensic units of psychiatric hospitals have committed a major crime such as murder. Mentally ill prisoners constitute around 1 to 2% of the patients in major psychiatric hospitals in India.

There are four options to develop the forensic psychiatric service in India:
1. Separate wards for mentally ill-prisoners inside the prison itself.
2. An exclusive forensic psychiatric hospital (special hospital).
3. A forensic psychiatric unit/ward inside a state psychiatric hospital with high security and constant care by mental health professionals.
4. Correctional settings for juveniles.

In the forensic ward of the psychiatric hospital, the emphasis should be on therapy and rehabilitation rather than control and containment.

As of now, mentally-ill prisoners are admitted to forensic units of psychiatric hospitals and are managed by psychiatrists. In some centers, the psychiatrists from the nearby hospitals visit the prisons periodically to treat the mentally-ill patients there.

Almost all the 37 state-run mental hospitals in India have a separate forensic psychiatric Unit in their premises and in some places the psychiatrists from the nearby hospitals visit the prison periodically to treat the mentally ill patients in prisons. The juvenile delinquents are kept under safe correctional settings.

What is currently not available is an exclusive forensic psychiatric hospital (special hospital) despite the Indian Mental Health Act, 1987 having made a provision for such an establishment.

As per the Care and Protection of Children Act of 2000 (Juvenile Justice Act, 2000), children who commit crimes, irrespective of the presence or absence of a psychiatric diagnosis, are to be detained in special correctional settings. Children exhibiting severe abnormalities such as violence and unmanageable behaviors may be sent to psychiatric hospitals with agreement from the Juvenile Justice Board.

The most feasible model for forensic psychiatric services in a developing country like India is to have forensic units in psychiatric hospitals with high security and constant care by well-trained personnel. The concept of exclusive forensic psychiatric hospitals poses additional costs, additional trained personnel and increases the stigma of mental illness.

FORENSIC PSYCHIATRIC SERVICES IN INDIA

Forensic psychiatric services in India are poorly developed compared to the West. Persons suffering from mental illness, who are also offenders are now considered as "mentally ill prisoners". Earlier, they were known as "criminal lunatics" but this terminology is not commonly used anymore. There are 37 state-run mental hospitals in India with a total bed number of around 20,000. The majority of these mental hospitals have a separate ward for mentally-ill prisoners.

The admission and discharge of a mentally ill prisoner in India is governed by the Indian Mental Health Act, 1987. Admission and detention of mentally ill prisoners in psychiatric hospitals in India can follow any one of the following three types:

1. Under-trial prisoners—Section 330 of the Code of Criminal Procedures 1973.
2. Not guilty by reason of insanity—Section 335 of the Code of Criminal Procedures 1973.
3. Sentenced prisoners—Section 30 of Act III of the Indian Prisoners Act 1900.

The World Health Organization (WHO) Expert Committee on Mental Health, in its fourth report (1955), suggested that "Mental hospitals should not be asked to take custodial care of dangerous criminals. They should be cared for in special establishments for criminals, if detained in mental hospital premises, security by the police should be provided in a specially created ward for mentally ill prisoners."

In India, no special forensic psychiatric hospitals exist. Mentally ill offenders are mostly cared in the forensic units of mental hospitals or in the forensic ward of general hospitals for a short term or inside the prison wards.

In India, especially in the State of West Bengal, indiscriminate detention of non-criminal mentally ill persons in jails was a regular occurrence. However, the Supreme Court declared on August 18, 1993 that "Admission of non-criminal mentally ill persons to jails is illegal and unconstitutional". This was a historic judgment. Mental health professionals had for many decades been demanding the abolition of the practice of admitting mentally ill persons to jails.

PSYCHIATRIC SERVICES IN PRISON—INDIAN SCENARIO

Psychiatric symptoms are common among many prisoners in the first two months of imprisonment but not all of them qualify for a diagnosis according to the International Classification of Diseases. Antisocial personality and substance abuse are usually the most common diagnoses. High rates of psychotic disorders exist in prisoners either under-trial, remanded or convicted. The prevalence of psychotic disorders among prisoners is almost similar to that seen in the general population.

The most common reasons for transfer of mentally ill offenders from prison to a psychiatric hospital are the following:
1. Violent and unmanageable behavior.
2. Potential danger to self or others.
3. Significant deterioration of a psychiatric illness.
4. Treatment refusal in a highly disturbed patient.

In India, opinions are divided between the mental health professionals and the prisoners with regards to the question in which place to detain mentally ill prisoners. Mental health professionals often prefer to keep these patients in prisons or if necessary in a forensic ward of a psychiatric hospital. Occasionally, they prefer to visit the prison periodically to give their opinion and take care of the mentally ill offenders. However, the majority of mentally ill prisoners in India prefer to stay in prison and are reluctant to go to a psychiatric hospital because they feel the comfort and facilities are much better in prisons than in the mental hospitals.

The plight of the mentally disordered offenders in India is pathetic. To quote Halleck (1986), "the insane criminals" has nowhere to go—no age or nation has provided a place for him. He is unwelcome and objectionable everywhere. The prisons thrust him out, the hospitals are unwilling to receive him. The law will not let him stay in his house, the public will not let him go aboard and yet humanity and justice, the sense of common danger and a tender regard for a deeply degraded man, all agree that something should be done for him.

The discharge of the mentally ill prisoners from psychiatric hospitals in India is carried out in one of the following methods:
1. Under-trial prisoners who are admitted to a psychiatric hospital through a detention order under Section 330 of the Criminal Procedure Code, 1973 are given active treatment in the psychiatric hospital. The visiting committee of the hospital—which meets every three months—monitors and assesses the mentally ill prisoners in psychiatric hospitals and recommends those fit for trial. At this point these under-trial mentally ill prisoners will be transferred to jail to await their respective court dates for trial. The fitness of mentally ill offenders for trial is mainly based on whether they are able to comprehend the

questions put to them, whether they are oriented to person, time and place, whether they are in a position to understand the charges against them and the court proceedings, whether they are able to instruct their lawyer and whether they understand what type of punishment they may receive.

2. Prisoners who are admitted under the Criminal Procedure Code 1973, Section 335 (not guilty by reason of unsound mind) will also be given active treatment in hospital and once their mental state has improved and their relatives are willing to assume responsibility, they will be discharged and sent back to the community. If no relatives come forward to take care of the individual, they are transferred either to a non-forensic ward of a psychiatric hospital or to a rehabilitation center outside as per the direction of the hospital visitors.
3. Sentenced prisoners who develop a mental illness in prison following conviction are admitted as per the Indian Prisoners Act. Once their mental state has improved, they will be sent back to prisons and are advised to continue regular follow-up.

MENTAL DISORDER AND CRIME

In a study of mentally ill offenders convicted of murder who were admitted to Government Rajaji Hospital, Madurai, 80% were males and 20% were females; 50% of them were diagnosed with schizophrenia and 40% of them were diagnosed as having a mood disorders; 10% had personality disorders (Krishnaram, 1988).

In a study of insanity related homicide, Rath, et al. (1990) found that around 47% of the mentally ill prisoners charged with murder were diagnosed with schizophrenia and around 20% were noted to have alcohol and drug related disorders. The other disorders diagnosed included epilepsy, bipolar disorder, and mental retardation.

In a study of 182 mentally ill offenders of the forensic unit of the National Institute of Mental Health and Neurosciences (NIMHANS), Bangalore, by Pratima (2002), it was found that the sample consisted predominately of males (92.8%) with a mean age of 39.

Around 13.3% were facing a charge/had been convicted for murder or attempted murder. Assault was the next commonest offence. Schizophrenia was the commonest diagnosis (41.5%) followed by mood disorders (23.2%), organic mental disorders (16.7%), and others.

In a study of psychosocial issues among prisoners by Suman, et al. in Bangalore, it is found that 30% of male prisoners and 55% of female prisoners had depressive symptoms and 20% each had somatic problems. It is also found that 74% were convicted for either homicide or abetting homicide, out of which, 30% of the homicides occurred during group violence. Many prisoners in this study were satisfied with prison conditions and treatment by prison officials. Men reported having a better social support than women prisoners.

An attempt to find an overall relationship between crime and mental disorders may be mistaken; the prevalence of serious psychiatric illness among the criminal population is low (Somasundaram, 1980). There is an underrepresentation of personality disorders, alcohol, and drug abuse among mentally ill prisoners in the psychiatric hospital in contrast to the high prevalence of personality disorders, especially antisocial personality disorder, and alcohol and other substance use disorders in prison-based studies.

PREVALENCE OF MENTAL DISORDERS AMONG PRISONERS IN INDIA

A recent unpublished study assessing the prevalence of mental health problems among prisoners in the State of Karnataka, suggests that around 60% of the total number of prisoners had some sort of mental health problems (according to the International Classification of Diseases, 10th edition (ICD-10) including mental retardation. The majority had antisocial personality disorder and alcohol and other substance use disorders. Other psychotic disorders, especially schizophrenia and mood disorders, were much less prevalent. The diagnostic category has been drawn as per This is in contrast to the prevalence of psychiatric disorders among prisoners detained in psychiatric hospitals. The majority of inmates of on forensic wards of psychiatric hospitals, suffer from schizophrenia (Somasundaram 1960, 1980; Nambi 2008). This is likely to be due to the non-referral of criminals with personality disorders to psychiatric hospital by the authorities. It is always a challenge to treat the mentally disordered with dangerous and severe personality disorders, whether it is in the prison or in mental hospitals. Some psychiatrists feel that severe antisocial personality disorders should not be considered as a clinical diagnosis meant for treatment and that psychiatrists should not take responsibility for this group. The Indian Mental Health Act of 1987 defines a mental disorder as a treatable condition. It is viewed that management of individuals with dangerous and severe personality disorder should occur in a separate forensic psychiatric speciality hospital or in a separate block inside the prison itself.

REASONS OF TRANSFER FROM PRISON TO HOSPITAL

In a study conducted in Tihar Central Jail, Delhi, Chadda (1998) reported there were about 300 women prisoners of around 9000 inmates (the actual capacity is only 2000). Around 80% of the prisoners were remand and under-trial prisoners, and 20% of them were prisoners serving their sentence. Among the 9000 inmates, only 72 male inmates were referred to the psychiatric clinic, i.e. less than 1%. Most of them (80%) were under-trial. Diagnostic categories included schizophrenia, depression, bipolar disorder, anxiety disorders, and malingering. Stress of imprisonment contributed to the illness only in a small percentage of patients. Among the admitted patients, the jail environment interfered with improvement. Frequent relapses were noted among the improved schizophrenic patients when transferred back to the jail.

HOSPITALIZED MENTALLY ILL PRISONERS IN INDIA—GENDER DIFFERENCES

In a 20 years retrospective study on the forensic ward in the Institute of Mental Health, Chennai, India by Nambi (1992), the followings findings emerged:

- Total number of admissions during 20 years 43,804
- Number of civil (noncriminal) mentally ill persons 43,267
- Number of mentally ill prisoners (Criminal Lunatics) 537
- Percentage of mentally ill prisoners in the total inpatient population of the psychiatric hospital 1.22%

MENTALLY-ILL WOMEN PRISONERS

The majority of female offenders are being sent to prisons not because of the seriousness of their offences, but because of the persistence of their nuisance. In India, female criminality is infrequent compared with that of males. This may be due to the lower recognition and identification and underreporting. The most common offences committed by women in India are stealing, shoplifting, prostitution, and drug peddling. Violent crimes are less common among Indian women. The most common psychiatric problems associated with offending in women include hysteria, premenstrual tension, drug abuse, and antisocial personality disorder. Rarely, women suffering from severe mental illnesses like schizophrenia and bipolar disorder commit major crimes like assault and murder. Very often Indian women are forced to indulge in crime as a self defense especially against their alcoholic husband's indulgence in domestic violence. In a Chennai based study (Nambi, 1992), it was found that out of 537 mentally ill prisoners admitted to a large state psychiatric hospital during a 20-year period, only 26 were females (4.84%). The most common crime among mentally ill women prisoners admitted to the psychiatric hospitals through a detention order was murder and the most common diagnosis was schizophrenia.

HOSPITALIZED MENTALLY ILL FEMALE PRISONERS—DIAGNOSTIC PROFILE

Diagnoses of women (as per ICD-10) on the forensic ward in the Institute of Mental Health, Chennai (Nambi, 1992) are shown in the (Table 13.1):

Table 13.1: Diagnoses of women (as per ICD-10) on the forensic ward

Diagnosis	*Percentage*
Schizophrenia	62.2%
Depression	7.6%
Mental retardation	7.6%
Personality disorder	3.8%
Other psychiatric disorders	18.8%

JUVENILE OFFENCES—INDIAN SCENARIO

In India, 15% of children have serious emotional disturbances (World Health Report, 2001). The facilities available to take care of them are inadequate. The high risk factors for developing juvenile delinquency (conduct disorder) in India are: Low socioeconomic status, parental pathology including death or separation of a parent, alcoholic father, unwed mother, antisocial personality in any one of the parents and birth trauma producing minimal brain damage and epilepsy.

Care and Protection of Children Act, 2000 (Juvenile Justice Act, 2000)

This act aims to regulate the provision of care, protection, treatment, development opportunities and rehabilitation of neglected or delinquent juveniles (Juvenile means a child, who has not completed age of 18).

The Juvenile Justice Act in India deals with three types of children:

a. Delinquent
b. Neglected
c. Uncontrollable.

Juvenile should not be confined to jails. Special facilities for treatment of children and juveniles like observation and juvenile homes and after-care institutions should be established in all the States. The offences committed by juveniles should be tried in juvenile courts and this act provides for the establishment of Juvenile Welfare Boards in all districts.

CRIME AND CHILDREN

The Indian Penal Code, 1860 provides some immunity against punishment to children. For example:

Section 82 states that nothing is an offence, which is done by a child under seven years of age.

Section 83 states that nothing is an offence, which is done by a child above seven years of age and below 12 years, who has not attained sufficient maturity of understanding to judge the nature and consequences of his conduct on that occasion.

PSYCHIATRIC DISORDERS AND CRIME

Drug Abuse and Crime—Indian Scenario

Unfortunately, there is an alarming increase in criminal activity associated with alcoholism and other substance use disorders in India, which has increased manifold during the last few decades. Apart from alcohol, the other common two drugs which are highly abused by many Indians, are Opium and its products and Cannabis. The amount of crime committed by addicts is vast. They include both major and minor crimes. In a study in Chennai (Nambi, 2008) around 80% of the "brown sugar" (heroin) addicts and multiple drug abusers were found to have a premorbid psychopathic personality based on the past history and criminal behavior. Around 70% of them had indulged in criminality like stealing, assault, etc. Another study in the Institute of Mental Health, Chennai (Nambi, 1998) regarding the prevalence of alcohol and drug abuse amongst mentally ill prisoners revealed that 50% of the mentally ill prisoners had abused alcohol and around 17% of the mentally ill prisoners had abused cannabis prior to their commission of crime. The consequences of the drugs and related problems and the association with crime has emerged as one of the foremost medical, psychological and legal implications in many of the metropolitan areas in India. In India, The Narcotic Drugs and Psychotropic Substances Act 1985, as amended in 1996, deals with all crimes and punishment related to narcotic drugs in India. The punishment envisioned is very stringent, but the implementation has so far not been very effective.

SUICIDE AMONG MENTALLY ILL PRISONERS

Approximately 14 suicides occur every hour of the day in India. More than one hundred and twenty five thousand individuals lost their lives by suicide in 2008 (National Crime Record Bureau 2008). Underreporting of completed and attempted suicides is very common in all parts of the country and the reasons are multiple. What is recorded in the official records of the National Crime Record Bureau is therefore only the tip of the iceberg.

It has been observed that social and economic causes have led most of the males to commit suicide, whereas emotional and personal causes mainly drive females to end their lives. Suicides because of "family problems" and illness accounted for 48.7% of total suicides. The common methods of committing suicide in India include self-poisoning (35%), self-immolation or fire-setting (killing oneself by setting fire after pouring kerosene or petrol over the body) (8.8%), drowning (6.7%) and hanging (32%).

Overcrowding, sensory deprivation, isolation, and poor contact and communication with relatives are some of the important causes of suicide among prisoners. Apart from these social causes we found that psychological reasons add to increase the number of suicides among mentally ill prisoners inside jail. Suicide among mentally ill prisoners is not at all uncommon in Indian prisons, but they are often underreported. Exact statistics about suicide among mentally ill prisoners in India are not available.

ETHICAL ISSUES OF THE MENTALLY ILL PRISONERS IN INDIA

One ethical issue to consider is the fact that there are no separate specialty hospitals for forensic psychiatric patients in India. Hence they are forced to stay inside the mental hospitals often or, worse, inside the prison, thereby the already existing stigma becomes worse. The WHO expert committee on Mental Health in its report (1955) suggested that the dangerous mentally ill criminals shall be kept in special establishments. Even the Indian Mental Health Act (1987) has made provision for the establishment of a special forensic psychiatric hospital.

There are only 37 state-run mental hospitals existing in India, where most of the mentally ill prisoners are kept and the problem of overcrowding is always present on the wards. Mental health is not provided with adequate budgets in many states and hence the facilities available are inadequate and the living conditions in these hospitals are not up to the standard.

In some of the mental hospitals in India, especially in the West Bengal State many wandering mentally-ill (mentally-ill non offenders) were detained inside the prison. Only in the recent past, after a Supreme Court Judgment in response to a Public Interest Litigation, these patients were released from prisons and sent to hospitals for treatment.

Persons who were acquitted because they have committed the crime under the influence of mental illness (as per Section 84 of Indian Penal Code) are difficult to discharge from mental hospitals to the community because either they do not have adequate social support or due to administrative procedural delay or due to the ongoing illness related risk of re-offending.

Prisons in India are still governed by the century old Prisons Act 1894 and the Prisoners Act 1900. The application of a century old law in the changed sociopolitical scenario is absolutely bizarre and it is out of tune with the entirely transformed picture of human society. During the past few decades, several organizations, intellectuals, and a committee setup for jail reforms have expressed their views on the importance of reviewing the laws.

The living conditions in many prisons continue to be poor, dehumanizing and in violation of basic human rights standards. There has been a plethora of recommendations for the improvement of these conditions both from the apex judiciary and by the National Human Rights Commission. But large chunks of these recommendations have not seen the light of the day. Overcrowding is the greatest practical hindrance to efforts of reforming the Indian prison system. Some prisons house as much as three times more inmates than their capacity. If the situation is so pathetic for all the prisoners in general, we can only begin to understand how mentally ill prisoners, suffering the double stigma, are treated inadequately and inhumanly inside prisons. It is time to think of better networking, effective prison reforms and their true application, education, and overall society's contribution to the improvement of prison conditions. We must seek solutions both inside prisons and outside in society for better care and improved quality of life for mentally ill offenders.

Some of the basic principles for the treatment of prisoners (as adopted and proclaimed by the General Assembly of United Nations Resolution 45/111 of December 14, 1990) are:

- All prisoners shall be treated with respect due to their inherent dignity and value as human beings.
- Prisoners shall have access to the Health Services available in the country without discrimination on the grounds of their legal situation.

India is still far away from achieving these standards.

CONCLUSIONS

Prisons in India are overcrowded institutions and the majority of them provide poor living conditions, lack of meaningful activity, endemic substance abuse, recurrent violence and sexual exploitation. Loss of freedom, separation from family and friends, uncertainty about the future, and the traumas of prison life all contribute to making living in prison a stressful experience. Psychiatric symptoms are common during the first two months of imprisonment. Thus the majority of psychiatric problems among mentally ill prisoners occur in under-trial and remand prisoners. Prisons that contain adequate mental health services are exceptional and inmates with mental health problems remain undetected because of the absence of trained prison staff. Mental health problems in India are more common in socially disadvantaged, minimally educated and unemployed persons. Personality disorder, alcoholism, and substance abuse are the most common diagnoses in studies conducted among prison inmates, whereas schizophrenia, alcohol-related disorders, mood disorders, organic mental disorders, and mental retardation are the common diagnoses in studies conducted in forensic wards of psychiatric hospitals. Although a complete range of mental disorders will be encountered by the prison doctors, suicide and self-injury, violence towards other inmates and paranoid syndromes are of special relevance in prison psychiatry in India.

Mental health facilities in Indian prisons are meager. Hence, arrangements should be made for visits of psychiatrists on a periodic basis, at least once a week. Prisoners with mental health problems should be kept separately or preferably shifted to psychiatric hospitals. However, due to overall shortage of trained manpower in mental health care, both in district hospitals and psychiatric hospitals, this may not become possible in the near future. Thus, there is a need to augment the mental health care system, both in terms of manpower and infrastructure. There is also a need to move from custodial care to a community mental health care approach (National Human Rights Commission recommendation on detention, 2008).

The problems faced by the psychiatrist treating mentally ill prisoners in India include a near total lack of any follow-up of their behavior in the community and whether they are continuing their treatment or not. In the Indian penal system, wide discretionary powers are vested with the courts in enquiring into the mental condition of suspected mentally abnormal offenders (Nair, 1992). This causes deterioration and relapse of already treated and improving mental disorder inside the mental hospitals. They are often shuttled between mental hospitals, prisons, and courts.

In summary, it is emphasized that there is an urgent need for improving the conditions in jails and developing separate forensic psychiatry specialty hospitals for better management and quality of care to the mentally ill prisoners in India.

SUGGESTED READING

1. Chadda RK, et al. "Clinical profile of patients attending a prison psychiatric clinic. Indian Journal of Psychiatry, 1998;40(3):260–5.
2. Chiswick D, Dooley E, et al. "Psychiatry in Prisons", Practical Forensic Psychiatry, (Seminars in the Royal College of Psychiatrists, 1995;243-71.
3. Halleck SL. The Mentally Disordered Offender. US Department of Health and Human Services, NIHM Publication, 1986;86-1471.
4. Krishnaram. Mentally Abnormal Offenders. A study of 15 convicts of murder. Proceedings of 21st Annual Conference of Indian Psychiatric Society, South Zone, 1988.
5. Mathiharan K, Tiphagne H. Resource Materials for Doctors and Psychiatrist, National project on preventing torture in India, 2006. Published by Peoples Watch – Tamil Nadu, India.
6. Murthy P, et al. Criminal offenders referred to Psychiatric Services—A 12 years experience in NIHMANS. Paper presented at the Indian Psychiatric Society, South Zone Conference, 2002.
7. Murthy S. Human Rights of "Mentally ill individuals—An Indian experience" commemorative brochure. 180 year Celebration of Institute of Psychiatry, Kolkata 1997.
8. Nair. judicial activism in giving the mentally insane offender his due, Cochin Law Review, 1992.
9. Nambi S. "A twenty years retrospective study of mentally ill female prisoners in a major state mental hospital in India", Paper presented at the Annual National Conference at Indian Psychiatric Society 1992.
10. Nambi S. Legal Aspects of Psychiatry—Indian Perspective, 2008. Published by Manashanthi, Mental Health Care Pvt Ltd.
11. Nambi S. Prevalence of alcohol and substance abuse among mentally ill prisoners", paper presented at the Annual National Conference of the Indian Psychiatric Society, 1998.
12. Narcotic Drugs and Psychotropic Substances Act, 1985 (with Amendments in 1996) Universal Law Publishing Company, New Delhi.
13. National Human Rights Commission—Recommendations on Detention (2008). www.nhrc.nic.in. Mental Health Act, 1987 (Act No 14, 1987), Commercial Law Publishers, India Pvt Ltd, Delhi 2007.
14. Rath NM, et al. A Study of Insanity Related Homicide. Indian Journal of Psychiatry, 1990;32(1):69-71.
15. Somasundaram O. Criminal responsibility—An overview. Indian journal of psychological medicine, 2001.
16. Somasundaram O. Murder in Tamil Nadu. Indian Journal of Psychiatry, 1980; 22:288-29.
18. Suman, et al. "Psychosocial Issues Among Prisoners: An Exploratory Investigation" Indian Journal of Social Psychiatry, 2007;23(1-2):57–63.
19. The Indian Penal Code 1860. Eastern Book Company, 1987.
20. The Juvenile Justice (Care and Protection of Children) Act 2000. Professional Book Publishers 2004.
21. Tiwari SC, et al. "A study of risk factors in recidivistic criminals". Indian Journal of Psychological Medicine, 2004;25(2):53-69.

14 Chapter

Marriage, Mental Health and Indian Legislation

Marriage has been since ancient times one of the most important social institutions-perhaps the greatest and most important of all institutions in human society. It has always existed in one form or another in every culture ensuring social sanction to a physical union between man and woman and laying the foundation for building up of the family-the basic unit of society.

Sociologists have offered several definitions of marriage:

1. 'Marriage consists of the rules and regulations which defines the rights, duties and privileges of the husband and wife.'—George A Lundberg
2. 'Marriage is more or less a durable connection between male and female, lasting beyond the mere act of propagation till after the birth of the offspring.'—Western Marck
3. 'Marriage is a contractual agreement which formalizes and stabilizes the social relationship which comprise the family.'

Marriage is a socially supported union between individuals in what is intended to be a stable, enduring relationship. It is the basis for the family and the institution defined by six social functions: regulation of sexual behaviour, reproduction, nurturance and protection of children, socialization, production, consumption, and the passing on of ascribed statuses such as race. Marriage and the family rest on many beliefs, the most important of which is kinship.

In the *shastras*, marriage was viewed as a sacrament. The relationship of husband and wife, once established through proper customs and rituals was believed to be irrevocable. In Hindu marriage, custom is sacrosanct, which is why a marriage ceremony is said to be complete only when the customary rites and rituals are fully performed. Of course, customs vary from place to place and society to society.

Since Hindu marriage is regarded as a means to establish relations between two families, utmost care is taken to ensure maximum cultural compatibility between the two. In Hindu 'exogamy', a person has to marry firstly outside his or her own gotra and secondly, avoid marrying a person who is a sapinda (*sapinda* means 'of the same body'). The former is called *gotra* exogamy, and the latter is called *sapinda* exogamy. In the Hindu tradition, the observance of custom is supreme and, if custom prevails, marriages between *sapindas* or within the prohibited degrees of relationship are also permissible. For instance, in Southern India, marriage between a maternal uncle and niece is valid, whereas in Northern India, it is unthinkable due to the absence of such a custom.

Other religions in India include Buddhism, Islam, Sikhism, Christianity and Jainism, which have their own variations of marriage customs. Among Muslim communities, the joint affirmation of the *nikah-nama* (or the marriage contract) is of prime importance. Most Muslims prefer marriage among relations; first cousins are considered most suitable, failing which alliances are sought among families with earlier matrimonial links. This is done to prevent the entry of foreign blood within the family and to retain the property inherited by a young couple.

The *nikah* or marriage service takes place at an hour that is ordained auspicious. The qazi or law officer presides over the ceremony, appointing two men as witnesses on the groom's side, to receive orders for the *nikah* from the bride's family. The amount of *mehr* (a compulsory amount of money given to the bride's family by the groom's family) is negotiated by the elders of the two families.

In Tamil Nadu, self-respect marriage has been introduced by the social reformer Periyar EV Ramasamy. The underlying principles of a self-respect marriage are; marriage is a personal contract between a man and a woman; nothing is sacred, sanctified, religious or divine in the union of man and woman. A contract may be withdrawn by either party or mutually. If marriage is contractual, devoid of religious sanctity, it ceases to be a necessary condition of social life. The male or female has the choice to marry, break away, or not marry at all. In a self-respect marriage, a contract upholds equality of sex, by implication, it means that chastity is not a unisexual virtue, but is common to both sexes. Since a contract is breakable, once it is broken, the man and woman may have any other partner by remarriage. Periyar also advises the couple to wait for five years before deciding on pregnancy, and to confine themselves to one or two children, irrespective of its sex and to forget about children if they do not conceive. The woman is not a childbearing machine, says Periyar. Pregnancy is a biological burden, which is an obstacle to a woman's freedom. There are a variety of marital patterns such as (i) monogamy, (ii) bigamy, (iii) polygamy, (iv) stable marital arrangements/companionship, and (v) same-sex marriage. In most cultures monogamy is ideal.

CONSANGUINEOUS MARRIAGES AND SAME-SEX MARRIAGES

Many workers in South India have reported a high prevalence of consanguineous marriages. Consanguineous marriages are still common in the states of Tamil Nadu, Andhra Pradesh and Karnataka. There is a strong association between consanguineous marriages and mental disorders.

A study of 147 patients at the Institute of Mental Health, Chennai, suffering from major mental disorders, found that consanguineous parents constituted 36%, and most of them were of second-degree consanguinity. A large series of 86 cases of primary microcephaly showed that in 70% of cases the marriages were consanguineous. A study of 100 mentally retarded children and adolescents attending the outpatient department of the Institute of Mental Health, Chennai, showed that in 28% of cases the marriages were consanguineous, and most of them were of second-degree consanguinity.

Same-sex marriage has been much talked about in recent times. Many countries abhor the basic concept of same-sex marriage; some countries have legalized it. Whether or not, same-sex union should be recognized has been discussed in many state legislatures in the West. In India, homosexuality and lesbianism are not only considered taboo, but also an offence. That does not mean that this practice is uncommon here. In India, there are organizations and support groups for the practice of homosexuality and lesbianism. One such organization is *Sangini*, a social and emotional support group for women attracted towards women. It is a support group for lesbian and bisexual women in India. It should be noted that gay and lesbian psychiatry is one of the specialty sections of the American Psychiatric Association.

Among same-sex common law couples, male couples outnumber female ones. In the United States of America, same-sex couples represented about 1% of all couples in 2000. In New Zealand, the proportion of same-sex couples increased from 0.4% in 1996 to 0.6% in 2001. In the 2001 Canada Census, same-sex couples represented 0.5% of all couples.

'Gay marriage is good for mental health,' is what the American Psychological Association said at its annual conference; last summer, when it passed a policy statement that same-sex couples should have the right to marry.

Marriage, variously defined as an institution, the bedrock of procreation and family life, a gamble, a life sentence or a heaven-programmed union between two people, is an ideal medium to gauge value shifts in society. Arranged marriages, not surprisingly, remain the most preferred option for most couples, but not arranged in the traditional sense. They are becoming flexible, adaptable, open-minded affairs, based on contemporary, practical and realistic factors. Match-making has come a long way from being the emotionally and socially loaded event 'fixed' by the aunt or the family pundit. It is now a modern industry chalked out on a bigger canvas with small middlemen playing a key role. Many marriages are fixed via matrimonial columns and matrimonial.coms.

REFORMS IN HINDU MARRIAGE CUSTOMS

The British succeeded in passing regulation XVII in 1829, which declared sati illegal and punishable by courts. The position of women in the nineteenth century was changing, thanks to the endeavors of social reformers like Raja Ram Mohan Roy and Ishwar Chandra Vidyasagar, and later in the twentieth century, in South India by social reformers such as EV Ramasamy Periyar. In fact, one of the distinguishing characteristics of modern society is the heavy reliance on law to bring about social change. In India, the first movement for women's marital rights centred on the three major problems of child marriage, enforced widowhood and property rights for women. The traditional concept of marriage has greatly changed now and Hindu marriage today has assumed more or less the nature of a contract for the mutual benefit of the parties concerned, duly aided by various legal provisions and reforms.

THE CONFLICT PERSPECTIVE OF MARRIAGE (WITH A SPECIAL EMPHASIS ON DIVORCE)

The increasing acceptance of divorce has dramatically altered the marriage situation. While couples still marry at the same constant rate, more than half of all couples married in the USA are now divorced. In India, even though the rate of divorce is not alarming, it is rapidly increasing-presently it is 5% to 7%. The vast majority of those divorced remarry, and the second marriage tends to last for the remainder of their lives. There are many in our society who believe that easy marriage and divorce cheapen the institution of marriage and threaten the structure of the family. This may or may not be true, but either way, laws in reality have very little impact on the rates of marriage and divorce. Laws are a reflection of people's needs, they make it easier for people to live with each other and try to ensure that everyone gets fair treatment. Society cannot dictate social and moral behavior through its laws. If laws do not fit, people will tend to disregard them. This is why so many people choose to live together in the West instead of marrying, as marriage does not fit their situation. Perhaps we would do better to make marriage fit the people, rather than trying to make people fit the institution.

DIVORCE

Is it a personal tragedy, a family embarrassment, or a social problem? Or, is it a new lease of life, a chance to start all over again, a chance to make something positive out of something that has turned negative? This is a matter of perspective, depending on how deeply one believes in the 'till death do us part' clause of the marriage contract. After months and even years of living with many differences and experiencing fights, frustrations, hurt and anger, a couple may seek divorce as the only viable alternative. At this point, marriage or relationship counselling may provide the couple with new skills in communicating and understanding each other.

Divorce is the emphasis on choice carried to its final limits as far as relationships go. People marry to prove their sense of commitment and to find security. In marriage, however, many find that commitment is situational and security is a figment of the imagination. The concept of divorce prevention revolves around making a mature choice of partner in the first place, making supreme efforts to grow at a parallel pace and continuing to foster the love relationship with care, respect and, above all, good communication.

Family disorganization occurs when statuses are not occupied or roles are not performed. Divorce, death and violence-themselves caused by social and ecological factors-are major causes of family disorganization. The greatest havoc wrought by divorce is the disruption of family life. Divorce in some cultures is no longer viewed as a last resort, but rather as an everyday occurrence. But where marriage is accepted as a sacrament, divorce is bound to be a sacrilege. There are many factors that are responsible for divorce. One of the most important causes has been found to be social change. The process of social change sets into motion a series of changes-in values, in customs, in ways of living, in roles of different people. Technological changes have led to urbanization. Urban society is highly heterogeneous as well as individualistic. The urban attitude is one of non-interference in the affairs of other people. Thus, the social life of urban people also exposes them to a variety of situations that can retract from the bond of attachment to the family. These situations therefore make divorce much easier.

The status of women in the family and society is another factor to be considered. The modern woman, because of her opportunities for education, training and employment, and creative activity has developed into a self-dependent and self-confident individual. This can lead to difficulties in adjustment in marriages, especially for women who have lived an independent and creative life before marriage. The scope for material prosperity has shifted social values from the spiritual and moral to the material. This change in values has encroached into the realm of marriage too. The wave of progressive liberalism and individualism has made insipid and outmoded the feelings of faithfulness and loyalty. The mass media has played an important role in changing such values. The influence of cinema, television and other media on the younger generation indirectly affects divorce rates. Besides social and cultural differences between the partners, infertility, and the social stigma attached to it, is also a cause for divorce.

MARRIAGE AND MENTAL HEALTH PROBLEMS

Marriage may be stressful for vulnerable people, which may lead to the development of mental health problems. The interplay between marriage and mental health problems has been dealt with in detail by Indian and International authors. Major mental health disorders may be the cause or effect of marital disharmony. Divorce-seeking couples have a high psychiatric morbidity in comparison to well-adjusted couples with more neurotic traits. The personality factors of divorce-seeking couples also differ from those of couples in stable marriages.

Studies consistently show greater distress among widowed/separated/divorced men and women. Greater distress is seen among married women as compared to married men, and greater distress in single women as compared to single men.

Community surveys in the West showed that women in all categories of marital status were more symptomatic than men in the same categories. After reviewing the epidemiological data, linking marital status with illness, it was seen that the 'effects of gender and marital status vary within ethnicity and psychological disorder.' An ICMR and DST study (1987) on severe mental distress found the highest common distress among housewives in both their urban as well as rural samples. All workers opine that those who were ever married, that is, married/widowed/widower or separated, suffered more than those who never married.

Though some authors feel that in terms of protection, marriage acts as a sort of insurance against psychological breakdown, it need not always be true, because marriage demands a sustained level of adaptation from both partners. The birth of a child, an abortion or miscarriage, economic stress, migration, episodes of illness, major career changes and any situation that involves a significant change in marital role can precipitate stressful periods in a relationship. Illness in a child exerts the greatest strain on a marriage; complaints of lifelong anorgasmia or impotence by marital partners usually indicate intrapsychic problems. Other problems that may induce a marital crisis also trigger off psychological disturbances. They include the discovery of an extramarital affair, onset of serious illness, announcement of intent to divorce, or problems with children or work, one or both members of the couple may be in therapy or may be psychiatrically ill, and one spouse may be seeking hospitalization for the other.

Women in India are less likely to receive mental health care because mental illness in the family, especially in a woman, is itself stigmatizing and an occasion for ridicule. Married mentally ill women are more likely to be sent back to their natal homes, abandoned, deserted or divorced. Clinical experience shows that the responsibility of care for the mentally ill woman is often left to her own family, than to her husband or his family.

SCHIZOPHRENIA AND MARRIAGE

There is evidence that marital status is significantly associated with first admission rates, age of onset, course and outcome of schizophrenia. Single males appear to be overrepresented in schizophrenia samples, including epidemiological studies such as the WHO's 10-country study. Since both overt schizophrenia and pre-schizophrenic impairments reduce the chances of marriage, married schizophrenics may represent a select group with a milder form of the disease. Alternatively, marriage itself (or living with a partner) may delay the onset of schizophrenia or cushion its effect. Neither of these two hypotheses can be definitely rejected on the basis of available descriptive epidemiological data. However, statistical analysis of the WHO data, in which confounding factors such as age, premorbid personality traits, and family history were controlled, found that married men experienced a statistically significant delay (1–2 years) in the onset of psychotic symptoms compared with single men.

Several workers examined the relationship between marriage and schizophrenia. Results from several studies have in common a low marital rate for schizophrenic patients compared with controls and other groups of mentally ill patients, a lower rate in women than in men, a poor clinical course and lower socioeconomic conditions among the divorced, and a clear evidence of selection for schizophrenia among those never married. Often, mental health professionals are faced with having to give advice regarding the marriage of a person suffering from schizophrenia. The answers to many of the questions posed by families are unclear, as there are little research data on which to base counselling on this important issue.

In a 10-year follow-up study, Thara and Srinivasan found that 'marital outcome in Indian patients is good with no significant gender differences'. The high marital rate (about 70% being married before the onset of the illness), presence of children, a shorter duration of illness at inclusion and the presence of auditory hallucinations at intake were all associated with a good marital outcome.

Being unemployed, experiencing a drop in socioeconomic level and the presence of flat affect and self-neglect for 10 years were all associated with a poor marital outcome.

For most women in India, marriage is a one-time event in life, which is glorified and sanctified and is associated with much social approval. It is also the ultimate fulfilment for most women. If this is endangered or broken by mental illness such as schizophrenia, the lives of these women are shattered beyond repair. After separation, almost all these women live with their parents, many of whom are aged. Social isolation and stigma is caused by this double disorganization, of chronic illness and a personal tragedy, stigmatized even now by society. It has brought to the fore the plight of women who, in addition to being affected by a serious mental illness, have also been abandoned by their spouses and left to fend for themselves in a world where few options are open to them. The social, psychological and cultural concomitance of being mentally ill and divorced/separated are particularly severe in the Indian culture. In addition to the stress of mental illness, hostility from family members and rejection from society in general, these women are ridiculed and ostracized for their divorced/separated status. Furthermore, for the families (primarily ageing parents), the emotional, financial and physical burden of caring for a severely mentally ill woman is extremely high. This once again emphasizes the need for educating and bringing greater awareness about mental illness among the people. Many relatives view that severe oddity of behaviour is something that would be set right by marriage. To this mistaken belief about marriage belongs the answer to all these ills. In a study of women with schizophrenia and broken marriages, Thara et al. found that the stigma of being separated/divorced is often more acutely felt both by families and patients than that of mental illness per se. Caregivers of these separated/divorced/deserted women suffer much more than the patients themselves. Feelings of disruption, loss, guilt, frustration, grief, disappointment and fear about the future of their daughter, all make them miserable. A striking finding from Thara's study was the holistic and very negative attitude of the other family members, such as the siblings, who often anticipating their role as future carers, distance themselves from the patients. This was true also of husbands and in-laws, who often feel cheated. In most arranged marriages, the fact of mental illness is often not disclosed or discussed with the family of the spouse. This is largely due to the fear that disclosure will lead to rejection of the woman. After marriage, in the case of an early relapse, an atmosphere of mistrust and suspicion is created in the family of the spouse that augurs poorly for the outcome of the illness. On the other hand, a psychotic episode after childbirth or after several years of marriage is considered more favourably and does not always result in separation/divorce. The children born to these women suffer from considerable neglect, emotionally and financially, which affects their future mental health.

The family is often considered to be a cause for the onset of schizophrenia. The deviant role relationship and disordered communication pave the way for disordered thinking. Two types of abnormal family patterns were reported:

Table 14.1: Mental illness, marital status and gender differences

							Separated					
			Single		*Married*		*Official*		*Unofficial*		*Widowed*	
Diagnosis	*Male*	*Female*	*Male*	*Female*	*Male*	*Female*	*Male*	*Female*	*Male*	*Female*	*Male*	*Female*
Schizophrenia (250)	155	95	65	18	86	56	3	8	6	9	2	7
Bipolar disorder (25)	17	8	4	—	7	3	—	—	0	2	—	—
Total 275	172	103	69	18	93	59	3	8	6	11	2	7

(i) Marital schew, in which one parent yielded to the other's (usually the mother's) eccentricities, which dominated the families; (ii) Marital schism, in which the parents maintained contrary views so that the child had divided loyalties. It was suggested that these abnormalities were the cause rather than the result of schizophrenia.

In a study of 275 patients at the Institute of Mental Health, Chennai mental illness, marital status and gender differences were analysed (Table 14.1). Table 14.1 shows that in the outpatient department of a mental hospital (i) persons suffering from schizophrenia outnumber those with bipolar disorder by 10:1; (ii) the majority of those seeking help are male (M:F = 3:2); (iii) nearly 26% of males and 6% of females are single; 30% of males and 23% of females are married; (iv) 10% of this patient population suffering from a major mental disorder are divorced/separated/widowed. Among these, the number of patients with schizophrenia is 13 times more than those with bipolar disorder.

MARRIAGE AND DEPRESSION

There has been considerable interest in the role of marital status as a risk factor for depression. For men, it appears clear that those married have the lowest rate of depression, while separated or divorced men have the highest rate of major depression. In women, the association is slightly less clear, but in the Epidemiologic Catchment Area (ECA) study, the same findings applied to women as well as men.[5] Understanding the nature of the association between marital status and rates of depression is more problematic. If personality is a risk factor for depression, then the same traits can interfere with the ability to marry or to stay married. There is little doubt that depression sometimes contributes to marital maladjustments and separation or divorce. Finally, the stress associated with divorce or separation can increase the likelihood of occurrence of an episode of depression.

In the context of marital relationship, previous research has indicated that for men, marriage confers protection against illness, while it appears to be associated with higher rates of depression for women. There has been some evidence that within marriage, the traditional role of the female is limiting, restricting and even boring, which may lead to depression.

Major depressive disorder occurs most often in persons without close interpersonal relationships or in those who are divorced or separated. Bipolar I disorder is more common in divorced and single persons than among married persons. However, this difference may reflect the early onset and the resulting marital discord characteristic of the disorder. Various social and interpersonal problems may also contribute to depressive relapse. Unhappy marriages seem to be important and a particularly relevant feature of marriage is criticism of the patient by the spouse. Women experiencing marital disharmony suffer from feelings of betrayal, humiliation and shame, which may pave way for developing a depressive disorder.

Children separated from their parents as a result of marital problems and divorce do subsequently have increased rates of depression. Children of divorced parents have more psychological problems than children of parents who are not divorced. It is not certain how far these problems precede the divorce and are related to disharmony between the parents or to the behaviour of one or both parents that contributed to the decision of divorce.

ALCOHOL AND MARRIAGE

Excessive drinking is liable to cause profound social disruption, particularly in the family. Marital and family tension is virtually inevitable. The divorce rate among heavy drinkers is high and the wives of such men are likely to be anxious, depressed and socially isolated. The husbands of battered wives frequently drink excessively, and some women admitted to the hospitals because of self-poisoning blame the drinking habit of their husbands. The home atmosphere is often detrimental to the children because of quarrelling and violence. A drunken parent provides a poor role model. Children of heavy drinkers are at risk of developing emotional and behavioural disorders, and of having poor academic performance at school.

Western studies have shown that almost 80% of domestic violence is due to alcoholism. Indian studies also corroborate this. Addiction seems to be the predominant cause in 50% to 60% of cases of domestic violence that have been reported. Marital relationships suffer most harshly from the ravages of addiction. It destroys all that is dear to the spouse, including family life, sexual relationship, economic resources, well-being of the children and status within the community. The wife witnesses the husband's addictive behaviour with increasing abhorrence; often she is also subjected to violence. Women affected by addicted husbands suffer from common difficulties and seem to develop similar behavioural patterns. Never married adults are at the most risk for alcohol and drug dependence.

MARRIAGE AND SUICIDE

Compared with the general population, people who have died of suicide are more likely to have been divorced, unemployed or living alone. Social isolation is a common factor among these associations.

Marriages reinforced by children seem to lessen the risk of suicide significantly. The suicide rate is 11 per 100,000 for married persons, double this rate is registered for those never married/single. Previously married persons, however, showed sharply higher rates than those never married, i.e. 24 per 100,000 among widowed and 40 per 100,000 among those who are divorced, with divorced men registering 69 suicides per 100,000 compared to 18 per 100,000 among divorced women.

Suicide research in India shows that one-fourth of the persons committing suicide are unmarried and the suicide rate is highest in the first year of marriage. Marital and family problems, which constitute around 50%, are more important than mere cruelty. The higher rate of married women committing suicide may probably be due to marital disharmony, dowry or ill-treatment by the in-laws.

ANTISOCIAL BEHAVIOR AND MARITAL DISHARMONY

Two types of behaviors point indirectly to the importance of parents' behavior and of enduring family relationships as a cause of antisocial personality disorder. First, there is evidence that parental separation usually follows a long period of tension and arguments that could themselves affect the child's development. Second, the behaviour of parents is an important cause of childhood behavioural disorders. For example, the association between separation and antisocial disorder in sons is determined by disharmony in marriage.

ANXIETY DISORDER AND MARRIAGE

Batra and Gautam found a high prevalence of neurotic disorders among divorce-seeking couples. The neurotic problems are encountered either as antecedents or consequences of marital disharmony.

A study comparing marital status in obsessive-compulsive disorder (OCD) patients with that in a matched group of patients with major depression found no significant differences between the two groups. A prospective study of 107 subjects with OCD found that being married significantly increased the probability of partial remission, with married persons being more than twice as likely to remit as unmarried ones.

Patients with schizophrenia are more likely to remain single and unmarried than patients in other diagnostic groups. This is particularly true of male patients and can probably be explained by the fact that women tend to be younger than men when first married and are less likely to have experienced an initial psychotic episode. From a cultural perspective, women are less active in initiating relationships, which may account for some differences.

Some researchers found low rates of fertility and reproduction among patients with schizophrenia. This finding can probably be explained by several factors including lack of interest in social relations, general apathy, loss of sex drive, and lack of opportunity for a sexual relationship due to hospitalization and institutionalization. Rates of reproduction in schizophrenic patients have probably increased since deinstitutionalization, although they are likely to remain lower than those found in the general population.

Some couples ask for help with sexual problems, which are the result and not the cause of marital conflicts. The sexual dysfunction may most probably be due to psychological disturbances such as anxiety and depression, or due to abuse of alcohol and drugs apart from other physical illness.

MARRIAGE, MENTAL ILLNESS AND THE INDIAN LEGISLATION

Every country and every religion has its own personal law. In India, under Article 44 of the Constitution, the state is bound by a constitutional mandate to secularize and homogenize family laws. The enactment of a uniform civil code was a goal to be achieved through a gradual process. The admixture of religion and ethics with legal precepts was naturally congruent. The practice of applying matrimonial law according to religious faith and beliefs has led to the prevalence of diverse matrimonial laws, besides one statutory law. As per Rule no. 3 of Order 32A of the Civil Procedure Code, it is the duty of the court to make efforts for settlement in matters concerning the family. As per Rule no. 4 of the same Order, a person, preferably a woman, who may or may not be related to the parties including a person professionally engaged in promoting the welfare of the family, may be utilized for the purpose of the settlement mentioned above. According to the Family Court Act, 1984, the Family Court was established with the view to promote conciliation in disputes concerning marriage and related matters. The Family Court may utilize the services of medical and welfare experts for conciliation. This Act reads that persons committed to the need to protect and preserve the institution of marriage shall be selected for appointment as judges and that women shall be preferred for such appointments. It is clear that the intention of law-makers is to prevent the fracture of a family. If a hard decision is inevitable it will be on a specific ground. The following Acts have a bearing on the legal aspects of marriage:

1. The Special Marriage Act, 1954
2. The Hindu Marriage Act, 1955 with amendment in 1976
3. The Dissolution of Muslim Marriage Act, 1939; The Muslim Women Protection of Rights on Divorce, 1986
4. The Parsi Marriage and Divorce Act, 1936
5. The Christian Marriage Act, 1872
6. The Indian Divorce Act, 1869
7. The Family Courts Act, 1984.

A family arises out of marriage. The single most important factor that influences the quality of family life is the quality of the marriage that supports it. Various socioeconomic changes and developments taking place in the society as a result of industrialization and urbanization have shaken the religious and moral foundations of the institution of marriage. Marriage, according to Hindus and Christians, is a sacred, indissoluble permanent union. Law-makers consider family to be a 'private sphere' and recognize the need to respect the privacy by minimizing interference with this institution. Till 1955, matrimonial relief was not available to Hindus and scarcely available to Christians.

The matrimonial relief that one can seek includes:

1. Decree for nullity
2. Restitution of conjugal rights
3. Judicial separation
4. Divorce.

Divorce or nullity is granted in cases where a socially accepted marriage is not legally accepted as a marriage, e.g. bigamy. There are two questions with reference to the marriage. Is the marriage a valid one? Is it possible for the relationship to continue? The conditions prevailing at the time of marriage decide its validity. An individual who is not capable of comprehending what is happening to him or her cannot give consent for marriage. The individual may not have the capacity for procreation. The relationship between the parties may be one that prohibited by religious codes. Such situations lay open to question the validity of marriage. Nullity of marriage means that the marriage is held null or void. In other words, a valid marriage does not take place at all. Conditions prevailing in the course of marital life determine the continuation of the relationship between the partners. For example, desertion, cruelty, adultery and mental illness may interfere with marital life and it may not be possible for the relationship to continue. Divorce means that the marriage was a valid one, but the relationship cannot be continued. Following the decree of divorce, the individual becomes eligible for remarriage.

MUSLIM LAW OF MARRIAGE AND DIVORCE

Under this section two Acts need to be taken into account:

1. The Dissolution of Muslim Marriage Act VIII of 1839
2. The Muslim Women (Protection of Rights on Divorce) Act, 1986.

A Muslim who is of sound mind and has attained puberty (presumed to have been attained on completion of 13 years, unless the contrary is proved) is qualified to marry. Under the Muslim marriage law, lunatics or persons of unsound mind and minors who have not attained puberty may be validly contracted into marriage by their respective guardians.

According to Muslim law, marriages are of three kinds: (i) *sahih* or valid; (ii) *batil* or void; and (iii) *fasil* or irregular. The Muslim law, unlike the Special Marriage Act, 1954 and the Hindu Marriage Act, 1955, does not classify any marriage as voidable marriage. A *sahih* or valid marriage is one that is contracted by observing all the conditions of marriage. If some of those conditions are violated, the marriage is batil or void. Those conditions are: consanguinity, affinity, forterage, marriage by a Muslim woman without divorce by a living husband. If some other conditions are violated the marriage is declared fasil or irregular.

Irregular (*fasil*) marriages are: (i) marriage contracted without witnesses; (ii) marriage with a fifth wife when four wives are present; (iii) marriage during the iddat period; (iv) marriage prohibited on the grounds of a different religion; (v) marriage prohibited as an unlawful conjunction.

Mutah marriage (*nikah-i-mutah*): A *mutah* marriage is recognized among the Muslims of the *Shia* section as a temporary marriage. Its duration can be fixed by an agreement between the two parties. The *Sunni* section does not recognize this kind of marriage.

The All India Muslim Personal Law Board (AIMPLB) has urged Muslims to avoid the practice of triple *talaq*, while its executive committee approved the draft of a model '*nikah-nama*' which contains guidelines for married couples. The AIMPLB said that Muslim couples should hesitate in giving *talaq*, particularly the triple *talaq*, which is considered to be a sin.

DISSOLUTION OF MARRIAGE AS PER THE MUSLIM LAW

A Muslim marriage can be dissolved by divorce by the parties without recourse to the court and on certain grounds by recourse to the court.

The law as ordained by the Holy Quran is that talaq must be for a reasonable cause and that it must be preceded by an attempt at reconciliation between the husband and the wife by two arbiters, one chosen by the wife from her family and the other by the husband from his family. If their attempts fail then talaq may be effective.

DISSOLUTION OF MARRIAGE WITHOUT RECOURSE TO COURT

Talaq: When divorce proceeds from a husband to his wife it is known as divorce by talaq. A Muslim husband of sound mind who has attained the age of puberty may divorce his wife whenever he desires without assigning any cause. The dictionary meaning of *talaq* in the language of law is 'taking off of the marriage tie by appropriate words'.

There are two kinds of *talaq* on the basis of effect:

1. Revocable (rujaee)
2. Irrevocable (bain)

There are three kinds of *talaq* based on the forms:

1. *Talaq absun*: This is done by a single pronouncement of divorce. If the marriage is not consummated, talaq can be pronounced in this manner.
2. *Talaq hasun*: This consists of three pronouncements made after an interval of a month. On the third pronouncement talaq becomes irrevocable.
3. *Talaq-ul-bidat*: Three pronouncements made at shorter intervals or even in quick succession. This mode is considered sinful.

Talaq may be through spoken words (oral) or by a written document (*talaq-nama*).

DIVORCE BY RECOURSE TO COURT (JUDICIAL DIVORCE)

According to the Muslim Marriage Act, 1939, a woman married under the Muslim law shall be entitled to obtain a decree for the dissolution of her marriage (based on mental health issues) on the following grounds:

1. That the husband has been insane for a period of 2 years.
2. That the husband was impotent at the time of marriage and continues to be so. Inability of the husband to consummate the marriage is one pattern of impotence.

Parsi Law: Parsi Marriage and Divorce Act, 1936, amended in 1988. A Parsi means a Zoroastrian and the Act is meant for this community. The Parsi Law does not prescribe any specific form of marriage; however, one essential ceremony must be performed in all Parsi marriages. This is the Ashirvad ceremony. No Parsi marriage shall be valid unless it is solemnized by the Ashirvad ceremony. Under the Parsi Marriage and Divorce Act, unsoundness of mind is not a ground for annulment of marriage.

GROUNDS FOR DIVORCE IN THE PARSI MARRIAGE ACT

Section 32: Any married person may seek divorce on the following grounds: That the defendant at the time of the marriage was of unsound mind and has been habitually so up to the date of the suit; provided that divorce shall not be granted on this ground, unless the plaintiff (i) was ignorant of the fact at the time of the marriage, and (ii) has filed the suit within three years from the date of the marriage.

Section 32 (b) (Amendment Act, 1988): That the defendant has been incurably of unsound mind for a period of two years or upwards immediately preceding the filing of the suit or has been suffering continuously or intermittently from mental disorder of such kind and to such an extent that the plaintiff cannot reasonably be expected to live with the defendant.

'Mental disorder' explained in this section is similar to that in the Special Marriage Act and the Hindu Marriage Act.

Christian Law of Marriage and Divorce and the Indian Divorce Act (The Divorce Act, 1869)

Dissolution of marriage: The Indian Divorce Act, 1869; amended in 2001.
On the demand of several Christian organizations, Section X of the IDA was amended by Act No. 51 of 2001. As per this amendment, the grounds for divorce are very much similar to those under the Special Marriage Act and the Hindu Marriage Act.

Section X (I) (II): Unsoundness of mind. This is a ground for divorce on two conditions: (i) The unsoundness of mind must be 'incurable' and medical evidence is required to prove it. (ii) It must be present for at least two years immediately before the filing of the petition. It is submitted that both the conditions must run together. If the respondent's unsoundness of mind was curable in the beginning, but later on became incurable, the period of two years will be counted from the date when the disease became incurable.

The Christian wife has some exclusive grounds for divorce: Section X (II): The three exclusive grounds for divorce that a wife can file are (i) rape, (ii) sodomy, and (iii) bestiality. Dissolution of marriage by mutual consent in now possible for Christians under Section X A of the IDA (Amendment Act), 2001.

Nullity of marriage: The grounds for nullity of marriage as per the IDA Section 19: Impotence, lunacy or idiocy are among the five causes for nullity.

Under Section 19 (3), it must be established that the respondent was a lunatic or idiot at the time of marriage.

THE SPECIAL MARRIAGE ACT, 1954

The Special Marriage Act is meant for any person in India and Indian nationals abroad, irrespective of the faith that the individual may posses. A marriage solemnized in any other form can be registered under this Act. The enactment of 1954 has been subsequently amended. The Marriage Laws (Amendment) Act, 1976 has brought about considerable changes in the grounds for divorce, judicial separation and nullity.

Conditions of Special Marriages

The section lays down five conditions of marriage:

- Monogamy
- Mental soundness (Clause b)
- Marital age
- Relationship (Clause d)
- Conditions of marriage in Jammu and Kashmir (Clause e)

Mental soundness: Marriage is tagged with lifelong responsibilities. The Special Marriage Act, therefore, provides that neither party:

- is incapable of giving a valid consent to it as a consequence of unsoundness of mind; or
- though capable of giving valid consent, has been suffering from mental disorder of such a kind or to such an extent as to be unfit for marriage and the procreation of children, or
- has been subject to recurrent attacks of insanity.

The condition of mental soundness for marriage does not mean that the person to be married must possess a high intelligence quotient. It only requires that he should understand the special nature of the relationship that marriage creates.

The present provisions of Section 4(b) are substituted by the Marriage Laws Amendment Act, 1976. The original provision was 'neither party is an idiot or a lunatic.'

According to the Marriage Laws (Amendment) Act, 1976, recurrent epilepsy was also a disqualification for marriage. Now that has been removed by the Marriage Laws (Amendment) Act (No. 39 of 1999) with effect from December 1999. Marriage in violation of this condition is void under section 24(I)(1).

GROUNDS FOR JUDICIAL SEPARATION

Section 23 provides for judicial separation on any of the grounds for divorce specified in section 27, sub-sections I and IA.

Unsound mind: That the respondent has been incurably of unsound mind or has been suffering continuously or intermittently from mental disorder of such a kind and to such an extent that the petitioner cannot reasonably be expected to live with the respondent.

GROUND FOR DIVORCE: SECTION 27(I)

A petition for divorce may be presented to the District Court either by the husband or the wife on the ground that the respondent, as per clause (e), has been incurably of unsound mind or has been suffering continuously or intermittently from mental disorder of such a kind and to such an extent that the petitioner cannot reasonably be expected to live with the respondent. In this clause:

- The expression of mental disorder means mental illness, arrested or incomplete development of the mind, psychopathic disorder or any other disorder or disability of mind and includes schizophrenia.
- The expression 'psychopathic disorder' means a persistent disorder or disability of the mind (whether or not including subnormality of intelligence) which results in abnormally aggressive or seriously irresponsible conduct on the part of the respondent and whether or not it requires or is susceptible to medical treatment.

HINDU MARRIAGE ACT, 1955

This is an Act to amend and codify the law relating to marriage among Hindus. This enactment of 1955 has been subsequently amended eight times from 1956 to 2003. The Marriage Laws (Amendment) Act, 1976 has brought about considerable changes in the original Act. The Hindu Marriage Act applies to Hindus, Buddhists, Jains and Sikhs. The Act of 1955 provided for four types of matrimonial relief: (i) restitution of conjugal rights, (ii) judicial separation, (iii) declaration of nullity and annulment, and (iv) divorce. Divorce was the most radical social reform. The dharmasashtras did not recognize divorce. By 1955, marriage came to be accepted as essentially a contract. The issue of divorce then comes as a natural consequence.

Adultery, desertion and cruelty were looked upon as 'matrimonial offences' which needed to be punished and divorce was used as an instrument for punishing people guilty of such offence. This was initially called the 'offence theory' of divorce. Later, insanity was added as a ground for divorce and came to be regarded as a 'matrimonial offence', though insanity or unsoundness of mind is a misfortune, not a cause for guilt. Since diseases like insanity could not be categorized as an offence, the 'offence theory' was renamed as the 'fault theory'. That is, if the respondent had 'some fault', which made continuance of cohabitation at most impossible, the petitioner was entitled to divorce.

Condition for a Hindu Marriage

Section 5: A marriage may be solemnized between any two Hindus, if the following conditions are fulfilled: (i) neither party has a spouse living at the time of marriage; (ii) at the time of marriage neither party (a) is incapable of giving valid consent in consequence of unsoundness of mind, or (b) though capable of giving valid consent, has been suffering from mental disorder of such a kind or to such an extent as to be unfit for marriage and the procreation of children, or (c) has been subject to recurrent attacks of insanity (the words 'or epilepsy' were omitted by Act 39 of 1999, Section 2); (iii) the bridegroom has completed 21 years and the bride has completed 18 years at the time of marriage; (iv) the parties are not within the degree of prohibited relationships; (v) the parties are not sapindas of each other unless the custom or usage governing each of them permits of a marriage between the two.

Section 5, Clause (ii): Mental Health

This clause requires that neither party to the marriage must be incapable of giving valid consent because of unsoundness of mind. The expression 'unsoundness of mind' has to be understood as lack of a state of mind or capacity to understand one's affairs or marital obligations.

ORIGINAL PROVISION

This clause has been amended by the Marriage Laws (Amendment) Act, 1976. The original provision was, 'neither party is an idiot or lunatic at the time of marriage'.

The term 'unsoundness of mind' in the present provision is more comprehensive. Idiocy and lunacy are types of unsoundness of mind. Idiocy is manifested by indecency of behaviour, dirtiness in habits or by vacancy of aspect or by inability to understand the most common rules of arithmetic. Unsoundness of mind is depravity or 'mania'. A person of dull or feeble intellect may not understand the nature of a marital relationship.

Unsoundness of mind is not the same thing as 'feeble mindedness' or 'dullness of intellect'. It is not a disqualification for marriage because a person of dull or feeble intellect may understand the nature of a marital relationship. In addition, neither party should be suffering from mental disorder of a type and to an extent as to render the party unfit for marriage and the procreation of children. A party could be said to be unfit for marriage if the party is not able to understand the nature and implication of a marital relationship. A party would be unfit for procreation if the party would not be able to look after or maintain the children from the marriage, or the children would be likely to be suffering from the same mental disorder or defect. The word 'and' between the expression 'unfit for marriage' and 'procreation of children' should be read as 'and/or'. The court can nullify the marriage if either condition or both the conditions contemplated exist. The word 'procreation' includes the capacity to rear children besides the capacity to beget them.

In the further alternative neither party should have been subject to recurrent attacks of insanity meaning 'subject to an increase of the acuteness or severity of unsoundness of mind recurring periodically in its course'.

A marriage in contravention of this condition is not void but voidable under section 12, sub-section (2), clause (b).

Grounds for Judicial Separation

On reading Section 10 and Section 13 together, relief of judicial separation would be available on the following grounds:

That the respondent has been incurably of unsound mind, or has been suffering continuously or intermittently from mental disorder of such a kind and to such an extent that the petitioner cannot reasonably be expected to live with the Respondent. See Section 13(1)(iii).

NULLITY

Unsoundness of mind or mental disorder or insanity- contravention of conditions specified in Clause (ii) of Section 5 to12(1)(b).

A marriage becomes voidable if the respondent was incapable of giving consent as a consequence of unsoundness of mind or, though the respondent was capable of giving valid consent, the respondent was suffering from mental disorder of such a kind or extent as to be unfit for marriage and the procreation of children; or the respondent has been subject to recurrent attacks of insanity. The Supreme Court held in R. Lakshmi Narayan versus Santhi that to brand a wife as unfit for marriage and procreation of children on account of a mental disorder, it needs to be established that the ailment suffered by her is of such a kind or to such an extent that it is impossible for her to lead a normal married life.

The unfitness for marriage and procreation of children contemplated here is one arising from mental disorder only, and not on account of any other disorder. Infertility or sterility as such is not a ground for annulment of marriage under Section 12 or for divorce under section 13.

In this case, the respondent was at the time of marriage suffering from schizophrenia. This disease of the mind affects normal behaviour. A person having this illness can be termed 'not sane'. Therefore, it was held that the case was covered by Section 12(1)(b) read with section 5(ii)(c) of the Act.

Section 13(1): Any marriage solemnized, whether before or after the commencement of this Act, may, on a petition presented by either the husband or the wife, be dissolved by a decree of divorce on the ground that the other party:

Section (iii) has been incurably of unsound mind, or has been suffering continuously or intermittently from mental disorder of such a kind and to such an extent that the petitioner cannot reasonably be expected to live with the respondent.

a. The expression 'mental disorder' means mental illness, arrested or incomplete development of mind, psychopathic disorder or any other disorder or disability of mind and includes schizophrenia.
b. The expression 'psychopathic disorder' means a persistent disorder or disability of mind (whether or not including subnormality of intelligence) which results in abnormally aggressive or seriously irresponsible conduct on the part of the other party, and whether or not it requires or is susceptible to medical treatment.

Section 13(1)(iii): Incurably of unsound mind or suffering from mental disorder. The expression 'incurably' of unsound mind cannot be so widely interpreted as to cover feeble minded persons or persons of dull intellect who understand the nature and consequences of the act and are therefore able to control them and their affairs, and their reaction in the normal way (AS Mehta versus Vasumathi (AIR 1969) Gujarat - 48; Parvathi Mishra versus Jagadananda Mishra (1994) 78 CLT 561. When there was sufficient evidence for the court to conclude that the slight mental disorder of the wife was not of such a kind and to such an extent that the husband could not reasonably be expected to live with her, divorce could not be granted (Rita Roy versus Sitesh Chandra, AIR 1982) Calcutta 138; 86 CWL 167. Each case of schizophrenia has to be considered on its own merits.

Table 14.2: A unsoundness of mind as affecting the capacity to marry

Hindu Marriage Act, 1955 (HMA)
A Hindu Marriage is voidable if either party:

- Is incapable of giving a valid consent as a consequence of unsoundness of mind, or
- Though capable of giving a valid consent as a consequence of unsoundness of mind, or Though capable of giving a valid consent has been suffering from mental disorder of such a kind or to such an extent as to be unfit for marriage and the procreation of children
- Has been subject to recurrent attacks of insanity.

The Special Marriage Act, 1954 (SMA)
Applicable to persons from any religion undergoing a civil marriage. Has provisions similar to the HMA except that a marriage under the SMA is void.

Indian Divorce Act, 1869
A Christian marriage is voidable if either party was a lunatic or idiot.

Parsi Marriage and Divorce Act, 1936
Unsoundness of mind is not ground for annulment.

Muslim Law
A person of unsound mind cannot contract a marriage and such a marriage if contracted is void. However, if the guardian of the person of unsound mind considers such marriage to be in his interest and in the interest of society and is willing to take up all the monetary obligations of the marriage then such a marriage can be performed.

Table 14.3: Unsoundness of mind as a ground for divorce

Hindu Marriage Act, Special Marriage Act and Parsi Marriage and Divorce Act
Respondent has been incurably of sound mind or has been suffering continuous or intermittently from mental disorder of such a kind and to such an extent that the petitioner cannot reasonably be expected to live with him.

Dissolution of Muslim Marriage Act, 1939
A muslim woman can seek divorce on the ground that her husband has been insane for period of two years.

Indian Divorce Act, 1869 Amendment, 2001 (For Chrisitians)
Unsoundness of mind is a ground of divorce on two conditions that is it must be incurable and it must be at least for two years immediately before the filing of the petition.

The medical evidence regarding the requisite degree of mental disorder is relevant, though not conclusive (Sharada versus Dharmapaul (2003) 4 SCC 493). In so far as granting the relief of divorce under section 13(1)(iii) of the Act is concerned, the nature and degree of mental disorder which meets the requirements has been clearly discussed and spelt out in one of the important cases (Ramnarayan Gupta versus Sreemathi Rajeshwari Gupta, Justice Venkatachaliah [Supreme Court 1998]). 'Each case of mental illness or schizophrenia has to be considered on its own merits.' Schizophrenia is what schizophrenia does. The judgment is significant because it gives importance to the effects and the impact rather that to the mere labelling of mental illness.

A Division Bench of the Andhra Pradesh High Court held in Hema Reddy versus Rakesh Reddy (2003) that psychological depression by itself is no ground for divorce under the Hindu Law.

IMPOTENCE

Impotence means the incapacity to perform sexual intercourse which is full and natural. Refusal to have sex is different from impotence. Impotence is different from sterility. Consummation means full penetration, not attempt to penetrate. Based on impotence at the time of marriage as per section 19(1) of the IDA and as per section 30 of the Parsi Marriage Act, and as per section 24(ii) of the Special Marriage Act and according to section 12A of the Hindu Marriage Law, the marriage becomes null and void.

According to section 2(v) of the Dissolution of Marriage Act, one of the grounds for dissolution of marriage is impotence. The institution of suit should be applied for within one year for nullity and after one year for divorce.

NAGGING BY SPOUSE: A GROUND FOR DIVORCE

In a recent judgment (December 2004), the Supreme Court held that a spouse can seek divorce if he or she is subjected to mental agony and cruelty due to constant nagging by his or her partner. This judgment invoked a lot of debate. Regarding this judgment, a magazine conducted a survey in Tamil Nadu: 56.25% supported the judgment and 37.5% opposed it; 65% of those surveyed accepted that they were nagged by their partners.

In a compilation of 61 cases of divorce, Dhanda found that divorce/nullity had been filed on the following facts: Hindu Marriage Act: 49, IDA: 11 and Parsi Act: 1. Out of 34 cases filed for divorce only 10 cases were granted divorce, and out of 30 cases for nullity of marriage, 12 cases were granted the same. In her compilation of 61 cases, Amita Dhanda found that schizophrenia forms nearly one-third of the diagnostic pattern of causes followed by mild mental disorder/ insanity/unsoundness of mind. The other categories are mental retardation, epilepsy and manic-depressive psychosis. In the Family Court of Chennai, during the past one year, nearly 5000 cases had been filed for dissolution/ nullity. Out of these only 45 cases were filed on the ground of mental illness. Of these, 42 cases were filed under the Hindu Marriage Act and 3 cases under the IDA. This finding indicates that in our culture the basis of mental disorder for filing a divorce suit is not significant.

Mental illness is a question of fact. It has to be proved in court. It is not a matter of interpretation. The law presumes that sanity and insanity have to be proved. The standard of proof is the preponderance of probabilities. It means that the probability of insanity should be more than the improbability of sanity. The court comes to a conclusion on the basis of not only medical evidence, but also other pieces of evidence. It will be of assistance to the court if the psychiatrist adds a description of the observable behaviour in the report. The burden of proving the insanity of the respondent rests on the petitioner. It is the responsibility of the psychiatrist to keep the documents sound. A certificate given by the psychiatrist is only a statement of opinion, and it attains the status of evidence only when its author undergoes cross-examination. The court need not accept the opinion of the psychiatrist and the medical evidence can be rejected.

The law should not discourage persons from seeking treatment for mental disorders, rather it should 'perform a promotive and facilitative role, it is suggested that an express legislative provision should be incorporated, which states that a past history of mental illness will be no bar to marriage; failure to disclose such past history or the fact of treatment would not amount to suppression of a material fact'. The psychiatrist must know that the intention of the court is similar to his/her. Both do not want to promote the incidence of broken homes. The decision of the court either preserves or breaks a family. The psychiatrist must be aware of the legal provisions, in order to meet the legal requirements.

In conclusion, it is important to recognize that although the legislation provides the constitutional and legal perspectives and sets standards for cases being settled through the process of law, the social problems of this nature have to be also worked through and resolved in many other ways. Legislation is necessary, but the promotive and harmony seeking approaches are equally important, and indeed are more likely to be useful.

SUGGESTED READING

1. Batra L, Gautam S. Psychiatric morbidity and personality profile in divorce seeking couples. Indian J Psychiatry, 1995;37:179-85.
2. Desai K. Indian law of marriage and divorce. 6th edition Nagpur: Wadhwa & Co; 2004.
3. Dhanda A. Legal order and mental disorder, New Delhi: Sage Publications, ew Delhi 2000;181-209.
4. Jablensky A, Sartorius N, Ernberg G, et al. Schizophrenia: Manifestations, incidence and course in different cultures: A World Health Organization ten-country study. Monograph. Psychol Med 1992, (Suppl. 20):1-97.
5. Nambi S. Presidential address, women and law in India, Oxford University Press, 2004.
6. Robins LN, Regier DA. Psychiatric disorders in America. The ECA study. New York: Free Press, 1991.

7. Testamentary Disposition of Property, The Legal Order and Mental Disorder. Sage Publications, New Delhi, Pgs. 267–78.
8. Thara R, Kamath S, Kumar S. Women with schizophrenia and broken marriages-doubly disadvantaged? Part I: Patient perspective. Int J Soc Psychiatry, 2003;49:225-32.
9. Thara R, Kamath S, Kumar S. Women with schizophrenia and broken marriages-doubly disadvantaged? Part II: Family perspective. Int J Soc Psychiatry, 2003;49:233-40.
10. Thara R, Srinivasan TN. Outcome of marriage in schizophrenia. Soc Psychiatry Psychiatric Epidemiol, 1997;32:416-20.

15 Chapter

Media, Mental Health and Ethics

Media coverage of psychiatric patients, issues and events plays an important role in shaping public attitudes and, therefore, public policy in the area of mental health. Unfortunately, persons with mental or emotional problems tend to be perceived as potentially dangerous. Consequently, negative stereotypes and unfounded fears based on misperceptions lead to resistance of community-based treatment programs as well as underfunding of mental health facilities. Media infrequently presents information on mental health and illness; when the disorder, it is often distorted. The task of mass media, in the context of mental health, is to reflect stories that are friendly, accurate and part of a long-term plan to create awareness about psychiatric illness and behavioral problems.

The following issues require consideration in discussing about Mental Health and Media.

1. Media coverage of mental health issues.
2. Evaluation of the communication between psychiatry and media in such forms as television, radio or press.
3. Media attitudes towards mentally ill.
4. Description in the media of specific treatment of a psychiatric patient, event, or mode of treatment.

Media coverage of mental health issues is often inadequate. Media in India has been focusing on mental health issues only recently and the coverage is often limited to issues like drug abuse, alcoholism, marriage counseling, stress management and mental hospitals. The coverage given to promotive factors of mental health, core issues of mentally ill, societal responses to care and rehabilitation of mentally ill, new and scientific treatment facilities in psychiatry, geriatric and child mental health are strikingly inadequate.

One of the most pressing needs in the area of mental health and illness is for a simple, informative, comprehensible and unbiased guide to help people to understand about the causes and treatment of mental illness. Many people including doctors, social workers and other professionals exhibit prejudice and even ignorance when it comes to psychological aspects of health and disease. It is important that relevant issues of mental health are adequately communicated by qualified mental health professionals. There are times in which a person not qualified in the area of mental health talks about mental illness management in media like television and often it is not surprising that such information is inaccurate, unscientific and unauthentic. It is equally important that the interviewer or journalist is knowledgeable so that his/her interact with the professional is meaningful. Sometimes important issues, explanations and contexts are often lost in the fight for space.

Media coverage may at times be distorted by an overemphasis on the bizarre symptoms of the mentally ill. Media reporters like the general public may have different attitudes towards the mentally sensationalistic sells. Reporters are often forced to take a sensationalistic approach to subject matter, because "that is what the public wants" and this is "what sells papers and advertising". Professionals time constraints and pressures force journalists to be sensationalistic.

The reporters may not be aware of the simple fact that mental illness management is scientific. There could be many causes for mental illness including organic, psychological and environmental. There are many myths and misconceptions surrounding mental illness. Certain treatment procedures like electroconvulsive therapy may be misunderstood and mistakenly believed to be abused by psychiatrists on their patients. The mental hospital may be picturized as degenerated places, where patients are uncared for and locked forever. Whereas a proper reporting of facts can lead to public awareness of underfunding of mental health facilities on the other hand, distorted sensationalistic version may create public antipathy towards psychiatry itself.

The following suggestions are made for improving media coverage of mental health issues:

1. **Education and communication:** Communication between professionals and journalists should be improved; professionals should speak at seminars or conferences of print or broadcast journalists on the implications of certain types of reporting, similarly, workshops should be organized for professionals on the art of communicating with media. More contact and exchange between the two groups would promote understanding and break down barriers of distrust and feelings of apprehension. It is recommended that psychiatric associations appoint liaison officers to deal with the media and that they approach the media with ideas, information, newsletters or press releases, rather than waiting to be questioned about the latest controversy. Similarly, newspapers should be encouraged to select medical reporters with a special interest in and knowledge about mental health issues to report on these issues.
2. **Accuracy:** Psychiatrists should get more involved in writing articles, book reviews, movie reviews to promulgate a more accurate portrayal of psychiatry. Psychiatrists should request live, rather than taped interviews, in order, to avoid misleading editing. Psychiatric associations should demand retractions and apologies if misinterpretations or inaccurate reporting take place.
3. **Positive image:** Attempts to counteract the frequently negative and pessimistic articles relating to mental illness must be made. Former patients who have been successfully treated should be encouraged to speak up about their positive experiences with psychiatry.

ADDICTION TO THE INTERNET AND ONLINE GAMING

No doubt the internet has become the powerful media today. As computer and internet use has become style of every day life, the potential for overt use is possible, which may lead to addiction. Research on internet addiction has shown that users can become addicted to it. Addiction to the Internet shares some of the negative aspects of substance addiction and has been shown to lead to consequences such as school failure, family, and relationship problems.

PUBLIC ATTITUDE, MEDIA AND MENTAL ILLNESS

"As far as media is concerned we must pray to be saved not only ignorance experience by the public, but also be saved from over zealousness, smugness of knowledge and professional militancy shown by the professionals. The worst we can do under the circumstances is to try and superimpose the media strategy (Specially from the west) of another country or to India.

When we discuss about altering the public attitudes through mass media, it could be presumed that there is an attitude or position prevalent in the society that is false/incomplete/mischievous and needs to be changed to true/complete/adequate information.

MOVIES AND MENTAL ILLNESS

Some of the popular movies dealing with mental illnesses as the core subject often give distorted views, negative attitudes and false propaganda which in turn accelerates the already existing stigma; example: "One who flew over the cuckoos nest" and many other Indian movies. But at the same time some of the movies give excellent narration about the nature, course and positive outcome of Mental illness and also emphasize the role of the caregiver in influencing the outcome, for example "The silence of the lambs", "A beautiful mind", "Iris", etc.

Regarding media and mental health, what is happening today is the lack of an appropriate scientific dissemination in the media or which may be worse. a dissemination of distorted information thereof. Violence in newspapers, magazines, movies, television programs and pornography within one's grasp—which deteriorates links.

Federico Fellini (1977) considered TV to be an invention that was not only strange but also devilish. "It has been born with the intention of informing but, due to a mysterious motive, it just failed. Instead of disseminating culture it destroys every thing, hurricane-like. It is as if war, religion, everything (the Almighty involved) were poured into a blender that will disintegrate all into tiny particles." In other words, TV has become a referent for the cliche of the medley culture pertaining to late modernism that construes life as a fragmentary projection, as a zapping session programmed by an unbalanced psychotic.

IMPORTANCE OF MEDIA ON HUMAN SEXUAL BEHAVIOR

With the advancement of technology, access to mass media has increased significantly. Over the years, the expression of sexuality has liberalized. But there are few studies of the selection, interpretation and application of sexual content in the media suggest that the mass media can affect awareness of, beliefs about, and possibly actual sexual behavior. More research is needed to say more precisely with which audiences, under what circumstances and with which content effects occur. Such research is especially relevant as access to increasingly explicit sexual material increases and other potential perspectives on sexually responsible behavior, such as parents, schools, and faith communities, remain relatively reticent.

With the available evidence, it can be said that mass media does not affect human sexual behaviour, especially young people. It is important for the broadcast and censorship media to promote healthy sexual behaviour. Mass media companies should incorporate messages regarding STDs and healthy sexual behaviors, including delaying sexual intercourse and using condoms.

Mental health is a matter of combined social and individual perception and thus heavily influenced by media. There are at least four important issues for which media have great importance in the arena of mental health. These are:

- Media influence the public awareness and perception of mental illness.
- Media has a strong influence on the stigma alleviation about mental illness.
- Media make a strong platform for advocacy for mental health promotion and
- Media may enforce negative impact on public information about mental illness and thus reinforce negative attitude (example of suicide reporting).

It is high time that whenever dealing with mental health problems, the media should observe a code of ethics. Because of the powerful influence of media on masses, wrong messages will have disastrous consequence. A media should be clear about what information they want to disseminate, the attitude of public and the real scientific background. Mental health professionals should also have equal responsibility. Their personal crusades on media professionals can ensure success of the programme. The lobby of psychiatrist should try to educate the reporters/ script writer/producer/actor/director about the trueness of symptomatology of mental illness.

SUGGESTED READING

1. Bhujang PM. Mentally ill and the law. Universal Publishing Corporation, Mumbai, 2003.
2. Blueglass R, Bowden P. Principles and practice of forensic psychiatry, 1990.
3. Chiswick D, Cope R. Practical forensic psychiatry. Royal College of Psychiatry, 1995.
4. Gunn J, Taylor P. Clinical, Legal and Ethical Issues in Forensic Psychiatry, 1993.
5. Nambi S. Legal Aspects of Psychiatry—Indian Perspective, 2009. Manashanthi Mental Health Care Publications 2008.

16 Chapter

Forensic Issues in Children

INTRODUCTION

"The development of children is the first priority on the country's development agenda, not because they are the most vulnerable, but because they are our supreme assets and also the future human resources of the country" these words underline the fact that the future of India lies in the future of Indian children.

As per 2001 census, India has around 157.86 million children, constituting 15.42% of India's population, who are below the age of 6 years, 75.95 million children are boys.

Sex ratio among children (0–6 years)—927 females for 1000 males. A significant proportion of these children live in economic and social environment which impedes their physical and mental development.

10–12% of < 18 years suffer from disorders in behavior, learning and development (ICMR 2001)—Mental and behavioral disorders in children and adolescents is—12.8% (WHO 2001)—Serious emotional disturbances in children and adolescents is 15%.

The medical profession and particularly the psychiatrists dealing with children have an increasingly crucial role to play in cases involving the welfare of children. His written report and oral evidence with reference to mental health issues in children are very important to safeguard the child's welfare.

Children with or without mental health problems at times come across legal issues, but not so common like adults. The children related offences may be of many kinds like children indulging in petty crimes or offences against children are in very many forms by adults including their parents. It is very essential for mental health professionals to recognize the legal issues centered around children and the various legislations in India to protect and safeguard the welfare of the children.

CRIME AND CHILDREN

Conduct Disorder

Antisocial behavior is inevitable in the course of development of children and is among the most common presenting complaints in the practice of child and adolescent psychiatry. Its relation to psychopathology is complex (Robins, et al. 1991, Rutter 1996). Conduct disorder is a medical (psychiatric) diagnosis: juvenile delinquency is a legal term and antisocial behavior or sociopathic or psychopathic behavior is a social term.

Conduct disorder is characterized by a pattern of behavior that violates the basic rights of others or age appropriate norms and rules of society. Conduct disorder is one of the most common disorders in child psychiatry. Conduct disorder constitutes around 30 to 50% of referrals in some child-guidance clinics. Various Indian community studies have reported prevalence of conduct disorder to vary from 0.2 to 13.5%. In US, the lifetime prevalence of conduct disorder has been estimated at between 6 and 16% per boys and 2 and 9% for girls. The ratio of boys to girls with conduct disorder is between 5:1. Conduct disorder is often associated with boys from urban/slum with poverty and with severe parental pathology like parental separation, alcoholic father, domestic violence, etc. The common comorbidity associated are attention deficit hyperactivity disorder (ADHD), substance abuse, and opposition defiant disorder, etc.

Sex Offences Committed by Juveniles

Sex offences committed by juveniles are especially a rising problem. Offences like rape and child molestation are not uncommon. Half of all adult offenders began their aberrant pattern of sex offending while juveniles. Hence it is vital to identify this type of offending at early age. In the past, juvenile sex offending has been minimized and many mental health workers looked upon these crimes as adolescent experimentation; but most adolescent sexual offenders detected have already committed multiple offences during their childhood. Perry and Orchard (1992) count many of the adolescent sex offenders in the following summary of facts.

- Their offending behaviors are not simply attempts to learn about sex.
- Not all offenders are male.
- They derive from all races, social class and levels of intellect.
- This sexual deviant behavior will not go away with simple maturity.
- Sexual assaults are not primarily sexually motivated behaviors.
- Sexual offences are largely planned actions.
- Adolescent offenders typically have committed more than one offence when apprehended.
- Not all adolescent sex offenders have been victims of sexual abuse.

Child Abuse by Adults with Mental Health Problems

Children with alcoholic fathers are often deprived of the love and affection and also they are lacking the care and protection and safeguard which a normal child deserves.

A husband often indulges in abusing his wife whom in turn displace her aggression towards children. In this type of families, child abuse, especially problems like child battered syndrome are not uncommon.

Antisocial personality disorder adults involve children to get ransom from parents by kidnapping, torturing, and at times even killing the kidnapped children. Children at times may be exploited by adults in indulging sexual offences, this especially so happen in children with below average intelligence or children hailing from pathological families. The girl children are forced to enter into prostitution and the male children are exploited for homosexual activity just to earn their livelihood. At times, children are exploited and utilized for drug trafficking.

Dilemma in Dealing with Children with Offence

In dealing with children with offences, there is always a dilemma—since the legal system adopt a "therapeutic" or "punitive" response to their behavior? For an adult, who committed a crime, this decision is made to prosecution, the procedure adopted is relatively straight forward except for some mentally ill offenders. But the crime committed by a child or adolescent. A juvenile below the age of 18 years, the procedures are different. They are referred to as juvenile offenders. A number of difficulties have surfaced over the years of children citing witnesses in criminal proceedings, especially in children giving the evidence in sexual abuse cases.

Mentally ill women at times because of their severe depression or because of their disturbance in thinking or perception even kill their children. Somasundaram (1973) in his study in Chennai on "Mothers who kill their children" analyzed the type of mothers who were detained as mentally ill prisoners in the mental hospital. Infanticide is the commonest crime by this type of women. Majority of the mothers who indulge in infanticide were found to be suffering from some mental health problems.

Mental Retardation and Crime

Mental Health Act, 1987, does not include mental retardation in its definition of mental illness. The Act defines mental illness as a condition that should be treatable and also it should exclude mental retardation, hence the concept of mental retardation is not found as an equivalent or not inclusive in mental illness as per Mental Health Act (1987), whereas mental retardation as a disability has been found a place has one of the six disabilities in (Disabilities Act, 1995). In the Rehabilitation Council of India Act, mental retardation is considered as one of the handicap. A child with mental retardation cannot be admitted in a psychiatric hospital as per MHA (1987). They can be admitted in special homes for mental retardation, but mentally retarded children with associated problems like behavioral disorder, psychosis, can be admitted in a psychiatric hospital. Mentally retarded children are prone to commit the following crimes:

1. Theft
2. Fire setting
3. Sexual offences
4. Drug trafficking
5. Prostitution

Child Abuse

Child abuse is a pervasive societal problem with enormous associated human and economic cause. Child abuse occurs at epidemic rates with victims of abuse comprising the significant protection of child psychiatric conditions. In US, each year, there are over one million substantiated reports of child maltreatment; 49% for neglect, 24% for physical abuse, 15%—sexual abuse, and 12% other forms of mal-treatment. Lifetime incidences of physical and sexual abuse among child and adolescent outpatient and inpatient. Cohorts have been estimated to be as high as 30% in children and 55% in adolescents.

Child abuse is of many kinds:

1. Physical
2. Sexual
3. Verbal
4. Emotional
5. Financial

A 13-State National Study by Ministry of Women and Child Development, (UNICEF, and Save the Children) notes that 69% of all Indian children are victims of physical, mental, or emotional abuse.

Physical Abuse

- Bruises or welts
- Burns, scalds, sprains dislocation, bites, fractures, especially in infants. Shaking injuries, e.g. retinal, hemorrhage. Inappropriate explanation of child's injury. Wariness of adult contacts (Table 16.1).

Table 16.1: Protection of children from abuse

Term	*Definition*
1. Abuse and neglect	Forms of maltreatment of a child
2. Child protection	Process of protecting individual children identified as either suffering, or at risk of suffering, significant harm as a result of abuse or neglect
3. Safeguarding and promoting the welfare of children	The process of protecting children from abuse or neglect preventing impairment of their health, and development and ensuring they are growing up in the circumstances consistent with the provision of safe and effective care which is undertaken so as to enable children to have optimum life chances and enter adulthood successfully

SPECIAL OPPORTUNITIES FOR SAFEGUARDING BOTH PHYSICAL AND MENTAL HEALTH IN CHILDREN

- Families living with poverty, crime, unemployment, or poor housing
- Families where there is domestic violence
- Families where a parent has a mental illness
- Families where a parent is misusing drugs or alcohol

- Families where a parent has a learning disability
- Families that face racism and other forms of social isolation
- Children abused through prostitution
- Fabricated or induced illness
- Investigating complex (organized or multiple) abuse
- Female genital mutilation
- Responding rapidly to an unexpected death of a child
- Children living away from home
- The abuse of disabled children
- Abuse by children and young people
- Bullying
- Children whose behavior indicates a lack of parental control
- Children acting as careers
- Child abuse linked to cultural beliefs for example in "possession" or "witchcraft" or related to spiritual or religious belief
- Children and families living in temporary accommodation
- Traveler families
- Migrant children
- Child victims of trafficking
- Unaccompanied asylum-seeking children.

ROLE OF PSYCHIATRIST IN CHILD ABUSE

- Psychiatrists need to acquire specialized knowledge.
- They should be alert to the fact that child abuse is highly prevalent.
- They should take initiatives to protect the child from continuing harm.
- They should take measures to diminish long-term effects.
- They should collaborate with multidisciplinary team that deals with child abuse.

CHILD SEXUAL ABUSE IN INDIA

Child sexual abuse is the use of a child for sexual gratification by an older or more powerful person. The offender is usually an adult, but could also be a more powerful child. Both girls and boys are vulnerable. Besides being a public health concern, it is a crime punishable by law. The damage is particularly severe in the context of sexual abuse. There is stigma and shame surrounding child sexual abuse. It usually leaves the child dealing with the harm in solitude, loss of confidence and belief in the human beings closest to the child. It can instill feelings of fear, suspicion, uncertainty and emotional isolation. He or she may never again feel safe or secure in the company of the person who perpetuated the violence. Sexual abuse of children is disturbing, aberrant, and very often an unimaginable crime; but the unfortunate reality is that, it exists. The United Nation Convention on the rights of the child specifies the right of every girl and boy to protection. Its Article 19, describes the child's right to protect from abuse and Article 34 describes the child's right to protection from sexual abuse in particular.

With regard to India, child sexual abuse is far more prevalent than society willingly acknowledges. This is because the focus has been more on basic survival needs of health, shelter, nutrition and education. Consequently, there has been very little attention paid on the sexual abuse of girls and boys and its impact. Besides, a very superficial understanding of the definition compounded by a paucity of knowledge. There seems to be hardly any awareness both among general public and professional human service providers regarding the extent and severity of sexual abuse in India.

An NGO based at Tulir, Chennai, along with save the children organization conducted a study in 2006 to find out the prevalence and nature of the child sexual abuse reveals the following facts.

- Out of the 2211 school-going child participants, 42% had faced sexual abuse in one form or other.
- The sexual abuse occurs in all types of family like joint family, nuclear family, and others.
- Severe forms of sexual abuse were present in 11%.
- The abusers are often considered to be dirty old men and "stranger danger" is commonly believed to be the biggest threat to children's safety.
- Majority of abusers are people who are known to the child.
- Majority of the children did not disclose because of fear of threat, fear of shame, fear of stigma, and fear of parental punishment.
- Child sexual abuse is one of the most fundamental violations of childrens rights and usually an underlying obstacle to their overall development.

RECOMMENDATIONS TO MINIMIZE CHILD SEXUAL ABUSE INCLUDE

- Awareness campaign among children.
- Initiate and institutionalize "personal safety education".
- Sensitize and train frontline workers, teachers, and professionals.
- Consider parents as main share holders and awareness campaign.
- Develop and disseminate rights based child friendly resource materials.
- Advocate for child friendly and holistic, legal procedure, protocol and services.
- Sensitize NGO's and society on child sexual abuse.

CHILDREN AND TORTURE

The term torture means any act, by which severe pain or suffering whether physical or mental is intentionally inflicted.

The "child", according to most international and legal standards, is anyone under the age of 18. The term juvenile also appears in human rights text, although, it is not exactly interchangeable. It usually refers to those who are able to be charged and try in the Juvenile Justice System.

The age of criminal responsibility usually different from the age of majority; it is commonly held to be the age at which a child can be expected and know right from wrong, understand the consequences of his/her actions, and be of sufficient emotional and intellectual maturity to understand and participate in hearings, trials, or other procedures within the appropriate Juvenile Justice Settings.

A HIDDEN PHENOMENON?

- Torture of children is "invisible".
- They are significantly under reported.
- The most common form of state torture against children is probably the beating of young criminal suspects in police custody.
- Juvenile criminal suspects will almost invariably be from the poorest or marginalized sectors of society, and discrimination against such groups often contributes to the lack of action against their torture or illtreatment.

MENTAL ILLNESS OR DISABILITY

A substantial proportion of children in detention suffer from some forms of mental illness or disability, ranging from retardation to psychotic disorders, which often go undiagnosed or untreated. Some have ended up in detention because of behavior resulting directly or indirectly from their mental illness, some have become mentally ill as a result of abusive conditions of incarceration. In many cases, the condition is exacerbated by substance abuse or addiction. These children are doubly vulnerable. Under International standards, all children in detention are entitled to medical treatment, but even basic medical care is lacking in many juvenile detention facilities and mental health provisions are frequently nonexistent. When treatment is inadequate or unavailable, mentally ill juveniles tend to suffer an intensification of their disability, which of itself may amount to cruel, inhuman, or degrading treatment. When the mentally ill are subjected to ill-treatment such as solitary confinement, confinement in a dark or soundless room or incommunicado detention, the effects of such illtreatment may be exacerbated, causing their condition to degenerate further. Children who suffer from mental illness may not be fully capable of forming or expressing opinions about their own treatment, or may express views harmful to their own well-being. The standard of "best interests of the child" in such cases must be carefully balanced against the child's evolving right to make their own decisions, and their right to be involved in all decisions affecting their own welfare.

THE PROTECTION OF CHILDREN UNDER INTERNATIONAL LAW

Both torture and ill treatment are prohibited by International Human Rights and Humanitarian Law, but children are entitled to even higher levels of protection. Article 19 of the children's convention obliges states, parties to protect children from "All forms of physical or mental violence, injury or abuse, neglect or negligent treatment, maltreatment, or exploitation including sexual abuse while in the care of parents, legal guardian, or any other person who has a care of a child."

Article 37 of the children's conventions forbids torture and cruel inhuman or degrading treatment adding that, "neither capital punishment nor life imprisonment without possibility of release, shall be imposed for offences committed by persons below 18 years of age." Implementation of the children's convention is monitored by the committee on the rights of the child. Children's conventions have been gratified almost by every country in the world. The convention definition of torture has a particular impact on how violence against girls is likely to be characterized and the girls are more likely to suffer, attack, or abuse in the home than in custody at school or the work place.

Torture of children is often invisible and a "hidden phenomenon" and signature under reported.

LEGAL PROTECTION OF CHILDREN IN INDIA

- The subject of children coming in conflict with law is receiving increasing attention of the society in recent times.
- Since their mental development, may not cope with the physical development, the children may not be able to control their emotions, stresses and impulses, which may lead to their delinquent behavior. Obviously the mind plays an important influence and the role of mental professionals in dealing with these situations is vital. Since the children are in impressible age, it is also essential that they are protected from evil influences of the criminal world and atmosphere. The juvenile delinquents, should be treated with more compassion and understanding, and they should be provided right kind of guidance and protection.
- Taking into consideration the mental development of a child, the Indian Penal Code provides the following immunity against punishment to children.

Section-82 (IPC)

"Nothing is an offence which is done by child under seven years of age".

Section-83 (IPC)

Nothing is an offence, which is done by a child above seven years age and under twelve, who has not attained sufficient maturity of understanding to judge the nature and consequences of his conduct on that occasion.

Thus determining physical and mental status (maturity) becomes vital in attributing the liability of child till the age of twelve.

Section-360 of Code of Criminal Procedures, 1973

Provides that a person below 21 years of age is known as the first offender and is not to be tried in a criminal court, through ordinary procedure. He is to be dealt with and corrected through special methods or treatment under law.

CHILD CARE AND PROTECTION AS PER CONSTITUTION OF INDIA

- Article 15(3)—ensures that there is no discrimination and access to all public facilities.
- Article 39(e)—protects child labor; (f)-opportunities in healthy manner and protect against moral and material abandonment.
- Article 45—state will provide early childhood care and education till 6 years of age.
- Article 47—State to raise level of nutrition and prohibit harmful intoxicating substance and drugs.

Criminal Procedure Code, 1973

Section 125 CrPc

- Any person having sufficient means neglects or refuses to maintain his children is punishable.
- Every person should protect his legitimate or illegitimate minor child whether married or not unable to maintain itself.
- (Not being married) attained majority, where such a child is, by reason of any physical or mental abnormality or injury is unable to maintain itself, his/her parents to safeguard them.

Admissions Under MHA, 1987

Section 16

Voluntary admissions in psychiatric hospitals—on request by guardian for admission of his/her mentally ill children. Involuntary admissions: Wandering mentally ill juveniles should be taken into custody by police and to be admitted as per MHA.

Discharges Under MHA, 1987

Section 18

- On request by guardian.
- On attaining majority while inpatient—intimate at the earliest and unless continuance is requested within a month.

CONSENT OF A MINOR

In general, minors so far have been considered as incapable of giving consent. Exceptions to this can be when minors seek birth control, treatment of STD, substance abuse and emergencies. Informed consent for adolescents seems like the right thing in the therapeutic setting. Patient, parent and therapist conflicts in consent. The debate continues as minors are becoming high income earners and self sufficient.

JUVENILE JUSTICE (CARE AND PROTECTION OF CHILDREN) ACT, 2000

Juvenile means, a child, who has not completed age of eighteen: This Act is the law relating to juveniles in conflict with law and children in need of care and protection, by providing proper care, protection, treatment by catering to their development needs and by adopting a child. Friendly approach in the adjudication and disposition of matters in the best interest of children and for their ultimate rehabilitation through various institutions.

The various objectives of this Act are:

1. Lay down basic principles for administering.
2. Justice to a juvenile: to bring the Juvenile Law in conformity in the United Convention on the rights of the child.
3. Both boys and girls below 18 years will come under this Act.
4. Speedy disposal of cases regarding juvenile or the child (within 4 months) lay down responsibilities for State Government, voluntary organization and local bodies. To create a Special Juvenile Police Unit with a humane approach. Establishing Juvenile Justice Board and Child Welfare Committees and homes in each district to minimize the stigma.

There are two parts of the Act:

I. For Juveniles in conflict with Law and the other for the juvenile or the child in need of care and protection.
II. Provision of rehabilitation and other social reintegration measures.

As per this Juvenile Justice Act, a child means:

- Who is found without any home or settled place.
- Who resides with a person (whether guardian or not) and such person.
- Has threatened to kill or injure the child.
    a. Has killed, abused, or neglected some other child.
    b. Who is mentally or physically challenged or ill-children.
    c. Who has a parent or guardian who is unfit or incapacitated to control the child.
    d. Who disorder not have parents or no one is willing to take care of and who is abandoned or who is missing or run-away child and whose parents are not found.
    e. Who is being or likely to be grossly abused, tortured and/or exploited for the purpose of sexual abuse or illegal acts.
    f. Who is found vulnerable and is likely to be inducted to drug abuse or trafficking.
    g. Who is being or likely to be abused for some other gains.
    h. Who is victim of harmed conflict, cruel commotion or natural calamity?
    i. Juvenile who is alleged to have committed an offence should be taken off by the juvenile police and the matter should be immediately informed to the Juvenile Justice Board.

The Juvenile Justice Board. Consists of the judicial magistrate, two social workers of whom of at least one shall be a woman and this Board has the power of a Metropolitan Magistrate laid down by the Code of Criminal Procedures (1973).

The child in need of care and protection will be taken care off by the child welfare committee appointed by the State Government. The Committee shall have the power to dispose off cases for the care, protection, treatment, development, and rehabilitation of the children and also to protect the human rights.

Juvenile offenders to be treated as per provisions of the act. Special observation homes are to be established either by government or with voluntary organizations for reception and rehabilitation of juveniles in conflict with law under this act.

Parents/guardians should be informed. Immediate bail to be granted whenever applicable.

The names of juveniles are not to be published without court permission.

Orders that may be passed include allowing to go home, participate in group counseling, to release on probation under someone's care, sending him to special homes.

No juvenile shall be sentenced to death or life imprisonment or committed to prison in default of payment of fine or in default of furnishing security.

A juvenile, shall not suffer disqualification, if any, attached to a conviction of an offence under such law.

Majority of the offence by juveniles are relatively trivial, more of a nuisance, than a serious threat. Most of the times they reflect petty, disorganized, impulsive and generally unprofitable crimes. Thefts, housebreaks, personal violence, drug and sex offences are common.

ADOPTION

Desire to have a child is a natural human instinct. Due to many medical and social reasons it is not always possible to have one's own children. Adoption is a method, universally used to satisfy that urge.

Adoption means to take a child of other parents as one's own child. The couple may adopt another's child for variety of reasons.

In order to legalize and to prevent misuse of the process the laws relating to adoption have been enacted.

The Hindu Adoption and Maintenance Act have the following provisions in reference to mentally ill persons.

Sections: 8.910 of the act prescribe that—

- A male (father) or a female (mother) of unsound mind cannot validly adopt a son or a daughter.
- Similarly a male (father) or female (mother) of unsound mind cannot validly give a son or daughter in adoption.
- If mother is of unsound mind, the father may dispense with the consent validly give a son or daughter in adoption.
- Likewise a mother may adopt or give in adoption a child without the consent of her husband, where husband is of unsound mind.

- Where both father and mother are of unsound mind, guardian may give a child in adoption.
- Among Christians and Parsis adoption was not recognized. However, based on custom and some court judgments the same is permitted. It is considered not valid for succession.
- Among Muslims adoption is not vogue. Mohammedan Law does not recognize adoption. Occasionally where adoption is a local custom, it is permitted.

CONCLUSION

Safeguarding, Child Protection and Mental Health

Safeguarding and child protection includes better understanding and recognition of children in distress and intervening wherever possible to prevent a range of adverse outcome. Achieving these goals will depend in part or greater awareness and more extensive training in psychosocial issues and forensic aspects of mental health of children.

Facts for Families

When a child tells an adult that he or she has been sexually abused, the adult may feel uncomfortable and may not know what to say or do. The following guidelines should be used when responding to children who say they have been sexually abused.

What to Say

If a child even hints in a vague way that sexual abuse has occurred, encourage or her to talk freely. Do not make judgmental comments.

Show that you understand and take seriously what the child is saying. Child adolescent psychiatrist have found that children who are listened to and understood do much better than those who are not. The response to the disclosure of sexual abuse is critical to the child's ability to resolve and heal the trauma of sexual abuse.

Assure the child that they did the right thing in telling. A child who is closer to the abuser may feel guilty about revealing the secret. The child may feel frightened if the abuser has threatened to harm the child or other family members as punishment for telling the secret.

Tell the child that he or she is not be blame for the sexual abuse. Most children in attempting to make sense out the abuse will believe that somehow they caused it or may even view it as a form stops.

What to Do

Report any suspicion of child abuse. If the abuse is within the family, report it to the local child Protection Agency. If the abuse outside of the family, report it to the police or district attorneys office. Individuals reporting in good faith are immune from prosecution. The agency receiving the report will conduct an evaluation and will take action to protect the child.

Parents should consult with their pediatrician or family physician, who may refer them to a physician who specializes in evaluating and treating sexual abuse. The examination doctor will evaluate the child's condition and treat any physical problem related to the abuse, gather evidence to help protect the child, and reassure the child that he or she is all right.

Children who have been sexually abused should have an evaluation by a child and adolescent psychiatrist or other qualified mental health professional to find out how the sexual abuse has affected them, and to determine whether ongoing professional help is necessary for the child too deal with the trauma of the abuse. The child and adolescent psychiatrist can also provide support to other family members who may be upset by the abuse.

While most allegations of sexual abuse made by children are true, some false accusations may arise in custody disputes and in other situations. Occasionally, the court will ask a child and adolescent psychiatrist to help determine whether the child is telling the truth or whether it will hurt the child to speak in court about the abuse.

When a child is asked as to testify, special considerations such as videotaping, frequent breaks, exclusion of spectators, and the option not to look at the accused– make the experience much less stressful.

Adults because of their maturity and knowledge, are always the ones to blame when they abuse children. The abused children should never be blamed.

When a child tells someone about sexual abuse, a supportive, caring response is the first step in getting help for the child and reestablishing their trust in adults.

SUGGESTED READING

1. Nambi S. Forensic issues in children. Indian Psychiatric Society, Tamil Nadu Branch, Souvenir, Annual CME, Trichy–21 December, 2010;74-88.
2. Psychological Intervention, Tanpsycon 2002—Souvenir, 17th Annual Conference, 13 and 14 July, 2002.
3. Responding to child sexual abuse. American Academy of Child and Adolescent Psychiatry Publication.

17 Chapter

Women, Mental Health and Legal Issues —An Indian Perspective

Psychosocial, cultural, economic and educational factors influence the mental health of men and women and as a result "there will be variations in their quality of mental health. Women have been deprived of opportunity and made to suffer inequalities. She is made as a mere chattel and placed at the receiving end, at the mercy of the male chauvinistic society. It is very pathetic to note even after adopting the constitution, the Indian women did not, so far, get their due share of justice—social, economic and political and equality of status and opportunity. For no fault of hers, she has been suppressed and oppressed in every walk of life. Her modesty has been outraged, time and again, within and outside the four walls of her house.

There are multiple sociocultural factors that affect the mental health of Indian women. This includes duality and contradictions in the female image, the deprivation of socialization, self-esteem, the complex dilemmas and stresses for women during her reproductive life starting from menarche to menopause and the deprivation or distortion of playing the primary role—all these life events that are a major source of frustration, misery, conflict and stress that take a toll on their mental health.

The emerging scenario of Indian Women's mental health is not very positive. The number of dowry deaths, female foeticide and infanticide, sexual abuse including rape, burning, domestic violence, neglect and humiliation of women and girls is steadily increasing over the years. As per the latest data, available from the National Crime Records Bureau, (NCRB, 2007), seven of the ten fastest rising crimes in India were those against women. Dowry deaths registered an increase of 15%, cruelty by husband and relatives by 14%, kidnapping and abduction of females by 13%, importation of girls by 12%, and sexual harassment by 11%. Rape and molestation cases grew by a more than 6–7%. Thus, there is clean evidence that in India, crimes against women are rising very fast which are influencing the increased rate of mental health problems among women.

PSYCHOCRIMINOLOGY AND WOMEN

- Crime by women.
- Crime against women.

Crime by Women

There is an obvious reduced rate of criminality among mentally ill women compared to mentally ill men. The following may be considered to be reasons for the above finding:

1. Criminality itself may be low among so called "normal females"; it is known that there are more male criminals than female criminals in prisons.
2. Recognition of mental illness among females may be low in prisons; mild or moderate mental health problems or so-called common mental disorders may go unrecognized for proper referral.
3. Major crimes are only usually considered in courts for implication of mental illness in crime. Minor crimes are usually not brought under section 84 IPC and they are dealt with as such by the court. In a study of mentally ill female criminals, this author found that among the mentally ill prisoners population, only 4.84% were females, compared to more than 95% of males. Schizophrenia is the most frequent diagnosis in the institutionalized female criminals. Nearly 70% of them are undertrial female prisoners admitted through section 330 of criminal procedure code. Majority of these mentally ill female prisoners (around 69%) have committed major crimes like murders and attempted murder. Majority of victims are children (Nambi, 2008).

The other crimes committed by female offenders with mental health problems include stealing, shop-lifting, drug trafficking and prostitution, etc. The majority of female offenders are being sent to prison not because of the seriousness of their offenses, but because of the persistence of their nuisances. Women, due to their premenstrual tension syndrome are more prone for aggression, violence and at times even criminal behavior.

Crime Against Women

Sexual Offenses

The Indian law recognizes 3 types of sexual offences:

1. Rape
2. Unnatural sexual offences
3. Obscene acts.

The Psychological Consequences of Rape: Include anxiety and fear, PTSD, Depression, suicidal ideations, sexual dysfunctions and at times substance abuse. The punishment for rape consists of 7 years of imprisonment, but which may be for life or for a term, which may extend upto 10 years and shall also be liable to fine. The consent to have sex is invalid in the following categories in the eyes of law.

- Consent obtained from a mentally ill person
- Consent obtained from an individual below 16 years and
- Consent obtained by impersonation, misrepresentation, intimiditation or threat to the life of the women.

The unnatural sexual offences include:

a. Homosexuality/lesbianism
b. Bestiality/sodomy
c. Sadism/masochism
d. Frotteurism
e. Voyeurism/exhibitionism, necrophilia, etc.

IPC 377-Unnatural sexual offences: Whoever voluntarily has carnal intercourse against the order of nature with any man, women or animal shall be punished with imprisonment for life, with imprisonment of either desertion for a life term or which may extend upto 10 years and shall also be liable to fine.

Psychiatrists especially those who are interested in forensic psychiatry, should realize the fact that more and more obscene sexual crimes like pornography and other sexual offending is increasing through the electronic media like internet, mobile phones. This type of cyber crimes are increasing day by day and the psychopathology of the offenders and victims especially the women are to be understood in a better manner to deal with these problems.

Section-354 indecent assault

Section-354 of IPC deals with this offence. A man who behaves indecently with a woman commits an assault. This shall be punishable with 2 years of imprisonment with or without fine. Indecent assault means outraging the modesty of a woman. Indian law has taken all the care about protection of the women from the sexual assaults on them, but had taken for granted that the Indian women always speak the truth. The other minor sexual offences against women include: Indecent exposure (exhibitionism), obscene telephone calls, (scatologia). These offenders mostly have other associated sexual deviation. This scatologia is an offence under telecommunication act.

Incest

The sexual relation between family members is forbidden by taboos, social norms and the law. Incest is a specific offence in many countries. The incest laws were passed in the hope of deterring the behaviour; but this has not happened. The vast majority of the cases don't come to the surface at all due to various reasons.

Sexual violence

Sexual violence is defined as the infliction of physical injury upon another person or threat there off. Sexual violence, as part of, or during sexual interference sexual violence can occur for a variety of reasons. They include socially isolated persons, hypersexuality, hostility towards women, frequent exposure to violent pornography, etc. Sexual assaults of women are very common. More than 22,000 cases were reported during the last one year alone. Many fold of these cases are not at all reported due to obvious reasons. Sexual violence against children are not uncommon.

Domestic violence

Psychosocial and legal aspects: Domestic violence means the violence that occurs within the family. It is a common social problem and a public health problem. This is considered to be one of the most important burning social problems and public health problem of the present day in India. In majority of the cases, the main aggressor is the spouse (husband). Domestic violence affects both mind and body. The United Nations defines domestic violence as "The violence in the family manifests itself as physical mistreatment often repetitive, which is inter-related to the exercise of mental torture, neglect of basic needs and sexual molestation". The important risk factors for domestic violence include alcoholic husbands, illiterate or poorly—educated couple, poor socioeconomic status, women with no income of their own and dowry problem.

In a Chennai study, it is found that 22% of women experience some sort of abuse. 15% experience verbal abuse, whereas 8% experience physical abuse and 3% experience sexual abuse. The perpetrators are primarily the husbands, parents and in-laws.

THE LEGAL PROTECTION FOR PERSON SUFFERING FROM DOMESTIC VIOLENCE INCLUDES

1. Constitutional Protection
2. Criminal Laws (Section 498 A of IPC) (Section 113 A and B of Indian Evidence Act). Section 306 IPC and
3. Dowry prohibition act of 1985.
4. Civil law—The protection of women from Domestic violence Act, 2005.

The Constitution of India through its Article 14 and 21 protects women. Article 14 embodies the idea of equality, which includes sex also (male or female). Article 21 embodies the right to live is not merely confined to physical existence, but it includes within its ambit, the right to live with human dignity.

Domestic Violence Criminal Laws

Section 498 A of IPC: Willful conduct of husband or his relative that is likely to drive the women to commit suicide or cause physical or mental trauma to her. This is the most widely used provision of criminal law against domestic violence. Harassment of women with a view to coercing her or any of her relative to meet any unlawful demand for property would be punished as cruelty.

Section 113 A And B of Indian Evidence Act—In this act, the presumption has to be abatement of suicide by a married woman has been introduced—for presumption to dowry death, Section 113 B is inserted.

Section 306 IPC: If a woman dies within 7 years of her marriage an inquest to be conducted as to the cause of death. Even it was a case of suicide, the husband and their relatives can be charged and prosecuted for abetment of suicide.

Dowry Prohibition Act of 1985

This act redefined the offence of dowry. It has been made cognizable, non-bailable and has been made more stringent. It is found that in India, 8% of suicide is related to dowry–related problems.

The Protection of Women from Domestic Violence Act, 2005

This is an act to provide far more effective protection of the rights of women generated under the constitution who are victims of violence of any kind occurring within the family and related matters.

As per the domestic violence act, violence against women has been grouped under 4 categories:

1. Physical violence.
2. Sexual violence.
3. Verbal and emotional violence.
4. Economic violence.

Anyhow, we have to understand that law alone cannot be a panacea to many of our social problems including domestic violence. Education, equal opportunities, attitudinal changes, modification of public opinion along with legislation can minimize the problem of domestic violence. Domestic violence laws are like double-edged weapon, should be used only protecting women and not taking revenge on men.

Suicide and Women, Legal Aspects

Sati is the self-immolation of widows which was widely prevalent in India during ancient times and it became a social problem after 18th century. *Sati* was abolished by the British Government in 1829 by Lord Bendick. According, to regulation XVII (those who encourage *sati* were guilty of culpable homicide).

Sati Prevention Act 1987: If any person commits *sati*, whoever abets the commission of Sati either directly or indirectly shall be punished with death or life imprisonment. Even those who glorify Sati are punishable.

SUICIDE BY YOUNG MARRIED WOMEN IN INDIA

Young married women due to adjustment problems with in-laws or due to domestic violence or due to dowry problems often commit/attempt suicide. As per section 304 B IPC, if a woman commit suicide within seven years of marriage, such death shall be called as "Dowry Death" and the husband and the in-laws would be punished if proved. Most of the dowry deaths (84%) were suicide committed by young women.

MARRIAGE, MENTAL ILLNESS AND INDIAN LEGISLATION

Every country and every religion has its own personal law. The ICMR and DST study (1987) on severe mental distress found the highest common distress among housewives. It is also found from other studies in India that married women have more psychopathology than married men. Women in the Indian Community are less likely to get Mental Health Care, because naming mental illness in the family especially in a woman is itself stigmatizing and an occasion for ridicule. Married Mentally Ill Women are more likely to be sent back to their parental homes, abandoned, deserted or divorced. Clinical experience reveals that the responsibility of care for the mentally ill women is often left to her own family than to her husband or his family.

The matrimonial relief that one can seek are:

- Decree for nullity
- Restitution of conjugal rights
- Judicial separation
- Divorce.

Divorce or nullity is granted in cases, where a socially accepted marriage is not legally accepted as a marriage.

The following Acts have to be gone through in order to understand the legal aspects of marriage in India.

1. The Special Marriage Act—1954.
2. The Hindu marriage Act—1955 with amendment in 1976.
3. The Dissolution of Muslim Marriage Act—1939. The Muslim Women Protection of Rights on Divorce—1986.
4. The Parsi Marriage and Divorce Act—1936.
5. The Christian Marriage Act—1872.
6. The Indian Divorce Act—1869.
7. The Family Courts Act—1984.

UNSOUNDNESS OF MIND AS AFFECTING THE CAPACITY TO MARRY

Hindu Marriage Act, 1955:

A Hindu Marriage is voidable if either party:

- It is incapable of giving a valid consent as a consequence of unsoundness of mind, or
- Though capable of giving a valid consent has been suffering from mental disorder of such a kind or to such an extent as to be unfit for marriage and the procreation of children
- Has been subject to recurrent attacks of insanity.

The Special Marriage Act, 1954

Applicable to persons from any religion undergoing a civil marriage. Has provisions similar to the HMA except that a marriage under the SMA is void.

Indian Divorce Act, 1869

A Christian marriage is voidable if either party was a lunatic or idiot.

Parsi Marriage and Divorce Act

Unsoundness of mind is not ground for annulment.

Muslim Law

A person of unsound mind cannot contract a marriage and such a marriage if contracted is void. However, if the guardian of the person of unsound mind considers such marriage to be in his interest and in the interest of society and is willing to take up all the monetary obligations of the marriage, then such a marriage can be performed.

UNSOUNDNESS OF MIND AS A GROUND FOR DIVORCE

As per the Hindu Marriage Act, Special Marriage Act and Parsi Marriage and Divorce Act, if the Respondent has been incurably of sound mind or has been suffering continuous or intermittently from mental disorder of such a kind and to such an extent that the petitioner cannot reasonably be expected to live with him, divorce can be obtained.

Dissolution of Muslim Marriage Act, 1939

A Muslim woman can seek divorce on the ground that her husband has been insane for a period of two years.

INDIAN DIVORCE ACT, 1869 AMENDMENT 2001 (FOR CHRISTIANS)

Unsoundness of mind is a ground of divorce on two conditions that is, it must be incurable and it must be at least for two years immediately before the filing of the petition.

Mental Illness and Marriage—Legal View

Legal insanity is different from medical insanity. It is not mere presence of symptoms, but inability to manage affairs is essential. Slight or occasional deviation from normalcy will not amount to legal insanity. As per law procreation means more than giving birth; it includes looking after children.

Protection of the Institution of Marriage

"It is the duty of the court to make efforts for settlement in matters concerning the family" - Rule No 3 of the order 32 A of Civil Procedure Code. Protecting and preserving the institution of marriage and preventing the fracture of a family is the intention of the law makers as well as medical health professionals.

NEED FOR A CHANGE IN THE ATTITUDE OF LEGISLATION AS WELL AS PUBLIC

The law should perform a promotive and facilitation roll. Past history of mental illness should be no bar to marriage. Failure to disclose past history illness or treatment would not amount to suppression of the fact.

Laws are generally protecting the family system. Law alone cannot be a panacea to many of our social problems. We need change in the attitude of society.

National Commission for Women was set up as statutory body in January 1992 under the National Commission for Women Act, 1990 to:

- Review the constitutional and legal safeguards for women
- Recommend remedial legislative measures
- Facilitate redressal of grievances and
- Advise the government on all policy matters affecting women.

CONCLUSION

Even though, many legal provisions are there in our country to protect the rights of woman, especially woman with mental health problems, but lack of education and awareness of legal and constitutional rights and the lack of means and support have reduced mentally ill woman to be meek and dumb. Unfortunately, in the mandate of the constitution, the personal laws are the laws with general or special application; all are man-made and did not effectively come to the rescue of mentally ill woman. A sincere effort has to be made to analyze various laws with judicial decisions relating to woman, especially woman with mental illness.

SUGGESTED READING

1. Batra L, Gautam S. Psychiatric morbidity and personality profile in divorce seeking couples. Indian J Psychiatry 1995;37:179-85.
2. Brahma A. Pattern of domestic violence amongst non-fatal deliberate self-harm attempters: A study from primary care of West Bengal. Indian J Psychiatry, 2008;50:6.
3. Desai K. Indian law of marriage and divorce. 6th edition Nagpur: Wadhwa and Co, 2004.
4. Dhanda A. Legal order and mental disorder, Sage Publications, New Delhi, 2000:181-209.
5. Heru AM, Stuart GL, Rainey S, et al. Prevalence and severity of intimate partner violence and associations with family functioning and alcohol abuse in psychiatric inpatients with suicidal intent. Journal of Clinical Psychiatry, 2006;67: 23–29.
6. Jablensky A, Sartorius N, Ernberg G, et al. Schizophrenia: Manifestations, incidence and course in different cultures: A World Health Organization ten-country study. Monograph. Psychol Med 1992; (Suppl. 20):1-97.
7. Srinivasaraghavan J. Domestic Violence, A community's response
8. Kumar S. Domestic violence and its mental health correlates in Indian women, Br J Psychiatry, 2005;187:62-67.
9. Myneni SR. Women and law, 2003.
10. Nambi S. Presidential address, women and law in India. Oxford University Press, 2004.

11. Revathi R. Laws Relating to Domestic Violence, Asia Law House , Hyderabad 2004.
12. Robins LN, Regier DA. Psychiatric disorders in America. The ECA study. New York: Free Press; 1991.
13. Surinder N, Sujatha K. 55th Annual Conference of the Indian Psychiatric Society, 2003.

18 Chapter

Ethicolegal Aspects in the Care of Elderly

ETHICS

- Set of rules laid down by got?
- Socially imposed rules?
- A set of principles?
- A person ought to do?
  - Ethics is the science of norms of behavior for any group; a code of conduct designed by a group of person in a particular society; it provides a frame work to guide ones own behavior in a particular setting.
  - They are relative and changing with time; ethics means moral duties; this duty cannot be unilateral.
  - "I will maintain the utmost respect for human life from the time of conception"—Code of Medical Ethics.
  - If so how about MTP? How about euthanasia?

Elderly are the Unwanted and the Neglected

- "Longevity is not in all cases a blessing"
- The old are not wanted in many houses
- They are even resented because of their failing capacities.

Most of the elderly are cheated out of their property rights, even pensions by their children, relatives and others.

The law has been unfair and unfavorable for aged parents, who can claim only ₹ 500/- as maintenance from their children.

Section 125 CrPc 1973 requires every person having sufficient means to maintain his/her parents, who are unable to maintain themselves.

The Hindu adoption and Maintenance Act, 1956—It is the obligation of a person to maintain aged or infirm parents.

Article 41 of the Indian Constitution—A directive principle of state policy, public assistance to the aged to the extent resources permit.

Boothalingam committee report on wages, income and prices—Stresses the need for providing social security for the destitute aged.

Elder abuse is much more common in India than what we think.
It becomes increasingly recognized by both medical persons and social agencies.

Types of Elder Abuse

1. Physical abuse
2. Neglect
3. Emotional abuse
4. Psychological abuse
5. Financial abuse
6. Sexual abuse
7. Abandonment.

Declaration of Hong Kong on the Abuse of the Elderly Adopted by WMA (1989)

1. The elderly have the same right to care, welfare and respect as other human beings.
2. It is the physician's responsibility to help prevent the physical and psychological abuse of the elderly.
3. Physicians will see that the elderly patients receive the best possible care.
4. If Physicians suspect ill treatment or unnatural death they will report to the relevant authorities.
5. The elderly should have their free choice of treatment and the doctor.

Assisted Suicide in the Elderly

Physician-assisted suicide as a health care option for the dying patients created a flurry of attention in recent days—another ethical dilemma.

Prescription of medication with the explicit goal of facilitating the patient's death is generally deemed to be unethical and illegal; public and professional opinion are changing in this issue.

Pain in the terminally ill can be treated with doses of analgesics that may depress respiration, but relieve pain.

When evaluating the persons who request physician assisted suicide, it is very important to rule out treatable disorders and attempt to give adequate treatment before proceeding further.

Euthanasia

The Act of deliberately ending the life of a patient, even at the patients own request or at the request of close relatives is unethical. (Declaration on euthanasia adopted by WMA, 1987). This does not prevent the physician from respecting the desire of a patient to allow the natural process of death to follow its course in the terminal phase of sickness.

Patients may have a right to die; that does not translate into physician having the right or obligation to kill.

Ethical Issues in the Care of the Demented

Ethical and legal issues frequently arise in the care of the demented and delirious. They are:

1. Reduced capacity to give informed consent.
2. Involuntary hospitalization.
3. End of life care and decisions and
4. Research protocols.

Diminished capacity due to cognitive impairment. Informed consent for medical treatment: Agreeing or declining depends on:

1. Information disclosure by the physician
2. Voluntary participation by the patient
3. Patient's competence.

Mildly delirious or demented are still capable of making informed decision.

Impaired cognition in severe cases prevents the patient to understand his illness and treatment.

Obtaining consent from a confused, early delirious state is unethical and illegal; nor it is proper to wait till the patient becomes fully delirious so that the procedure can be done without his consent.

In dementia patients, it is necessary to confer with family members about the procedures.

Physician should assist patients and family members in deciding when the treatment is likely to be futile.

LEGAL ISSUES IN DEMENTED ELDERLY

Civil rights—Severely demented are deprived of their basic civil rights because of their severe impairment in cognition.

Admission procedure—Severe demented elderly with behaviour problems cannot be admitted in a Psychiatric Hospital on voluntary basis. As per MHA1987, they can be admitted under special circumstances. After a period of 90 days, if relatives do not turn up for discharge, it is illegal to detain them. But it is highly unethical to discharge patient and send him out of hospital without social support.

Crime, fitness for trial and criminal responsibility—Mentally ill prisoners suffering from severe dementia, if they commit a crime, They are incompetent to stand for trial. They come under McNaughton Act (Guilty but insane).

DEMENTIA, DISABILITY AND INCOME TAX EXEMPTION

- Very often dementia is considered to me a permanent disability.
- The disability in dementia can be assessed and quantified by IDEAS (Indian Disability Evaluation and Assessment Scale).
- After obtaining a disability certificate from a psychiatrist, caregivers of persons with dementia can avail Income Tax exemption to the tune of ₹ 40,000/- per annum (Income Tax Act Section 80 DDB; Income Tax Rules 11 DD).

HOMICIDE AND BRAIN DAMAGE

Nature of organic mental disorder	Mentally disordered homicidal offenders (N = 533)	Mentally disordered non-offenders (N = 3392)	
Organic cerebral degenerative disorders	40 (7.5%)	452 (13.3%)	X2 = 14.2 pO.001
Late acquired brain damage	43 (8.0%)	350 (10.3%)	
Epilepsies	29 (5.4%)	177 (5.2%)	
Other disorders	50 (9.4%)	614 (18.1%)	

These figures are quoted from Hafner and Boker, 1973

DEMENTIA AND CRIME

A Case Example: A 54-year-old married woman, formally noted for unusual intelligence and social pose, became lazy, quarrelsome and tactless. Somewhat, later she began to cheat at bridge and on a shopping expedition stole a box of chocolates from a shop counter, showing no concern for the subsequent expostulations. During the next 4 years, she was apprehended five times for similar blatant shoplifting. Finally, language deterioration and memory impairment brought her to medical attention.

CRIME AND DEMENTIA

Only 6 person of the sample of 533 mentally abnormal offenders had dementia (Hafner and Boker, 1973).

It is likely that dementing patients with all, but the most serious antisocial behavior can be contained within the health care system and that those with social ties still are Roth (1968) outlined the likely associations between senility and offending, in particular, the link between disinhibition of behavior and sexual offending.

Deutsch, et al. (1991) described physical aggression in nearly one-third of patients with Alzheimer's disease attending a research clinic in the USA (Johns Hopkins).

HUNTINGTON'S CHOREA—FORENSIC ISSUES

Huntington's chorea is commonly associated with antisocial behavior (around 38%), violence, inappropriate sexual behavior, cruel and callous behavior. Huntington's chorea is of particular interest to the forensic psychiatrist, principally, because of the prevalence of criminal and antisocial behavior.

Criminal or deviant behavior is most likely to occur during the prodrome or in the early stage of the illness. Social deterioration may be an early feature and may give rise to antisocial and criminal behavior.

CRIMINAL OFFENCES IN PATIENTS WITH HUNTINGTON'S CHOREA

(Dewhurst, et al. 1970)

Assault	14
Offences against property	13
Cruelty to Children	9
Malicious damage	2
Blackmail	1
Arson	1
Total	40

DEMENTIA—A DEATH IN LIFE

Though wise men at their end know dark is right, because their words had forked no lightning they.
Do not go gentle into that good night.
. . . .
And you, my father, there on the sad height,
Curse, bless, me now with your fierce tears, I pray.
Do not go gentle into that good night.
Rage, rage against the dying of the light.
—Dylan Thomas
"Do not go gentle into that good night"

ETHICAL AND LEGAL ISSUES IN DEMENTIA

Declining mental capacity in dementia:

- Dementia is a neuropsychiatric disease
- Devastating emotional consequences for the patient/family
- Characterized by;
  - Decline in intellectual functioning severe enough to interfere with personal ADL
  - Decline in social and occupational functioning
  - Gross disturbance in judgement and decision making:

Prevalence of dementia in Indian Population

Authors (Years)	**Rate/100,000**
Shaji, et at. (1996)	
Kerala (Rural)	3.4 %
Rajkumar, et al. (1997)	
Chennai (Urban)	2.7%

Rajkumar, et al. (1997)
Tamil Nadu (Rural) 3.5%
Chandra, et al. (2001)
Ballabhgarh (Rural) 1.36%
Roy T, et al. (2006)
Kolkata (Urban) 1.02 %

There are nearly 3 crores of persons with dementia in India and nearly 21 lakhs persons with dementia in Tamil Nadu.

ETHICAL ISSUES IN THE CARE OF THE DEMENTED

Ethical and legal issues frequently arise in the care of the demented. They are:

- Reduced capacity to give informed consent.
- Involuntary hospitalization.
- End of life care and decisions and
- Research protocols.
- Diminished capacity is due to the cognitive impairment.
- Consent is a concurrence of will (Sec. 13. Indian Contract Act)
- Informed consent for medical treatment, Agreeing or declining depends on:
  - Information disclosure by the physician.
  - Voluntary participation by the patient.
  - Patients competence.

Mildly demented are still capable of making informed consent.

Impaired cognition in severe cases prevents the patient to understand his illness and treatment. It is necessary to confer with family members about the procedures.

Physician should assist patients and family members in deciding when the treatment is likely to be futile.

ETHICAL ISSUES IN DEMENTIA

The growing dementing population will intensify the ethical issues that emerge in clinical practice and research.

- Issues in early disease: Genetic testing, use of drugs in mildly affected and diagnostic disclosure.
- Research issues: Informed consent process, conflicts of interests and research design issues such as the use of placebos.
- Issues in later stages: Concern about appropriate therapeutic goals and end of life care.

In early stages of dementia, the family members should be encouraged to seek the patients guidance in making long-term legal and financial decisions, while the patient can still comprehend and make decision, planning may include:

- Establishing durable power of attorney for financial matter
- Including a family member's name in bank accounts
- Financing of home health or institutional care
- Completing or updating of patients last will and testament
- Planning a living will.

CAPACITY

Capacity is a legal qualification of capability (Section 92 Indian Evidence Act), a position enabling one to do something (Section 466 IPC)

Durable powers of attorney: A formal instrument by which one person empowers another to represent him or act instead for certain purposes—can be considered for health care and for management of property matters.

Guardianship: One who has or is entitled to the care and custody of the persons or property or both of a person legally incapable of managing his own affairs. Guardian to be appointed by the court as per MHA.

COMPETENCE

Competence means having legal sufficiency

- It is the doctors (psychiatrists) responsibility, whether the demented person is legally competent to understand (comprehend) what is involved and to consent to it or refuse.
- Patient with dementia may be competent in the early stages.
- If patient is not found to be competent and certified so, consent to be obtained from a relative or care giver.

GUIDELINES SUGGESTED IN CIVIL MATTERS

Families should be encouraged to discuss these issues openly with the patients in the course of AD.

Whereever possible, advance directives should be drawn up when the patient is legally competent (in the early stages).

- The Patient can give a power of attorney.
- Through a living trust—a patient designates another person as a trustee to manage property while the patient is living.
- To appoint a guardian or manager through the court.

SUGGESTED READING

1. Agarwal AK. Ethics in Psychiatry. Indian Journal of Psychiatry, 1994;36:1-5-11.
2. Agarwal AK, Gupta SC. Ethical issues in Psychiatry. Souvenir of the Annual Conference of Indian Psychiatric Society and World Psychiatric Association held at Jaipur, (1993, 1998).
3. Appelbaum PS. Privacy in psychiatric treatment: threats and responses. Am J Psychiatry, 2002;159:1809-18.
4. Oyebode F. Clinical errors and medical negligence. Advances in Psychiatric Treatment, 2006;2:22-27.
5. Gutheil TG. Paranoia and progress notes: A guide to forensically informed psychiatric record keeping. Hosp Community Psychiatry, 1980;31:479-82s.
6. Handbook of Psychiatry, Bhugra D (ed), 2005.
7. Hippocrates, the 5-4 century, BC.
8. Nambi S. The ethical and medicolegal aspects of elderly with special reference to Dementia, I Annual National Meet of Indian Association for Geriatric Mental Health, Scientific Convention Centre, Lucknow, 2005;20-22.

19 Chapter

Forensic Aspects of Alcoholism and Drug Addiction

These are days of increasing social stress, escalating violence, uncontrolled drug and alcohol problems and changing patterns of crime. An association between drug dependence and crime is no longer disputed. After a long controversy about the relationship between crime and addiction, recent research has unequivocally demonstrated that habitual criminality is an integral part of established addiction.

The amount of crime committed by addicts is vast. In the USA, it is estimated that narcotic addicts commit over 50 million crimes per year. Much of the crime relates to the need to purchase drugs, but the range of offences is wide. National differences in social, legal and treatment approaches to the problem of drug abuse have not effected variations in this general association of addiction with crime. In studies, from many countries association between crime and the addiction emerges as a repeated universal finding.

THE INCIDENCE OF DELINQUENCY IN ADDICTS

Bingham (1937) survey of 1000 narcotic addicts found 80% had no conviction before addiction, but 67% had been convicted before their first narcotic offence. The inference that addiction created criminal behavior was not supported by a police survey of 200 narcotic offenders (Leinhouser, 1943). A 12-year follow-up study of 100 New York addicts (Vaillant, 1966) found 52% convicted before addiction and 96% convicted by the end of the follow-up period.

British studies of hospital heroin addicts (Bewley and Ben Arie 1968, Willis 1969) found a record of conviction in 80% of those patients. British studies of young drug clinic attenders (Gordun, 1973 and 1983; Mott and Ruthod, 1976) consistently report pre-drug conviction rates between 30% and 50% and subsequent conviction rates of over 90%. All these surveys indicate high incidence of a criminal record in established drug users. In an American study of 354 narcotic addicts (Shaffer, et al. 1984) delinquency was admitted by every addict in the sample.

DELINQUENT ANTECEDENTS OF DRUG ABUSE

An American Study of 1328 heroin addicts in treatment programs (Taylor and Albright, 1981) confirm that criminality precedes drug use and observes a strong relationship between the extent of predrug crime and the number of postdrug convictions. Early delinquency is not only a common precursor of drug abuse, but is linked with a higher incidence of continuing conviction and a poorer prognosis for drug abstinence (Gordon, 1983).

AGGRESSION, VIOLENCE, AND DRUG ADDICTION

Influencing Factors

- The expectations of the user.
- The personal response to intoxication or withdrawal effects.
- Social setting.
- Interpersonal issues.
- The comorbidity of major mental disorder.

The Prevalence of Substance Abuse and Crime

The ECA Report: Prevalence of violence behavior per 10,000 individuals.

- 2.27% for those with no mental disorder.
- 6.98% in major mental illness.
- 19.72% for substance abuse disorder.
- 22.02% for comorbid responder.
- Follow-up of 1136 patients after discharge.
- One year prevalence of violence.
- 18% for patients with major mental disorder.
- 31% for those with substance abuse (MacArthur Violence Risk Assessment Study).

Drug Addiction and Crime

- The association between drúg dependence and crime is no longer disputed.
- Habitual criminality is an integral part of established addiction.
- The association between crime and addiction emerges as a repeated universal finding.
- The amount of crime committed by addicts is vast.

How Often Addicts Commit Crime?

- A record of conviction in 80% of the British studies of hospital heroin addicts. (Will is 1969).
- An American study of 1328 heroin addicts in TT program confirms the criminality precedes drug use.
- Around 80% of the brown sugar (heroin) addicts and multiple drug abusers have a premorbid psychopathic personality. Around 70% indulge in increase rate of crime (Chennai Study).
- Around 70% of the mentally ill prisoners (criminal lunatics) abuse drugs before their crime. (Nambi, 1992).

Offences Related to Substance Abuse

Violent offences—involving changes in mental state.
Acquistic offences—related to high economic cost of illicit drug use.
Other offences—against legislation to control, drug use or drunken driving.

Types of Crime and Addiction

1. Drug related (cultivation, manufacture, supply, and possession, etc.).
2. Non drug related (stealing, homicide, attempted suicide, sexual crimes, forgery, gambling, violence, etc.).

The Nature of Delinquent Behavior

An addictive habit predisposes the drug user to two main offences; possession and/or supply of drugs, and larceny related to the need to purchase drugs. Offences committed by the addicts are of two types.

- Drug related, and
- Non drug related, with the implication that drug-related offences (possession, supply, and larceny) are an inevitable aspect of the life style, of the street addict. More recent studies note that the range of offences committed by addicts is extremely wide, extending far beyond a mere need to obtain drugs and encompassing serious and distinctive offences.

An FBI analysis in 1966 of the average criminal carrier of an addict over a 12-year period found 60% of conviction was for non-drug offences. 26% of heroin addicts had a conviction for violence and 74% were convicted for larceny.

A 4-year follow-up study (Savage and Sinyson, 1981) of 1155 American Narcotic Addicts, using self report data categorizes three types of post-treatment criminality.

Type I: Illegal support from robbery, burglary or drug dealing crimes against the person or crimes for profit.
Type II: Illegal support from prostitution, pimping, gambling or minor offences.
Type III: Drug arrests for possession only.

In a study of 243 Baltimore narcotic addicts (Ball, et al. 1983) using self report data, the main offence behavior emerged as theft (38%) followed by drug dealing (27%), pimping and gambling (26%) confidence games and forgery (8%) and violence (2%). Although the range of offences was wide for the addict group individuals tended to specialize and pursue one or two main types of crime, supplemented by other types only occasionally.

Certain users commit crime to support their daily habits, crimes which they otherwise would probably not committed.

TYPOLOGY OF CRIMINAL ACTIVITY IN ADDICTS

Drug addicts are not a homogenous group, either in their choice of drugs, their lifestyles or their criminal behavior. Some addicts avoid illegal activity altogether while others commit multiple even violent crimes persistently. Criminal activity in addicts may maintain a stable level or wax and wane with time or with variations in the extent of their dependency.

CANNABIS AND CRIME

The link between cannabis use and offending are complex. Abuse itself may give rise to offences, there may be a more general tendency to criminality and violence among addicts, and trafficking in illegal drugs, including cannabis is widely recognized to be associated with crime. One has only to think of the mafia and the smuggling of drugs from Colombia into the USA or from Pakistan into Europe to realize this. However, it is widely believed that cannabis takers are much less delinquent than other drug abusers such as takers of heroin, cocaine, and morphine. Indeed, Kraus (1981) found that criminal involvement was less among cannabis takers than among opiate and sedative – drug abusers. On the law and predisposes to taking harder drugs. Thus in India (Chopra and Jandu, 1976) cannabis drugs are generally used by the poorer sections of society with a high percentage of criminals and other disreputable individuals. Moreover, most of their money is spent on cannabis, forcing them to steal. Other individuals have personality problems and exhibit irritability, violent behavior, however, many cannabis abusers prefer to live alone and become violent only when they are, or believe they are, about to be attacked. Another use for cannabis in India is to stupefy the prospective victims of crime.

ALCOHOL AND CRIME

The link between alcohol and crime has been recognised for many years. Since World War II, attention has been particularly focused on the role that alcohol may play in the carrying out of a subsequent criminal event and also the frequency of alcoholism in criminal populations and in the relationship between alcohol and aggression.

- "That which hath made them drunk hath made me bold"
  Lady Macbeth—Macbeth, Act 2 Scene 2 (Shakespeare).

HOW ALCOHOL INFLUENCE VIOLENCE OR CRIME?

- May be a direct precipitant of crime through toxic or disinhibiting effect.
- A facilitator for offending arising from social relations or desires.
- May precipitate a psychiatric disorder.
- May result in an increase in crime to support the habit.
- Alcohol abuse and offending may be related by a common etiology.

TRENDS IN ALCOHOL CONSUMPTION RELATED TO CRIME RATES

Lanke (1975 and 1976) who showed that during the period 1960–73, a high statistical correlation occurred between violent crime rates and alcohol consumption. When there is less alcohol available, the frequency of social interaction is reduced, which may result in a decrease in personal crime, which is much more likely to arise in the social setting.

DRINKING PRECEDING CRIMINAL EVENTS

A large number of studies have attempted to examine this relationship (e.g. Greenberg, 1982). A whole variety of different types of crimes have been examined. These include homicide, sexual crimes, marital assaults, sexual crimes against children, crime against property and crimes of violence.

HOMICIDE

Gillies (1976) in a study of homicide in the West of Scotland carried out psychiatric examination on 400 individuals. His consideration was that 58% of males had been intoxicated at the time of their crimes and 30% of females. Homicide squad of the Philadelphia Police Department over a five-year period reviewed the records of 588 cases for evidences that alcohol was present in the victim of the offender. They concluded that in 44% of these cases alcohol was present in both victim and offender, in 11% of cases in the offender-only, and in 9% in the victim only.

Sexual crime: Amir (1967) in a well-known study, which used analyses from the files of Philadelphia Police Department found that alcohol was present in the rapist and victim in 21% in the victim only in 9.6% and in the offender only in 2.9%.

Personal violence: The last decade has seen increasing publicity drawn to assaults by men on their female partners. Gayfold (1975) using self-reporting questionnaires and personal interviews, examined 148 women who claimed serious physical assault by their husbands. In 44 of the cases wives concluded that violence occurred regularly when husbands were drunk.

Child molestation: Another recent area of concern is child molestation. Rada (1976) administered a questionnaire to 405 mentally ill sex offenders of all types. The results showed that 49% of child molesters stated that they were drinking at the time of the commission of the offence, of whom one third were drinking heavily.

Violent crime: In relation to violent crime Acts including marital assaults, Gerson (1978) in a Canadian Study found that in 35% of the acts, the offender alone had been drinking, In 29% of the cases studied, victim alone and in 36% both had been drinking.

Greenberg (1982) considers that the essential first question is whether alcoholism increases the chance of criminal behavior because of the effects of intoxication or whether it is the condition of alcoholism itself.

Alcohol and aggressive behavior: It is commonly suggested that alcohol use is related to aggressive behavior. Alcohol intoxicated subjects initiated higher levels of attack than those without alcohol only in threatening situations.

Alcohol and driving offences: It is not surprising that alcohol, is associated with driving accidents, as relatively low blood alcohol concentrations have been shown to impair performance on the type of tasks used in driving skills, for example, motor function, reaction time and sensory function tests. Alcohol related accidents do not occur randomly but peak at night and weekends, the periods when drinking is at its heaviest.

DRUG AND CRIME—THE CHENNAI SCENE

Alcohol, alcoholism and related problems have been prevalent since time immemorial, though in the last 2 decades consumption of alcohol has increased tremendously in an alarming fashion due to the changes in the prohibition policy in Tamil Nadu. There are mushrooming of illicit arrack sale and distillation, which by themselves is crimes, became prevalent in the recent past in Tamil Nadu. There is obvious relationship between illicit liquor and power politics.

Cannabis abuse is also very much prevalent in many parts of the state due to increased cultivation and trafficking from the Western Ghats. As observed in other parts of the World, cannabis abuse is not so commonly associated with criminality when compared with narcotic drug abuse.

Unfortunately, the alarming increase in criminal activity associated with drug addiction has increased manifold during the past ten years after the commencement of the ethnic conflict in the neighboring Srilanka refugees, especially the youth belonging to the militant groups began to push the drug, heroin, into Tamil Nadu. For them the crude form of heroin i.e. brown sugar spells magic. It gave big and quick money to lead their day to day life and also to purchase arms and ammunitions. Heroin being a costly drug as of today costing about ₹ 140 per gram they began to realize that the need for money was more in order to perpetuate and support the habit. Hence heroin addicts indulged in more acts of felony, brutal violence and robbery for the money which they needed very badly. The irony of the situation is that inspite of heavy drugs trafficking, the enforcement of laws is meagre due to the involvement of money power and politics here as in any other part of the world.

On an average per year 1500 drug addicts are admitted in the Institute of Mental Health, Chennai. Alcohol related problems including alcohol dependence constituted the majority. About 635 persons were admitted in 1993 with drug related (excluding alcohol) problems, among which 473 were multiple drug abusers, 140 were heroin addicts and cannabis dependants were 22. Majority of the multiple drug abuse group consist of intravenous drug users.

Around 80% of the brown sugar (heroin) addicts and multiple drug abusers were found to have a premorbid psychiatric personality. Around 70% of them indulged in increased rate of criminality like stealing and assault, etc.

In another study in Institute of Mental Health, Chennai about the prevalence of alcohol and drug abuse amongst mentally ill prisoners (criminal lunatics) out of 30 patients, 15 of them have abused alcohol and 5 persons abused cannabis prior to their commission of crime.

In 1980s and 90s, there was an alarming increase in the number of injection drug users in Chennai. Commonly used drugs are liquid preparation of brown sugar (heroin), injection, buprenorphine (tidigesic) and injection pentazocine (fortwin). These narcotic analgesics are abundantly available in the street corners of Chennai and peddlers sell them at a cost much higher than the actual.

The consequences of the drugs and its related problem and its association with crime has emerged as one of the foremost medical, psychological and legal implications in the State of Tamil Nadu, especially in its capital Chennai in the recent past.

DRUG ABUSE, INDIAN LAWS, AND LEGISLATION

- No single prevention program has succeeded in curbing drug abuse. Hence, a multidimensional approach is aimed at.
- Controlling the supply of drugs.
- Suppression of illicit trafficking.
- Prevention and reduction of demand.
- Treatment and rehabilitation.
- The awareness of the need to enforce legislative measure dates back to the Opium Act of 1857. The next major effort to identify and control potentially.
- Harmful drugs occurred only in 1930 when the Dangerous Drug Act of 1930 was introduced. It was only in 1985, with the enactment of the Narcotic Drugs and Psychotropic Substances Act (NDPSA) that the seriousness of the drug problem was taken cognizance of.
- The Opium Act of 1857 amended in 1878.
- The Dangerous Drug Act, 1930 amended in 1933, 1938 and 1957.
- The Narcotic Drugs and Psychotropic substances Act, 1985 (NDPSA)
- NDPSA (amendment) Act, 1988.
- Substance abuse was found to be very high in the inmates of forensic ward. Alcohol 25% cannabis 10% and multiple substance use was found in 17.5% of cases. (Dr Farooq Ahmed Khan), et al. Addiction in criminal ward offenders.
- Persons with alcohol dependence are at increased risk for violent and aggressive behavior. The violence should be assessed during the evaluation. Violent behavior can occur as part of alcohol intoxication or as a manifestation of assisted psychopathology such as depressive agitated state, antisocial personality disorder or agitated withdrawal delirium. Assessment of the risk of violence includes a review of history of past violence, drug abuse, threats to specific people and the availability of weapons.
- The presence of impaired impulse control, coping ability with aggressive urges. The ability to contract for safety and treatment should also be carefully examined.

Substance Use Disorders and Violence

Aggression in particular and impulsivity put people at risk for substance abuse. If one can modify these, he may reduce the risks for substance abuse and other antisocial behavior. Predictors of drug abuse include the aggressive child at the highest risk for substance abuse, subsequent criminal behavior and violence.

The Narcotic Drugs and Psychotropic Substances Act (NDPSA)—1985

An Act to consolidate and amend the law relating to narcotic drugs to make stringent provisions of the control and regulation of operations relating to narcotic drugs and psychotropic substance, to provide for the forfeiture of property, derived from or used in illicit traffic in narcotic drugs and psychotropic substances, to implement the provisions of the International Conventions on Narcotic Drugs and Psychotropic Substance and for matters connected therewith.

NDPSA—Six Chapters

1. Preliminary—Title, Definition, etc.
2. Authorities and Officers Central and State Government Authority, NDPSA Consultative Committee:
    - National Fund for control of Drug abuse.
3. Prohibition, Control and Regulation.
4. Offences and Penalties.
5. Procedure and powers to search, seize, and arrest persons involved:
    - A forfeiture of property derived from illicit trafficking.
6. Miscellaneous.

NDPSA—Salient Features

Entrustment of responsibility to the central government to combat abuse and trafficking of illicit drugs.

To coordinate with State Governments and drug enforcement authorities for implementation of the international conventions.

To arrange for identification, treatment, education after care, rehabilitation and social reintegration and social reintegration of addicts.

Constitution of special courts for trial of drug offenders.

Penalties as per NDPSA

For offences—10 year RI, extendable upto 20 years, fine ₹ 1 lakh to 2 lakhs.
Subsequent—15 years extendable upto 30 offences years RI, fine ₹ 1.5 lakh to 3 lakhs.
For ganja—5 Years RI, fine ₹ 50,000.
For possessing drugs—One year imprisonment or a fine or both small quantities (small quantities) heroin 250 mg, ganja for personal use 500 gm, opium 5 gm etc.

The person has to prove the Mens Rea (that is he had no such mental state with respect to the offences).
There is also a provision for detoxification under court order.

NDPSA (Ammendment Act) 1988

- Seizure of property derived from illicit drug trafficking.
- Provision of National fund for the control of drug abuse.
- Stringent punishment instituted.

Death penalty for subsequent conviction in respect of specific quantities of drugs.

 - Cocaine LSD, THC–500 gm
 - Amphetamine, Methaquione–1500 gm
 - Morphine–1 kg
 - Opium–10 kg
 - Pure heroin, codeine–1 kg
 - Hasish–20 kg.

NDPSA an Appraisal

- Major part is devoted to "Supply Side" issues, overshadowing the treatment related issues.
- Release for treatment appears to be at the discretion of the judge. How much it may be relevant?
- The treatment and rehabilitation programs are not given due priorities.
- The Act looks upon the drug addict as a delinquent rather than a diseased person.
- Misuse of this Act for political purpose may be possible.

SUGGESTED READING

1. Ball JC, Shaffer JW. Neuco DN. The day-to-day criminality of heroin addicts in Baltimore—a study in the continuity of offence rates: Drug and alcohol dependence, 1983;12(2):119-2.
2. Ball JC Roseuh, Friledman EC, Neuco DN. Re-impact of heroin addiction upon criminality. National Institute of Drug Abuse Research Manograph, 1979;27:163-69.
3. Barton WI. Drug histories and criminality surveying of inmates of state correctional facilities, 1980;15(2):233-58.
4. Brocco K. Association among alcoholism, drug abuse, and antisocial personality:A review of literature psychological reports 1984;55:4-55-740.
5. Bluglass R, Paul (ed). Principles and practice of forensic psychiatry. Churchil Livingstone, first edition, 1990.
6. Gordon AM. Drugs and Delinquency and 10-year follow-up of drug clinic patients. BJP, 1983;142:169-73.
7. Gordon AM. Pattern of delinquency in drug addiction. BJP, 1973;122:205-10.
8. Joye H, Son L, Ruiz P, Millman RB. Substance abuse—A comprehensive textbook. second edition, 1992.
9. Kumar KA (ed.). Facts of substance abuse—An update. 1991.

10. Muthalagan J, Nambi S, Bashyam VSP. Prevalence of alcohol and drug abuse in the institutionalized mentally ill criminals, Paper presented at 25th Annual Conference of IPS, South Zone, Salem, 1992.
11. Sethi BB, Tiwari SC, Kumar P, Trivedi JK. Drug abuse in India: An overview with special reference to cannabis. Indian Journal of Psychiatry, 1984;26(1).
12. Shaffer JW, Neuro DN, Kinlock TW. A new classification of narcotic addicts based on type and extent of criminal activity—Comprehensive psychiatry, 1984;25:315-28.
13. Southern Zonal Branch 27th Annual Conference, Dharwad, October, 1994.
14. The Narcotic Drugs and Psychotropic Substances Act, 1985 (61 of 1985).

20 Chapter

Ethical and Legal Aspects of Suicide and Euthanasia

One person commit suicide every five minutes and one attempted suicide is made every minute in India. (National Crime Research Bureau, 1996)

There is a gross underreporting of suicide and attempted suicide in India. Few reasons are:

1. Fear of punishment.
2. Stigma attached to suicide.
3. Ignorance and many other social causes.

In India, 1,10,000 people die by committing suicide every year. In the last two decades the suicide rate has increased by 64% from 6.4% per 1,00,000 to 10.5% per 100,000 in 2002. The majority of suicides in India are committed by persons below the age of 30 years.

Suicide literally means the deliberate termination of one's own physical existence. Suicide (Felo de se) is where a man of age of discretion and compos mentis voluntarily kills himself. In England, at some point of time deliberate suicide by a sane person was a felony punishable by forfeiture of the offender's goods and chattels to the Crown by an ignominious burial in the highway with a stake driven through the body and without Christian rites of sepulture. As to English Law on the point, although, suicide is no longer an offence in itself, it is an indictable offence, punishable by 14 years imprisonment, for any person to aid, abet, counsel or procure the suicide of another or an attempt by another to commit suicide. In England, suicide is no longer a crime.

In India, attempt to commit suicide is constituted an offence punishable under section 309, IPC. Although completed act was not a crime, surprisingly, attempt to commit the act was made an offence.

It may be found that Article 21 of the Constitution of India reads that no person shall be deprived of his life or personal liberty except according to procedure established by Law. The concept of reasonableness must be projected in the procedure contemplated by Article 21. The fundamental rights have their positive as well as negative aspects. For example, the freedom of speech and expression includes freedom not to speak, and to remain silent, and if this is so, logically it must follow that right to live as recognised by Article 21 will include also the right not to live or not to be forced to live, include a right to die or to terminate one's own life. The blanket prohibition on the right to die on pain of penalty, it was pointed out is not reasonable. The judgment was overruled by the Supreme

Court in AIR 1996, SC 946 (Five judges bench) Gian Kaur vs State of Punjab and others.

In a case (AIR 1994 SC 1844) (P Rathinam vs Union of India), the constitutional validity of Section 309 was challenged and the Supreme Court held that the provision punishing the attempt to commit suicide is cruel and irrational and is violative of Article 21 of the constitution and it deserves to be effaced from the Statute Book to humanize the penal laws. This decision has subsequently been overruled in AIR 1996 SC 946.

Gian Kaur vs State of Punjab and others and it has been held that the attempt to commit suicide is an offence and provisions of punishing this offence as laid down in Section 309 are not unconstitutional.

On appeal, the Supreme Court set aside the order of the High Court and following the decision in Lokendra Singh vs State of MP (1996 AIR SCW 1336: AIR 1996 SC 946), upheld the validity of section 309 and said that the criminal case initiated on charge of attempt to commit suicide required to be decided on merit.

The accused in another case had jumped into the well after throwing her children inside the well but nobody had seen her doing this. (Kavitha vs State of Tamil Nadu, AIR 1998 SC 2473: 1998(6) SCC 108).

Hunger strike attempt to suicide by: As to the peculiar difficulty about suicide by starvation, if a man openly declares that he will fast to death and then proceeds to refuse all nourishment until the stage is reached when there is imminent danger of death ensuing, he could be held guilty of the offence of attempted suicide. But when the evidence falls short of the conclusion that a stage had been reached that there was imminent danger of death the charge under section 309 IPC cannot be sustained.

Plea for abolition of section 309; It should be stated in this connection that in many countries attempt to commit suicide is regarded more as a manifestation of a diseased condition of mind deserving of treatment and care rather than as an offence to be visited with punishment.

The persistence of this law leads to following difficulties: (AR Lakshmanan, 2008).

- Emergency treatment for those who have attempted suicide is not readily accessible as they are referred by local hospitals and doctors to tertiary centres as it is termed as medicolegal case. The time lost in the golden hour will save many lives.
- Those who attempt suicide are already distressed and in psychological pain and for them to face the ignominy of police interrogation causes increased distress, shame, guilt, and further suicide attempt.
- At the time of family turmoil dealing with police procedure adds to the woes of the family.
- It also leads to a gross under-reporting of attempted suicide and the magnitude of the problem is not unknown. Unless one is aware of the nature of extent of the problem effective intervention is not possible.

- As many attempted suicides are categorized in the guise of accidental poisoning, etc. emotional and mental health support is not available to those who have attempted as they are unable to access the services.

SUICIDE—ABETMENT AND ATTEMPT

Section 306: Abetment of Suicide

Section 306 of the Indian Penal Code penalizes abetment of suicide. It reads as: "306. Abetment of suicide—If any person commits suicide, whoever abets the commission of such suicide, shall be punished with imprisonment of either description for a term not exceeding ten years, and shall also be liable to fine."

8.02 The constitutionality of Section 306 was challenged in Smt Gian Kaur vs State of Punjab. Upholding the constitutionality of section 306, the Supreme Court held that section 306 enacted a distinct offence which is capable of existence independent of Section 309. The Court observed:

(SI) Section 2(1) of the Act imputes criminal liability complicity in another's suicide. It reads: "2 (1) A person who aids, abets, counsels or procures the suicide of another, or an attempt by another to commit suicide, shall be liable on conviction on indictment to imprisonment for a term not exceeding fourteen years."

II Section 309 – Attempt to Commit Suicide

8.03 Section 309 of IPC punishes attempt to commit suicide with simple imprisonment for a term which may extend to one year or with fine or both.

8.04 The Law Commission in its Forty-Second Report had examined whether attempt to commit suicide be retained as a penal offence. The commission referred to the *dharmasastras* which letgitimized the practice of taking one's life in certain situations and also referred to the Provisions of Suicide Act 1961 in Britain which decriminalized the offence of attempt to commit suicide. After examining these views, the Commission recommended that Section 309 is harsh and unjustifiable and it should be repealed.

"Section 309 IPS deserves to be effaced from the statute look to humanize our penal laws." (Mr Justice BL Hansari, 1994).

In 1994, Supreme Court of India declared section 309 of the IPC as constitutional and stuck down this section.

The Supreme court examined the constitutional validity of Section 309 in P Rathinam vs Union of India with reference to Article 14 and 21 the Court considered the decisions of the Delhi, Bombay, and Andhra Pradesh High Courts and disagreed with the view taken by Andhra Pradesh High Court on the question of violation of Article 21. Agreeing with views of the Bombay High Court, the Supreme Court observed.

On the basis of what has been held and noted above, we state that Section 309 of the Penal Code deserves to be effaced from statute book to humanize our penal laws. It is a cruel and irrational provision, and it may result in punishing a person again (doubly) who has suffered agony and would be undergoing ignominy because of his failure to commit suicide. Then an act of suicide cannot be said to be against religion, morality or public policy and an act of attempted suicide has no baneful effect on society. Further, suicide or attempt to commit it causes no harm to others, because of which, State's interference with the personal liberty of Section 309 violates Article 21, and so, it is void. May it be said that the view taken by us would advance not only the cause of humanization, which is a need of the day, but of globalization also, as by effacing section 309, we would be attuning this part of criminal law to the global wavelength."

But this law of Supreme court was overruled by a larger Bench in Smt Gian Kaur vs State of Punjab wherein Verma J, (as he was) speaking for the court, held that P Rathinam's case was wrongly decided. The court observed.

In 1996 – a five judge constitutional bench of the Supreme Court again revoked the earlier provision of Section 309, the right to life, as guaranteed under Article 21 of the constitutions did not include the right to die. Hence person who attempts suicide would continue to be an offence and punishable. Person who attempts suicide require assistance in his personal and psychosocial life, not punishment. Penal deterrents are better suited to criminal acts and not to Act of distress.

The Supreme Court's decision in Smt Gian Kaur has thus categorically affirmed that right to life in Article 21 does not include the right to die. Consequently Section 309 which penalizes attempt to commit suicide is not unconstitutional.

In my opinion, this is an issue which is in the exclusive domain of the parliament to determine. The recommendation of the Law Commission is already on the record (156 Report of 1997).

When a man commits suicide he has to undertake certain positive overt acts and the genesis of those acts cannot be traced to or be included within the protection of the "right to life" under Article 21, the significant aspect of "sanctity of life" is also not to be overlooked. Article 21 is a provision guaranteeing protection of life and personal liberty and by no stretch of imagination can "extinction of life" be read to be included in "protection of life". Whatever may be the philosophy of permitting a person to extinguish his life by committing suicide, we find it difficult to construe Article 21 to include within the "right to die" as a part of the fundamental right guaranteed therein. Right to life is a natural right embodied in Article 21 but suicide is an unnatural termination or extinction of life, and therefore, incompatible and inconsistent with the concept of "right to life". With respect and in all humility, we find no similarity in the nature of the other rights, such as the right to "Freedom of speech", etc. to provide a comparable basis to hold that the "right to life" also includes the "right to die". With respect, the comparison is in opposite, for the reason indicated in the context of Article 21. The decisions relating to other fundamental rights wherein the absence of compulsion to exercise a right was held to be included within the exercise of that right, are not available to support the view taken in P Rathinam qua Article 21.

Attempted suicide is:
- A cry for help
- A disease of hope
- An Act of despair.

Are we justified in punishing this emotionally disturbed person under Indian Penal Code?

The Mental Health Professionals consider attempted suicide is a psychological crisis to be taken care of and not a criminal behavior to be punished. Hence the Indian Psychiatric Society and other organizations working for the prevention of suicide strongly make an appeal to the government of India to remove the Section 309 Indian Penal Code which labels the attempted suicide as the criminal behavior. The legal commission of India also recently comes out with the recommendation to the Government of India favoring removal of penal action for suicidal attempt.

Suicide By Young Married Women in India

Young married women due to adjustment problems with in-laws and dowry problems often commit/attempt suicide.

Section 304 (Indian Penal Code)—when death of women is caused by burns, bodily injurious or occurs otherwise than under normal circumstances within seven years of marriage, such death shall be called as dowry death. Most of the dowry deaths (84%), were suicide committed by young women. Dowry deaths contribute 2.7% all suicide in India. (Accidental death and suicide in India, 1995).

Suicide: Epidemiology

- Suicide is considered to be the commonest cause of unnatural death.
- Over the last few years there is an alarming increase in the rate of suicide and attempted suicide in India.
- One percent commit suicide every five minutes and one attempted suicide is made every minute in India.
- Over hundred thousand Indians commit suicide every year.
- There is any ugly rise of suicide among females and young people. "National Crime Research Bureau"—1996.

Suicide in India

There is a gross underreporting of suicide and attempted suicide in India.
Few reasons are:
- Fear of punishment.
- Stigma attached to suicide.
- Ignorance and many other social causes.
- Suicide counters such as family, social, ethical, religious, economic, and moral factors tend to minimize the self destructive behavior.

Some Ancient Concepts

- The Hindu religion has lot of philosophical ideas about death.
- The *dharmashastras* (Book on the codes of living in Ancient India condemn suicide.
- *Yama Smriti* (600 BC)—those who die by suicide should be defiled, and if his attempt was successful, his sons and friends should pay the fine.
- The ancient Hindu living principle allowed some suicides.

Some Ancient Methods

- *Sati*
- Drowning in the holy rivers
- Mahaprasthana (Great journey of life towards the North direction)
- Sitting on mountain towards the North direction till death—"Vadakkumthala"
- Fasts unto death
- Throwing themselves before the running temple car (chariot).

Misconceptions

- Suicide happens without warning.
- All the suicidal individuals are mentally ill.
- People who talk about suicide will not commit.
- People who commit suicide are fully intended to die, etc.

Cultural Factors in Suicide and Attempted Suicide

- Culture defines basic attitude towards life and death and also towards suicide in society.
- In India religion is still a meaningful and protective factor for many individuals in a suicidal crisis.
- Cultural variations in attempted suicide has been documented from India, Srilanka and Pakistan.

ATTEMPT TO COMMIT SUICIDE IS PUNISHABLE IN INDIA: SECTION 309 INDIAN PENAL CODE

"Whoever attempts to commit suicide and does any Act towards the commission of such offence, shall be punished with simple prisonment for a term which may extend to one year or with fine or with both".

Abetment of Suicide of Child or Insane Person

Section 305—Indian Penal Code

If any person under 8 years of age, any insane person, any delirious person, any idiot or any person in a state of intoxication commits suicide, whoever abets the commission of such suicide shall be punished with death or imprisonment for life or imprisonment for a term not exceeding 10 years, and shall also be liable to fine.

Section 306—Indian Penal Code

"If any person commits suicide, whoever abets the commission of such suicide, shall be punished with imprisonment either description for a term which may extend to 10 years and shall also be liable to fine."

Section 309 IPS Stuck Down on 28 April 1994

"Section 309 IPS deserves to be affected from the statute look to humanize our penal laws" (Mr Justice BL Hansari, 1994). "It is cruel and irrational provision and it may result in punishing a person (doubly) who has suffered agony and would be undergoing ignominy because of his failure to commit suicide".

Attempt to Commit Suicide—Section 309

(Indian Penal Code), Law, Claw, or Flaw?

In 1994, Supreme court of India declared section 309 of the IPS as unconstitutional and stuck down this section.

In 1996—a five judge constitutional bench of the supreme court again revoked the earlier provision of section 309 the right to life, as guaranteed under Article 21 of the constitutions did not include the right to die. Hence attempt to commit suicide would continue to be an offence and punishable.

Person who attempt suicide require assistance in his personal and psychosocial life, not punishment. Penal deterrants are better suited to criminal Acts and not to acts of distress.

Attempted suicide is:

- A cry for help
- A disease of hope
- An Act of despair.

Are we justified in punishing this emotionally disturbed person under Indian Penal Code?

SELF IMMOLATION—A POLITICAL SACRIFICE?

- Highly emotionally charged followers of political leaders kill themselves by self-immolation. This is frequent happening in Tamil Nadu.
- Indirectly they get the blessings and appreciation from politicians.
- This type of suicide is glorified as martyrdom.

SUICIDE BY YOUNG MARRIED WOMEN IN INDIA

- Young married woman due to adjustment problems with in laws and dowry problems often commit/attempt suicide.
- Common method—self-immolation.
- Section 304 B (IPC) when death of a woman is caused by burns, bodily injuries or occurs otherwise than under normal circumstances within seven years of

marriage, such death shall be called as dowry death. If it is shown that before death the husband is guilty unless proved otherwise and will be punished.

- Most of the dowry deaths (84%) were suicide committed by young women. Dowry deaths contribute 2.7% all suicides in India. (Accidental deaths and suicide in India, 1995).

SATI—SELF-IMMOLATION OF WIDOWS LEGAL ASPECTS

Widely prevalent in India during ancient times, it became a social problem after 18th century.

Some Causes

1. To prove the world that she was the most loyal and chaste woman.
2. An Act of bravery where she got public acclaim when she committed *sati*.
3. Because of the taboos and ill treatment meted out to the widows.
4. *Sati* was abolished on 4th December 1829, by Lord Bentick according to regulation XVII (those who encouraged *sati* were guilty of culpable homicide).

***Sati* Prevention Act 1987:** If any person commits *sati*, whoever abets the commission of *sati* either directly or indirectly shall be punished with death or life imprisonment. Even those who glorify *sati* are punishable.

Risk and Protective Factors

Cultural, social, psychological, biological.

Situational Factors

- Recent stressors availability and lethality of methods.
- Intent to commit suicide.
- Suicide attempt.
- Death or survival.
- After—effects.

MAJOR PUBLIC HEALTH CONCERNS IN THE FIELD OF SUICIDE

- Suicidal ideation and suicide attempts are surprisingly common in the general population.
- The rapid rising, rate of suicides among adolescents and young adults.
- Unemployment as a major risk factor for suicide.
- Easy access to lethal suicide methods such as psychotropic drugs and organophosphorous compounds.
- High alcohol consumption and increasing substance misuse.
- Under treatment of major psychiatric disorders such as depression and schizophrenia.
- Suicide model projected by the mass media.

Euthanasia and Assisted Suicide in India

- Euthanasia the Act of deliberately ending the life of a person at his request is highly unethical and rejected by many Indians.
- The assisted suicide in which the doctor provides the patient with lethal prescriptions who is suffering from serious or terminal illnesses to commit suicide.
- This is also considered to be unethical and condemned by the medical profession in India.
- No specific laws to deal with euthanasia and assisted suicide in India.

THE STANDARDS OF REASONABLE AND PRUDENT CARE IN SUICIDAL PERSONS

The Essential Steps Required

- An evaluation of suicide risk should be done with all psychiatric patients, regardless of whether they present with overt suicidal complaints.
- Measures to identify the correct statistics regarding the epidemiology of suicide.
- Creating awareness about the causes and prevention of suicide to public as well as health care professionals.
- Public health education through mass media.
- Identifying the high-risk groups.
- Creation of crisis intervention centres and counselling centres at vulnerable places.

WHO IS RESPONSIBLE TO TAKE CARE OF THE PERSONS WITH SUICIDAL TENDENCY

- Government
- NGO's
- Health Care Personnel
- Teachers, Group leaders, Politicians, Religious heads and Bureaucrats
- Media and above all.

ISSUES IN FAILURE IN CARE OF SUICIDAL PERSONS IN INDIA

- Non-availability of the correct statistics.
- Failure to identify assess and manage persons with suicidal tendency.
- Failure to have a national suicide policy and national suicide prevention program.
- Failure to control the sale of organophosphorous compounds and psychotropic drugs.
- Failure to have suicide prevention clinics and crisis intervention centers.
- Lack of trained counsellors.
- Inadequate mental health professionals.

LIABILITY AND MALPRACTICE WITH REGARDS TO SUICIDE/ATTEMPTED SUICIDE

- Negligence involving suicide—three categories.
- Failure to diagnose properly (that is to assess the potential for suicide).
- Failure to treat (i.e. use reasonable treatment interventions and precautions).
- Failure to implement (i.e. carry out treatment properly and not negligently).
- All these above are likely to render a doctor (psychiatrist) liable if patients is harmed because of a suicidal attempt.
- The law tends to assume that suicide is preventable if it is foreseeable.

Euthanasia and Indian Court

Euthanasia or Mercy Killing means and implies the intervention of another human agency to end the life. Mercy killing is not suicide and attempt to mercy killing is covered by section 309, IPC, it is homicide though, in English Law. "Mercy killings" are treated as manslaughter and this enables the judge to reduce or extinguish the sentence, there is no such parallel provision in Indian Law. Thus, mercy killing due to impairment of mental faculty is no exception under the Indian Law.

Euthanasia means "a gentle and easy death" and, has come to mean "the good death of another" or "Mercy Killing".

Euthanasia has been defined as "the bringing about of a gentle and easy death for someone suffering from an incurable and painful disease or in an irreversible coma." (Pearsal and Trumble, 1996)

There is a lot of controversy amongst the lawmakers, physicians including psychiatrists and between the family members and caregivers of the terminally ill—whether euthanasia is allowed or not. The Royal Dutch Medical Association Policy permits euthanasia for competent patients who persistently request it and who are experiencing unbearable suffering that cannot be relieved otherwise with the present day knowledge. It accounts for nearly 2% of all deaths in Netherlands, where the indications include intractable suffering and in April 2001, that country became the first legalized the practice fully. Since, approval of the death and with Dignity Act, initially in 1994, and again in 1997, the State of Oregon in USA has allowed Medically Assisted Suicide, where the physician may provide a patient with lethal drugs, but may not actually abandon them. Increasingly, mental health professionals are being challenged to consider their role end of life decisions.

Several critical issues for psychiatrists have been raised with the advent of "Physician-Assisted Suicide" (PAS), which is the deliberate participation of medication to or counseling of ill patients so that such patients may use this medication or information to end their own life (Cohen, et al) 1994.

While psychiatrist specializing in geriatric psychiatry or Liaison Psychiatry may have regular experience in the management of patients in the end stages of dementia or other terminal conditions, most general psychiatrists have little experience of euthanasia related issues.

Advocacy for Euthanasia

There are few advocacy organizations in India and outside claiming that Euthanasia for the incurable, painful, or irreversible illnesses should be permitted. They claim that law should also recognize, the principle of personal autonomy and self determination, the right of every human being to have his or her wishes respected in decisions involving his or her body. It is essential to recognize that every human being is, in principle, master of his or her own destiny. He or she may, of course, for moral or religious reasons, impose restrictions or limits on his or her own right of self determination. However, these limits must not be imposed on the individual by the law except in cases where the exercise of this right is likely to affect public order or the rights of others.

Even if one is religiously opposed to euthanasia, it does not follow that one has the right to insist, through criminal law, that others follow one's religious belief. Current attitudes on ethical issues in India are worrisome and they should concern others who believe in personal privacy and freedom of choice. It is tiresome listening to moralists, who believe they have a profound understanding that the rest of the people do not; and that their moral code, having the stamp of Almighty, is beyond reproach.

Fixing the cause of death may be important from a legal point of view for it may determine whether criminal charges are brought against the doctor, but one should not immediately think that this notion can be used to show a moral difference between active and passive euthanasia. The reason why it is considered bad to be the cause of someone's death is that death is regarded as an Evil – and so it is. However, if it had been decided that euthanasia – even passive euthanasia is desirable in a given case, it has also been decided that in this instance death is no longer an evil than the patient's continued existence and if this is true, the usual reasons for not wanting to be the cause of somebody's death do not apply.

Is there a difference between a person who, at a dying persons request prepares a poison and leaves it on the bedside for him to take and a person who helps the patient to drink it or who administers it directly at the request of a dying person who is unable to take it himself is there, in short a real distinction between killing and letting die. Those who are in a chronic persistent vegetative state, where no form of treatment could restore to cognitive life – comatose with respirator or just that quality of life has deteriorated as badly or fit candidates for euthanasia. It is wrong to prolong the suffering of the person needlessly. If the crucial issue concerning euthanasia is the intentional termination of the life of one human being by another, then, how can it be consistent to forbid "Mercy Killing" and yet deny that the cessation of treatment is the intentional termination of life? What is the cessation of treatment if it is not the intentional termination of life of one human being by another? The so called distinction between active and passive euthanasia does not provide a useful moral distinction. Even if the patient is not competent to make the decision to stop treatment it may be made by a surrogate acting accordingly to patient's wishes. One consequence of such rulings is the increased interest in so called Living Wills.

Individuals have the right to decide about their own lives and deaths. Denying terminally ill patients the right to die with dignity is unfair and cruel. The golden rule requires that we allow Active euthanasia for terminally ill patients who request it in certain situations.

PSYCHIATRIC ASSESSMENT FOR PATIENTS WHO DEMAND EUTHANASIA AND/OR PHYSICIAN-ASSISTED SUICIDE (PAS)

Psychiatric assessment is mandatory for patients who request Euthanasia or PAS. In some jurisdictions, but not in others. In assessing patients request for Euthanasia and PAS, the primary role of the psychiatrist is to identify and treatment psychiatric illness, if anything. The psychiatrist may also be expected to provide an assessment of the patients decision making ability and to support staff in their own decision making process. These are all important issues in light of the prevalence of depression in this patient group and also the potential for distress and division among staff members.

WPA Guidelines on Euthanasia

The physician's role, first and foremost, is to promote health, reduce suffering and protect life. The psychiatrist, whose patients may include those who are severely incapacitated or incompetent to reach an informal decision, should be particularly careful about actions that could lead to the death of individuals who cannot protect themselves because of disability, and should be vigilant to the possibility that a patient's views could be distorted by mental illness such as depression. In such situations, the psychiatrist's role is to treat the illness.

The Ethical and Legal Aspects of Euthanasia

The right to die is one of the most controversial and illusive issues facing the legal and ethical angle of suicidology. In fact, the increased control that has been gained over biological life because of progress in medical treatment will force a confrontation with the subject.

Euthanasia refers to the practice of allowing the person to die with assistance, often by a medical doctor. Assisted suicide is not performed by another person, rather, the means are provided by which the person can end his own life. These distinctions are critical, especially, if one looks at the diversity of global views.

Euthanasia, the Act of deliberately ending the life of a person even at his own request is considered to be highly unethical and is rejected by many Indians. In physician-assisted suicide the doctor provides the patient with lethal prescriptions thereby assisting the individual to commit suicide. The individuals involved may be suffering from serious or terminal illnesses. Physician assisted suicide like euthanasia is considered to be unethical and is condemned by the right to decline medical treatment is a basic right of the patient and the doctor does not Act unethically even if respecting such a wish results in the death of the patient.

There are no specific laws to deal with (euthanasia) assisted suicide in India.

Euthanasia and Indian Court

There have been five cases of Euthanasia pleas in India all of which have been rejected by courts.

- ***In 2002, Kerala High Court*** did not allow BK Pillai, down with a disabling illness to die.
- ***In 2004, in Hyderebad***, the patient of muscular dystrophy sought permission to die on the plea that it would enable him to donate his vital organs. The court rejected his plea for euthanasia.
- ***In 2006, in Jaipur***, a retired principal with a severe cardiac problem sought the Rajasthan Highcourt, the permission to end his life in case his health deteriorates, the Rajasthan High Court rejected the plea.
- ***In 2004, in Chennai***, a 45-year-old person with schizophrenia appeared to the court through free legal aide service for uthanasia. The Member Secretary of the free legal aide cell did not forward to the court and advised him to go for treatment.
- ***In 2011, The Supreme Court***, rejected a Euthanasia plea on Aruna Shanbaug, a nurse worked in the Bombay hospital was bedridden for 38 years after a brutal sexual assault in 1973.

Euthanasia Timeline

fs• In 1996—A two-judge bench of the Supreme Court in P Rathinam vs Union of India rejected his plea for Euthanasia and said that it would be permitted only by legislation.
- April 27, 2005—New Delhi seminar on "End-of-life issues" by Indian Society of Critical Care Medicine, where then Law Minister HR Bhardwaj agrees that a framework was needed for withdrawal of life support to dying patients and entrusts Law Commission to come out with a legal paper.
- April 28, 2006—Law Commission suggests a draft bill on passive euthanasia. It says pleas must be made to High Court which should decide it after expert opinion.
- December 16, 2009—Supreme Court notice on Pinky Virani's plea to permit euthanasia for Aruna Shanbaug.
- March 2, 2011—Supreme Court reserves verdict on Virani's plea.
- March 7, 2011—Supreme Court allows passive euthanasia, recommends decriminalization of attempt to suicide.

Laws on Euthanasia Abroad Need Study

New Delhi: The Supreme Court on Monday (March 8, 2011) Times of India, broke new ground with a judgment allowing passive euthanasia. "We agree that the approval of the High Court should be taken in this connection. This is in the interest of the protection of the patient, protection of the doctors, relatives and next friend, and for reassurance of the patient's family as well as the public." Justice Katju, a voracious reader, quoted a famous couplet of 18-century poet

Mirza Ghalib: "*Marte aati hai par nahin aati* (one dies longing for death, but death, despite being around is elusive)."

"Euthanasia is one of the most perplexing issues which courts and legislatures all over the world are facing today. This court, in this case, is facing the same issue, and we feel like a ship in an uncharted sea, seeking some guidance by the light thrown by legislation and judicial pronouncements of foreign countries, as well as the submissions of learned counsels before us". He said.

An important idea behind this distinction (between active and passive euthanasia) is that in passive euthanasia the doctors are not actively killing anyone. They are simply not saving him. While we usually applaud someone who saves another person's life, we do not normally condemn someone for failing to do so, he added.

On euthanasia, the Bench referred to a constitution bench judgment in Gian Kaur vs State of Punjab (1996 (2) SCC 648), which held that both euthanasia and assisted suicide were not lawful in India. The Constitution Bench had ruled that right to life under Article 21 of the Constitution did not include right to die. It also said euthanasia could be made lawful only by legislation.

Justice Katju said as the Supreme Court in Gian Kaur's case had connected that "the debate even in such cases to permit physician assisted termination of life is inconclusive", no final view on the issue of euthanasia had been taken. It laid down the law and the procedure on passive euthanasia. The law commission's 196th report to the government on April 28, 2006 had comprehensively dealt with the issue of euthanasia in a 435-page analytical volume which included a draft Bill. The recommendation was identical to what the apex court ruled on Monday.

The Commission, headed by retired Supreme Court Judge M Jagannadha Rao, had said: "We have thought it fit to provide an enabling provision under which the patients, relatives, next friend, or doctors or hospitals can move a Division Bench of the High Court for a declaration that the proposed action of continuing or withholding or withdrawing medical treatment be declared lawful or unlawful."

"As time is essence, the HC must decide such cases at the earliest and within 30 days. In UK, decisions are sometimes made within half-an-hour and if there is grave urgency and reasons are given later. Such speedy procedure has to be followed because courts are dealing with life and death situations". It is said, however, the Commission had said "Living Wills" by which a person records how he wanted to die and Medical Power of Attorney to be illegal. It feared such instruments could be easily abused and created unwanted litigation.

The ONUS is on us

The attitude of psychiatric residents on the legislation of euthanasia and their opinion about psychiatric evaluation of terminally ill patients asking for euthanasia was assessed. 85% respondents endorsed the view regular legalization of euthanasia, half of the respondents agreed that euthanasia and be considered in comatose and terminally ill cancer patients while only 18.33% felt that euthanasia may be considered in any psychiatric condition. Psychiatric evaluation of the terminally ill as long for evaluation is favored.

SUGGESTED READING

1. Lakshmanan Justice AR. (Former Judge, Supreme Court of India, Chairman, Law Commission of India), Suicide prevention, SNEHA, Key Note Address, 2008.
2. Vijayakumar L. Suicide and its prevention – The urgent need in India, Indian Journal of Psychiatry, 2007;49(2):81-84.
3. Nambi S. Legal aspects of psychiatry – Indian Perspective Manashanti Mental Health Care Pvt Ltd, 2008.
4. Kallivayalil R A, Varghese PP. Suicide prevention: A handbook for community gatekeepers.
5. The Onus is on us. Jada, et al. Indian Journal of Psychiatry, 2002;44.

21 Chapter

Psychological and Legal Aspects of Domestic Violence

INTRODUCTION

Women occupy a unique position in the society due to the importance in the procreation of the human race. However, patriarchy and traditional patterns of life have neglected women to a position of insignificance. Women suffer this discrimination in silence. They are the victims of violence like female foeticide, infanticide, child marriage, dowry, purdah, sati, and slavery.

The gender based violence haunts a woman at all stages of her life. The birth of a daughter is considered as bad luck. A growing girl child is considered to be a burden for the family. A female child at the tender age is subjected to sexual exploitation. The married woman is subjected to myriad forms of violence of varying proportions. The aged and infirm woman is unwanted and neglected.

Despite the enactment of a plethora of laws, the status of women has not improved. The home has become the least safe place for women, whereas, it has become the safest place for men to commit violence against women. It is unfortunate that even after 55 years of Independence, the position of women has not changed. Even though the Constitution of India affords equality of status and opportunity to all its citizens, Indian womanhood is still tied up by the rusted chains of religious customs and traditions. According to the statistics in 2001 census, the female sex ratio is 933:1000. This reflects society's preference for a male child and an indication of the low status accorded to women. The incidents of wife battering, harassment by her husband and in-laws, dowry deaths, suicides, kitchen accidents, occur on a large scale. The victims are not able to raise their voice nor protest against violence. The violations of their rights are still not considered as gross violations of human rights. Even now, the exact statistics of wife battering or dowry deaths are not known as many cases go unreported.

The moment a woman complains of domestic violence, she is thrown out of the house. There is still a major deterrent to her resistance. The sufferings of a woman are still not considered as a serious matter. To allow them to suffer silently and in secret would harm their dignity and health. Therefore, domestic violence is to be viewed not merely as a private problem, but as a social problem. More so, it is a public health hazard.

There are other equally compelling reasons why this issue cries out for urgent and fervent public attention, they are:

- Domestic violence spreads menacingly into the next generation. Children of the violent fathers are often physically abused along side their mothers.
- Children of violent parents are more apt not only to repeat the behavior with their own offspring, but to commit violent acts in the larger society.
- It is a matter of public health. Violence debilitates women and girls physically, psychologically, and socially sometimes with lifelong results.
- Women's aspirations and achievements are powerfully inhibited not just by the injuries of physical attacks, but by the implicit threats of male violence.

DOMESTIC VIOLENCE THEORETICAL PERSPECTIVE

Women have always been an object of gross and severe violence at the hands of man. The biological weakness of a woman makes her an easy prey to all and sundry. She is often a victim of physical and mental violence not only outside her home, but also inside it. Every society accepting the importance of equality of sexes has therefore, made affirmative provisions against gender discrimination. However, inspite, of the enactment of these provisions, equality between men and women continues to be an elusive goal. Hence, women are deprived of basic freedom and thereby are easily exposed to exploitation.

Violence and its perpetuation are often related to conflicts of caste, class ethnicity, communalism, fundamentalism, and terrorism. All these factors cumulatively have a negative impact on women. Of all types of violence against women, domestic violence is of the most serious type because it is caused silently within the four walls of a house. It is a global phenomenon and has been on the rise constantly spreading its tentacles far and wide.

Definition of Domestic Violence

Domestic violence means the violence that occurs within the family. UN gives the most comprehensive definition of family violence—accordingly, violence in the family manifests itself as physical mistreatment, often repetitive, which is interrelated to the exercise of mental torture, neglect of basic needs, and sexual molestation.

Violence is the foremost social stressor on women's mental health. Women globally, particularly Indian women live in a social environment, where violence is an immediate reality, overriding sociodemographic difference of cultural background, class, education, occupation etc. Feminist definitions of violence use "Power" and "Domination" as their operative constructs and explains male violence against women. Violence is now days considered to be a criminal behavior, perpetuating fear, misery, injury, sickness and possibly death in the victims. Traditional definition of violence includes "Unjust" or "Unwanted exercise of physical force".

Domestic violence means the violence that occurs within the family. It is the common social problem and a physical health problem also. Domestic violence is considered as one of the important burning social problem of the present day in India. Globally and in India also, the main aggressor is the husband and the victim is the wife. Domestic violence affects both mind and body.

Domestic violence is not something new; but an age-old phenomena. In the past, mostly it was hidden behind the four walls of the house. Those within do not wish to speak about and those outside do not want to hear it. Social practices, customs, beliefs, myths, and patriarchy are the important causative factors for domestic violence in India. The other names to some extent similar but not exactly the same for domestic violence are:

1. Intimate partner violence.
2. Violence against women.

The causes of violence can be classified as follows:

- Biological determinants—like hormonal factors, neurotransmitters.
- Intrapsychic determinants—like personality characters of both victims and perpetuator.
- Behavioral approach—social conditioning.
- Cognitive approach—accepting others anger, faulty processing of social information.
- Social—family and social situations.

There are many definitions for domestic violence. Some of them are:

1. "Violence in the family manifests itself as physical mistreatment, often repetitive, which is inter-related to the exercise of mental torture neglect of basic needs, and sexual molestation." (UN)
2. Any Act or threatened Act of violence, including any fearful detention of an individual, which—
   - Results or threatens to result in physical injury.
   - Committed by a person against another individual to whom such person is related by blood or marriage or otherwise legally related or with whom such person is lawfully residing. (USA Law on family violence)
3. Any Act, omission or commission or conduct of the respondent shall constitute domestic violence in case it—
   - Harms or injures or endangers the health, safety, life limb, or well-being, whether mental, physical of the aggrieved person or tends to do so and includes causing physical abuse, sexual abuse, verbal, and emotional abuse and economic abuse.
   - Harasses, harms, injures or endangers the aggrieved person with a view to coerce her or any other person related to her to meet any unlawful demand for any dowry or other property or valuable security.

- Has the effect of threatening the aggrieved person or any person related to her by any conduct mentioned in clause.
  - Or clause.
  - Or injures or causes harm, whether, physical or mental to the aggrieved person (DVA, 2005).

The Risk Factors for Domestic Violence

The risk factors involve the following:
1. Alcoholic husbands.
2. Illiterate or poorly educated couple.
3. Poor socio-economic status.
4. Women with no income of their own.
5. Dowry problems.

Reason for the Increased Incidence of Domestic Violence

Many of the accused women never expose their problem outside. Even when women speak out about their problems, they are not taken seriously by society.

Women who ask for justice are labeled by the community as arrogant. The future of the family becomes questionable, when husband gets punished for his violent behavior. Like a volcano that keeps seething fire within, women suppress their suffering within, while showing a calm face outside.

How to Identify Women Exposed to Domestic Violence

It is the trauma inflicted on the women is the evidence for the domestic violence. The trauma may be physical and/or psychological or emotional.

Physical Trauma

Injuries are usually caused by hands, legs, and sometimes by firewood. The injuries are commonly seen in the head, neck, hands, legs, and genitals. Sometimes burns and fractures may be detected. On seeking medical help, often women suppress the fact and gives flimsy reason as the cause for the injures.

Psychological Trauma

The symptoms include:
a. Fear and anxiety.
b. Depression, suicidal ideas, acute stress reaction and symptoms of PTSD and loss of appetite and loss of sleep.

In a study on domestic violence, the International Center for Research on Women, ICRW in multiple centers in India conclude:
a. Eighty-five percent of men admit that they had indulged in violent behavior against their wives, physical, emotional or sexual, at least once in the last 12 months.

b. Fifty-seven percent of men with 6–10 years of individuals admitted to have sexual abuse with their wives.
c. Thirty-two percent of men admitted to committing violence on their pregnant wives.

The men indulged in violence as a tool to establish their power over the weaker sex.

In a study of violence against women, Sathyanathan, et al. (1996), the following findings emerged.

• Total sample size	332
• Women experienced abuse	76 (22%)
• Verbal abuse (individuals to criticism)	51 (15%)
• Physical abuse (slapping, biting, and kicking)	25 (8%)
• Sexual abuse (forced sex)	3%
• The perpetrators	12%
• (Primary) Husband	4%
• Parents and in-laws	2%

THE PSYCHIATRIC ASPECTS OF DOMESTIC VIOLENCE

The mental health problems related to domestic violence are varying in nature. Many women accept this as normal phenomena in our culture. Some overtly react through their physical aggression. Many suffer in silence for a few. The psychological symptoms emerge as subsyndromal or diagnosable disorders.

Initial responses may be fear, shock, numbing and denial. Ongoing and repeated abuse may read to symptoms of anxiety and depression.

Feelings of worthlessness, hopelessness, and despair may set in and at times acts are not uncommon. Sleep disorder, loss of appetite, fatigue, substance abuse are also common. Many women become isolated and experienced intense shame, blame themselves, and feel guilty suicide attempts often are a cry for help. Chronic headaches, abdominal pain, back pain, chest pain and other multiple vague/somatic complaints which can be labeled as Somatization disorder can occur. Some women having earlier hysterical or attention seeking personality may also get possession attack. Adjustment disorder with depression or anxiety is not uncommon.

Domestic violence is defined as a spectrum of abuse that includes physical, psychological, economic, and sexual harm with the intent to control another person's behavior. It is a persistent pattern of behavior occurring over a period of time that can occur at any point during the life cycle such as during childhood, adulthood, or advanced age.

All over the world 90 to 95%, of domestic violence is committed by men against women. Recognizing this, the UN passed the following declaration on the elimination of violence against women (VAW) in 1993.

Article 1: VAW means any act of gender based violence that results in or is likely to result in physical, sexual or psychological harm or suffering to woman including threats of such acts, coercion, or arbitrary, depravation of liberty whether occurring in public or private life.

Article 2: VAW shall be understood to encompass, but not limited to the following: Physical, sexual, and psychological violence occurring in the family including battering, sexual abuse of female children in the household dowry related violence, marital rape, female genital mutilation and other traditional practices harmful to women, non-spousal violence related exploitation.

- Physical, sexual and psychological violence occurring within the general community including rape, sexual abuse, sexual harassment, and intimidation at work in educational institutions and elsewhere, trafficking in women and forced prostitution.
- Physical, sexual, and psychological violence perpetrated or condoned by the State wherever it occurs.
- Violence against women takes place at various stages of life. Sex selective abortions and effects of battery during pregnancy on birth outcomes, female infanticide, child marriage, female genital mutilation, incest, prostitution and pornography are all examples of how a female could be affected prior to adolescence. During adolescence and adulthood women potentially face date violence, economically coerced sex, incest, sexual abuse at the work place, rape, sexual harassment, forced prostitution and pornography, trafficking, dowry abuse, and honor killing. Elderly women maybe subjected to forced "suicide" or "homicide" of widows and *sati*.

Domestic Violence around the World

In a study of random sample of women in London, United Kingdom 25% have been punched or slapped by a partner or ex-partner in their lifetime (Mooney, 1995). Studying representative sample of women aged 20 to 24 and their partners in two districts of Uganda, 41% of the women report being beaten or physically harmed and the same percentage of men report beating their partner. (Blanc, 1996). In a study from Israel involving systematic random sample of 1,826 married Arab women 32% report at least one episode of physical abuse by their partner during the last four months. (Haj Yahia, 1997). In a study from Columbia involving 6.907 women ages 15–49 years, 19% reported physical assault by their partner in their lifetime (DHS III Survey, 1995).

Domestic Violence in India

There were 972 females to every 1000 males in 1901, however, this has declined to 927 females to every 1000 males by 1991. Narasinham (1994) found 7,999 of 8000 aborted fetus in Maharashtra were female, the exception was a Jewish woman who wanted a daughter. George (1995) found 41% of the early neo-natal female deaths in rural Tamil Nadu appeared to be due to infanticide. About 12 to 15% of maternal deaths are related to domestic violence. Early marriage of girls continues to be an issue; nearly 12% were married by age 12, 26%

married by age 15 and 24% married by age 18. Narayana (1996) reported that 18 to 45% of married men ages 15 to 65 from five different districts of Uttar Pradesh acknowledged physically abusing their wife. In a community based study involving 450 women in Gujarat, 42% experienced physical beatings and sexual abuse and 23% experienced abusive language, belittlement, and threats. It is interesting to note that 56% of women believe that wife beating is justified.

Unfortunately, the cycle of domestic violence continues from generation to generation in the following way. An abused boy/boy child witnessing his father beating up his mother grows to be an abusive husband and an abusive girl/girl child witnessing her mother being battered grows to be a battered woman herself.

Domestic Violence: A Community's Response

Domestic spousal violence against women has far-reaching mental health implications. In a study in Chennai, 9938 women's survey 40% reported to have poor mental health. Logistics, regression showed that women reporting "Any violence, i.e. "slap" ,"hit", "kick", or "beat" (OP 2.2, 95%, CI – 2.0 to 2.5) or "All violence" all of the four types of physically violent behavior (OR 3.5, 95% CI – 2.94 to 3.51) were in increased risk of poor mental health. These findings indicate a strong association between domestic spousal violence and poor mental health, and underscore the need for appropriate interventions.

It is very important to identify and treat domestic violence in those with mental illness, especially, suicidality, love, hate, suicide and murder can come together in about half of all murders committed by domestic partners and serious mental illness contributes to the risk.

Both deliberate self-harm (DSH) and domestic violence are serious social malady with major public health implications. Stressful high situations and multiple types of victimization in the family are some of the factors responsible for both. The timely psychosocial intervention may definitely reduce morbidity and mortality from DSH assisted with domestic violence in the context of community mental health program.

LEGISLATIVE RESPONSE TO THE PROBLEMS OF DOMESTIC VIOLENCE AGAINST WOMEN

International Instruments to Curb the Violence Against Women

The UN General Assembly recognize the urgent need for the universal application of women's rights regarding equality, security, liberty, integrity, and dignity by its resolution.

The UN is also a concern that violence against women is an obstacle to the achievement of equality. Article 55 and 56 of the UN charter cast a legal obligation on the UNO to promote respect for the principle of equality and observance of human rights.

Article 5 of the Universal Declaration of Human Rights states that no one shall be subjected to torture or cruel inhuman or degrading treatment or punishment. This principle has been accepted in the Constitution of India. There has been three UN World Conferences on women. One in Mexico in 1975, the second in Copenhagen in 1980, and the third in Nairobi. As per the third combination, strategies were framed to promote gender equality and opportunity for women. They were based on three objectives such as equality development and peace.

- ***Vienna Declaration (1993):*** The declaration calls for action to integrate the equal status human rights of women into mainstream of the UN System. Stresses the importance of working towards the elimination of violence against women in public and private life.
- ***Beijing Conference*:** This conference provided a platform for action concentrating on some of the key issues identified as fundamental obstacles to the advancement of majority of women in the world. The conference mainly concentrated on issues like documentation against women, violence against women and the like. This convention on elimination of all forms of documentation against women (CEDAW) was a landmark document in three ways.
  - It framed violence against women within the dialogue on human rights.
  - It identified female as the primary risk factor for violence.
  - It broadened the definition of gender violence to include all aspects of women's life.

Constitution of India and Protection for Women

- ***Article 14:*** Article 14 of the Indian constitution embodies the idea of equality expressed in the preamble. Thus the difference in treatment between men and women by the State is totally prohibited on the grounds of religion, race, caste, sex, or place of birth.
- ***Article 21:*** Article 21 embodies the right to live is not merely confined to physical existence, but it includes within its ambit the right to live with human dignity.

Criminal Law Domestic Violence

Female Feticide: Female infanticide, prenatal sex selection are considered as criminal acts. The prenatal diagnostic techniques (Regulation and Prevention of Misuse Act, 1994) came into existence from 1996 in India to prevent female feticide.

Dowry death, murder and suicide: Because of dowry problems, more often, women are harassed, abused, forced to commit suicide and sometimes burnt alive in a brutal manner for not bringing sufficient dowry. Until 1980s, women's death by the fire had been put down as suicide and even these suicides were rarely seen as being due to dowry harassment. Sudha Goel case is the first case in which Supreme Court in 1985 sentenced the husband and mother-in-law of the deceased to life-imprisonment. This has become such a menacing reality and with a view to combat the increasing menace of dowry deaths, suicide, a new section that is Section 304-B and for the presumption as to dowry death, Section 113-B is also inserted in Indian Evidence Act, 1872. Section 304-B of IPC 1860, deals with dowry death. It reads as where the death of a woman is caused by any burns or bodily injury or occurs otherwise than under normal circumstances within seven years of her marriage and if it is shown that soon before her death, she was subjected to cruelty of harassment by her husband or any relative of her husband for/or in connection with any demand for dowry, such death shall be called "Dowry Death" and such husband or relative shall be deemed to have caused her death.

Section 306 IPC deals with abetment of suicide which runs if "any person commits suicide, whoever abets the commission of such suicide shall be punished with imprisonment of either description for a term which may extent to 10 years and shall also be liable to fine.

IEA section 113 A deals with the presumption as to abetment of suicide of a married woman and section 113-B relates to presumption as to dowry death. Both the provisions are a departure from the normal rule of evidence and a presumption arises against the accused in a case, where the death of the victim occurred unnaturally within a period of seven years of the marriage. In such cases, the burden shifts to the reference to show that she died in natural circumstances. The offences of dowry under section 304-B or suicide section 306 are cognizable, nonbailable and noncompoundable, triable by court of session.

Criminal Offense of Cruelty: Is dealt in Section 498-A of IPC. Section 357 CrPC provides for compensation payable to the victim by the accused. It is only a discriminatory civil remedy provided under the CrPC.

Marital Right: According to Section 377 IPC, whoever voluntarily has carnal intercourse against the order of nature with any man, women, or animal shall be punished with imprisonment for life and shall also be liable to fine. However, this provision has rarely been used in the matrimonial context. In India, the exception to Section 375 IPC explicitly says that sexual intercourse by a man with his own wife not being under 15 years is not rape. Thus if the wife is above 15, then forcible intercourse even without her consent is not rape. This is unreasonable. There is a lacune in the legal provision with regard to marital rape. This need to be changed.

DOMESTIC VIOLENCE—HOW TO HELP?

Domestic violence not be completely eradicated at present; but efforts to be taken to reduce the severity of the problem.

Women

- Try to find ways to get free from domestic violence.

- Female education—Finding employment—independent decision making—guidance to other women.
- Vocational training.
- Through these they can reduce their complete dependence on males.
- Efforts to prevent attempted suicide.
- Males: Create awareness about the punitive laws for domestic violence.

Males

- They should come forward to minimize male chauvinistic behavior.
- Avoiding dependence on alcohol.
- Realizing that in the long-run they and their children will be the victims, eventually.

Community

Organizing a self-help group to get support and to help in better coping strategy. The principle of parity between male and female is to be established. The harmful cultural norms should be changed. Feminist organizations should uphold the affected women and special institutions to help female victims.

THE PSYCHOSOCIAL IMPACT OF DOMESTIC VIOLENCE

- Domestic violence undermines women's confidence and sense of self-esteem at every level, physically and psychologically.
- It destroys women's health and denies their women rights and participation in social activities.
- Domestic violence deprives of the women of her earnings. Creates a sense of insecurity, the fear of sexual abuse prevents her from going out and taking a job.

Domestic Violence—Prevention (Psychosocial)

- Education and economic independence of women in some extent to prevent domestic violence.
- Women should come out of their problems they suffer in silence at home. The ICRW conducted a TV program in four channels titled "*Bol*" (speak out) on DV—which has created an awareness among women folk.
- Early recognition and effective treatment should be given to husband's abusing alcohol.
- The role of media in creating awareness about the psychosocial and legal implications of domestic violence.

Domestic Violence—Legal Perspectives

- Domestic violence implies unjustifiable force both physical and mental cruelties perpetrated on the women at home.

- Domestic violence a wide variety of violence spanning from sex determination (to do a way with the female child), dowry harassment and bring to neglect and ill-treatment.
- When a suffering women prefers to come out of her wedlock she is viewed with suspicion, she become the object of criticism, a victim of social bias and prejudices. She has to compromise with her husband and in-laws. She has to suffer in silence.
- Hence, domestic violence is considered to be a human right violation.

Laws Relating to Domestic Violence

- International instruments to prevent the violence against woman
  - Vienna Declaration (1993)
  - Beijing Conference (1995)
  - Convention on Elimination of all forms of Discrimination Against Women (CEDAW) (1981)
- Constitution of India and Protection for Women
- Criminal Law—Domestic Violence
  - Female Foeticide—Prenatal Diagnostic Techniques
  - Dowry Death: Murder and Suicide—304B IPC, 306 IPC
  - Section 113 A and B of Indian Evidence Act
  - Criminal Offence of Cruelty Section 498 A of IPC,
  - Marital Rape Section 377 IPC
  - Dowry Prohibition Act 1986
  - Civil Law—The Protection of Women from Domestic Violence Act, 2005.

INTERNATIONAL INSTRUMENTS TO PREVENT THE VIOLENCE AGAINST WOMAN

a. **Vienna Declaraction: (1993)**
   Calls for action to integrate the equal status and rights for women – working towards the elimination of violence against women in public and private life.
b. **Beijing Conference: (1995)**
   Identified the fundamental obstacles to the advancement of women – focused the issues like discrimination against women, violence against women, etc.
c. **Convention on elimination of all forms of Discrimination Against Women (CEDAW): (1981)**
   It framed violence against women within the dialogue on human rights – It identified female as the primary risk factor for violence. It broadened the definition of gender violence to include all aspects of women's lives.

Constitution of India and Protection for Women

Article 14

It embodies the idea of equality expressed in the preamble. Thus the difference in treatment between men and women by the state is totally prohibited on the grounds of religion, race, caste, sex or place of birth.

Article 21

The right to live is not merely confined to physical existence but it includes within its ambit the right to live with human dignity.

DOMESTIC VIOLENCE—CRIMINAL LAW

- Section 113-A and B of Indian Evidence Act: In this Act the presumption has to abetment of suicide by a married women has been introduced–for presumption to dowry death section 113-B is inserted in IDA.
- Section 306 IPC: If a women dies within 7 years of her marriage an inquest to be conducted as to the cause of death. Even it was a case of suicide, the husband and their relatives can be charged and prosecuted for abetment of suicide.
- Dowry Prohibition Act 1985: This act redefined the offence of dowry. It has been made cognizable, non-billable and has been made more stringent.

DOMESTIC VIOLENCE–CRIMINAL OFFENCE OF CRUELTY

- Section 498-A of IPC.
- Willful conduct of husband or his relative that is likely to drive the women to commit suicide or cause physical or mental trauma to her.
- This is the most widely used the provision of law against DV.
- Harassment of a woman with a view to coercing her or any of her relative to meet any unlawful demand for property would be punished as cruelty. The offence will be cognizable.

MARITAL RAPE AND OTHER SEXUAL VIOLENCES

Section 377 IPC: Whoever voluntarily has carnal intercourse against the order of nature shall be punished.

OTHER SEXUAL VIOLENCE

- Forced sexual intercourse.
- Forced to watch pornography or other obscene material.
- Forcibly compel to entertain others.
- Any other act of sexual nature, abusing humiliating, degrading or otherwise of violating dignity.

DOMESTIC VIOLENCE—CIVIL LAW

- The Protection of Women from Domestic Violence Act, 2005
  (Act No. 43 of 2005, date 13.09.2006)
  (Wef 26.10.2006 vide So No. 1776 (E), date 17.10.2006)
  - "This is an Act to provide for more effective protection of the rights of women generated under the constitution who are victims of violence of any kind occurring within the family and for matters concerned therewith."

THE PROTECTION OF WOMEN FROM DOMESTIC VIOLENCE ACT, 2005

5 Chapters

- Chapter 1—Preliminary
- Chapter 2—Definitions
- Chapter 3—Power and Duties of Protection Officers (PRO Service Providers, Government, etc.)
- Chapter 4—Procedure for obtaining orders for relief
- Chapter 5—Miscellaneous penalty for breach of protection, not discharging duty or cognizance offence committed by PRO. Power of Central Government to make rules.

Types of Protection Given Under this Act

- Section 18—Protection Order
- Section 19—Residence Order—Providing the safe and secure shelter to live
- Section 20—Monitory Relief Order
- Section 21—Custody Order—custody of the child/children to aggrieved person or her relatives
- Section 22—Compensation order

Different Types of Violence as per Domestic Violence Act

- Physical violence
- Sexual violence
- Verbal and emotional violence
- Economic violence.

Protection Officers

- To be appointed by the State Government for every district.
- A Liaison Officer between the victim and the magistrate.
- Responsibility to safeguard aggrieved women, protect their rights and prepare application under Section 12.
- May be government officers or members from NGO's with 3 years experience in social sector; tenure—minimum 3 years—preferably woman.

DOMESTIC VIOLENCE—CONCLUSION

- DV is to be considered as a public health problem; It is the human rights violation.
- Constitutional provisions and other laws are generally protecting family system.
- Law alone cannot be a panacea to many of our social problems including DV.
- Education, equal opportunities, public opinion, attitudinal changes along with legislation can minimize the problem of DV.

- DV Laws are like double edged weapon; should be used only for protecting women and not taking revenge on men.

SUGGESTED READING

1. Brahma A. Pattern of domestic violence amongst non-fatal deliberate self-harm attempters. A study from primary care of West Bengal. Indian J Psychiatry, 2008;50:6.
2. Heru AM, Stuart GL, Rainey S, Eyre J, Recupero PR. Prevalence and severity of intimate partner violence and associations with family functioning and alcohol abuse in psychiatric inpatients with suicidal intent. Journal of Clinical Psychiatry, 2006;67: 23–29.
3. Kumar S. Domestic violence and its mental health correlates in Indian women. Br J Psych, 2005;187:62-67.
4. Myneni SR. Women and Law, 2003.
5. Nambi S. Legal aspects of Psychiatry—Indian perspective, 2009. Manashanthi Mental Health Care Publications, 2008.
6. Revathi R. Laws relating to domestic violence. Asia Law House, Hyderebad, 2004.
7. Srinivasaraghavan J. Domestic violence: A Community's response Annual National Congress of the Indian Psychiatric Society.
8. Surinder N and Sujatha K. 55th Annual Conference of the Indian Psychiatric Society, 2003.

22 Chapter

Medical Record Keeping in Psychiatric Practice

MEDICAL RECORDS IN PSYCHIATRIC PRACTICE

Information has been defined as "that which helps decision making". When one has to decide about a patient's management, the relevant information consists of clinical data (presenting symptoms, signs, laboratory results) and clinical knowledge (general facts about disease, how to interpret laboratory results, how to choose therapies, so on). Thus, we see that clinical data vary from patient to patient, while clinical knowledge applies to many patients. For the purpose of clinical knowledge, one can rely on journals, books, and bibliographic systems. For information about individual patients, medical records are essential.

The medical record has medicolegal, economic, educational, investigational and historical functions. Psychiatrists often are skeptical about the utility of these procedures and are irritated by having to comply with them.

However, it has been found that physicians who are informed about the various purposes of demands of accountability develop sensibility about what to be put in index record. Medical record is an important document, which contains information about the client's clinical data and all other clinical knowledge pertaining to him/her. The clinical data is the identification data of the client such as name, age, sex, date of birth, address, etc. Each client is given a separate identifying number. (Registration Number).

Significance of Medical Records

The purpose of the patient's medical record may be classified as follows:

Medical purposes: To assist in the physician's diagnosis, making process, and to serve as a record for teaching medicine.

Legal purposes: To document insurance claims for the patient and to serve as legal proof in case of malpractice, claims for injury or compensation, case of homicide or for disability certification.

Reimbursement: The medical records serve as a document based on which the patient can use it for claiming reimbursement.

The uses of the records for billing and legal purposes are secondary and should not interfere with good patient care.

Clinical Data

There are four major groups of clinical data:

- Subjective
- Objective
- Assessment
- Plan.

Subjective data consists of the patient's symptoms, clinical history, past medical history, and allergies. Objective data include the clinical signs observed. Assessment includes a diagnostic formulation, problem list, and casual explanation of findings. Plan includes diseases that must be ruled out and further course of action that has to be taken.

Errors in clinical data are bound to happen. This may be due to bad history taking, denial or less experience. Deliberate misrecording by the physician in order to avoid litigation is constantly increasing and is a cause of serious concern, and many psychiatrists follow defensive practice.

Medical Records

Medical records must be accurate, complete of what has been observed and done. The purpose of a medical record is to store, archive, and facilitate quick retrieval, so that, the psychiatrist can quickly answer questions like.

1. When did the problem start?
2. Has there been any thought or perceptual disturbance?
3. Has any medical illness been ruled out?
4. What is the clinical diagnosis? And
5. What was the treatment that was meted out?

Many medical records are evolving to be user friendly, physician oriented, that aids in the medicolegal scenario. The other functions of a medical record include the clinical research, auditing, education, health service management, and the most important function being that it serves as a medicolegal document.

The Components of an Ideal Medical Record

An ideal medical record must consist of all the information and each data should be entered only once. It should be accurate, complete, unambiguous, and portable. Only authorized persons should be allowed to enter the data and an accurate summary of the patient's record should be made. A copy of patient's summary must be retained and one copy must be sent to the source of referral. Retrieval should be fast, accurate and simple. Trained persons must be available. They must not erode the confidentiality or the doctor-patient relationship. Most of the record systems have been paper based, which has some disadvantages like they are bulky, they may be photocopied with chances of tampering are present, records can be missed, etc. As technology has advanced people are now resorting to paperless data.

Putting Additional Sheets in Medical Records

Every sheet in medical records, in both inpatient and outpatient department, must have the name of the patient and must be numbered serially. Medical records of the inpatients must be in continuity and timing of entries in proper sequence. The failure or neglect of a patient to follow advice or conduct investigations should be recorded specifically. Clinicians must update themselves with recent medical literature.

Correcting/Deleting Entries in Medical Records

Do not erase or put white ink on entries made in medical records. Instead, circle the wrong entry and write the correct entry besides it. Hospitals must formulate and implement appropriate protocols to ensure that only those doctors and nurses who are duly authorized and fully conversant with the patient's case, make entries in medical records. Take proactive steps to correct post procedure complaints/complications and duly record both, and the steps taken.

Stealing or Snatching of Medical Records by Patients/Relatives/Attendants

Instances of patients snatching or stealing medical records are becoming common. In such an eventuality, it is imperative to inform the local police station in writing, duly acknowledged and probably send a legal notice. Do not attend or attempt to treat a patient who is outside the scope of a speciality. Consultants must visit the patient at requisite intervals and must promptly state their opinion in writing.

Improving Conventional Records

Firstly, a problem-oriented medical record system (POMR) can be adopted. The contents are organized according to the presenting problems and the summary of the active and inactive symptoms are maintained. It has its own pitfalls.

Secondly, some departments use problem-focused proforma to act as a checklist and thus achieve standard and legible records, but the data format might not be acceptable to all the staff as it might be understandable, but filling up the proforma can become tedious.

Thirdly, the records can be handed over to the patient, but, unfortunately, the psychiatric patients brought their records in less than 50% of their review with the psychiatrist.

Fourthly, the arrangement of the records serially in a hanging file is found to be suitable.

In order to reduce bulk of the records, we can do microfiche filming. Micro filming may destroy dates which is printed in color or written faintly and so data retrieval becomes difficult. A document archival system has been introduced in which the documents are scanned by the computer and can be stored in an optical disk.

Computerized Medical Records

Computer-based record has been called as "an essential technology for health care". With the advent of the microcomputer in the 1980s, computer has become a common place in all healthcare settings.

Components and Techniques

A computer's concentration never fails, their logic and patience are inexhaustible and they excel at repetitive task. The hardware of a typical clinical data system includes:

1. Data input device
2. Data output device
3. Central processors
4. A temporary memory
5. Permanent memory in the form of a floppy, CD-ROM, or a pen-drive. "Local area and networking" usually link computers from the same building. "Wide area networking" allows faster links and greater choice of services such as file transfer through internet, etc.

Methods of Data Entry

Writing on paper is the most familiar way of recording data, but, transferring them to the computer is labour intensive and time-consuming. Many clinicians resent having to type the data. Keyboards are noisy and hazardous to health. Another method of data entry is through Windows, Icons, Menus, and Pointing device, "WIMP". An accuracy of 97% of limited vocabulary of 1000 to 2000 words is attainable after "training" to an individual's voice.

Inpatient Medical Records

The parts of the medical history follow the standardized sequence, differing only in small details. The detailed order can be as follows:

Identification data, chief complaints, a detailed history of the presenting complaints, past medical or psychiatric illnesses, family history, birth and developmental history, premorbid personality, sexual history, a complete physical examination, a complete mental status examination, laboratory and imaging studies, case summary, diagnostic formulation, and a diagnosis, assessment or problem list.

Plan

For each problem and the patient as a whole, we need to develop a plan. The plan for each problem has three parts:

1. Differential diagnosis
2. Therapy to be given
3. Education for the patient and the family.

Physician's Signature

Each medical record should be accompanied by the physician signature and the date and time of signing as proof of authorship. In the hospital record, the physician's initials alone are not inadequate. The complete written signature should be legible. All the dates should include the day, month and year. Progress notes of inpatients are made daily and whenever necessary.

Database: A database stores all the data in a form that computers can read. The following are some of the criteria for selecting a database program.

1. Can run on different operating systems (Windows, Macintosh).
2. Can use industry standard Structured Queering Language (SQL).
3. Allows import and export of data.
4. Allows data to be arranged and rearranged in different ways.
5. Will support use by a number of users simultaneously.
6. Supports a distributed data model.

The computerized record system has various advantages over the conventional record system. It has better quality of documentation, problem-oriented flow sheet, and summaries. It helps faster order of clinical tests in a prefilled form. It helps us as a reminder of our activities. It may provide an access for research and planning. If the database can handle images and sounds, multimedia, there will be an added advantage.

DEVELOPMENT AND IMPLEMENTATION

A system analyst captures users' needs on paper and writes detailed specification for the programme, which is turned into a computer programme by a programmer. The system is tested and operators are trained. Finally, a maintenance correction may be required. There is initial resistance to the installation of the computer in every institution. The anomalies which were previously suffered by human beings are exposed and the system usually slows down the productivity after the initial flaw thorn effect until the training and implementation is complete, after which there is no turning back.

It must not be forgotten that the system users are the key element in any computerized system. The clinician may distrust the system believing it to be the need of the administrators. Some clinicians may fear the junior doctors may outshine them because of their computer literacy. It is therefore very essential to empower ourselves in computer knowledge and to involve the clinical staff in all stages of development of the system.

Specialists in the burgeoning field of telemedicine envision enhanced development of interactive visual consultation from any remote source.

CONCLUSION

Medical records have to be tailor made according to each individual clinician and institution. The clinician has to judge what features are needed in their system in order to correct the balance between ease of data retrieval and security and to say whether the huge costs of a hospital-wide system with hundreds of terminals are warranted or not. Some institutions may have only a case register computerized (age, sex, diagnosis), some may computerize the whole recording and retrieval system. As professionals, we must decide what kind of clinical data system we need before the computer programmer installs the program. Finally, we must have a positive attitude towards computerization and must be motivated to update our knowledge on the computer daily.

SUGGESTED READING

1. Medical law Cases for Doctors, the Medical Law Reporter for Indian Doctors, Unichem, Issue 4.
2. Zhang Jun. Textbook of Diagnostics, Medical Records and Diagnostic Framework, 52nd Annual National Conference of the Indian Psychiatric Society and Indo-British-American Symposium, ANCIPS- 2000 Souvenir, Kochi (Kerala).

23 Chapter

Psychiatrist in the Court

PSYCHIATRISTS AND THE JUDICIARY

There is a need for perfection in knowledge and applications of law in clinical practice, which attained unprecedented importance. Psychiatry has become established as a medical speciality and psychiatrists now have achieved the status of an expert for the purpose of assisting the law in performing its role. Based on a plea of insanity, a psychiatrist can give evidence convincing a judge or judges that the crimes were committed as a result of his mental illness. Thus one can see that the psychiatrist owes a peculiar duty to himself and to his speciality to create an image of an individual, who is honest, truthful and objective.

Subpoena: The attendance of the witness can be assured by serving upon them in person, a witness summons (subpoena). The expert will be in contempt of court and liable to a penalty for non-attendance. Expert witnesses are professionals who know the importance of attending court.

THE PSYCHIATRIST AS A WITNESS

- As a witness to fact.
- As a professional witness (when the accused may happen to be his patient).
- As an expert witness. In most situations, the psychiatrist is involved as an expert witness. He is there because of the expertise he can provide to assist the court in understanding matters which are outside the courts competence or experience. He should not resent it as an intrusion on his time or be intimidated by the prospect.

Before going to court, prepare yourself: In all cases it is advisable to go over the case-files and documents briefly beforehand to refresh the memory. In criminal cases, it may be helpful to see the accused again before the proceedings start. This is particularly important where the issue is fitness to plead, i.e. for undertrials. Psychiatrists are expected to come to court with all his documents relating to the case. It is better off with more than less. Past reports, case notes, lab reports, anything that the court could ask for should be kept ready. It could save his trip back to court.

Witness in various courts: In the following courts, the psychiatrist may be summoned to give evidence.

- Civil courts
  - For assessing the mental capacity.
  - To clarify the earlier report.
  - Family court.
- Criminal courts.
- Others—Consumer protection commission: Negligence/malpractice.
  - NHRC/SHRC—Violation of human rights.
  - Any other enquiry commission

Giving evidence in criminal proceedings: Mostly psychiatrist report/certificate are not followed by a request to give oral evidence. The court accepts as it is, but in some situations, the (court feels that oral evidence is further required in the following instances. If the report is unclear, ambiguous, or equivocal and clarification is needed.

If the court finds it difficult to accept a opinion and requires persuasion.

- If the court has several reports with conflicting opinions, each of which needs to be evaluated.
- In specific cases where oral evidence is sometimes requested or may be obligatory. For example:
  - In support of a defense of criminal responsibility.
  - When the court is evaluating the future risk of the public.
  - In consideration of fitness to plead.

PSYCHIATRIST AS AN EXPERT IN THE COURT

The rule that an expert's opinion is admissible is to provide scientific information that is outside the experience or knowledge of the judge. It is not normally permissible for a psychiatrist to comment on the intent of the accused person; that is the role of a judge to decide. Psychiatric evidence may be given to show that a witness suffers from a disease, defect or abnormality of the mind that affects the reliability of his evidence. Despite these basic rules, exemptions and inconsistencies are common in jurisdiction throughout the world.

PSYCHIATRISTS IN THE WITNESS BOX

The performance in the witness box and the impression that the witness makes on the court are obviously, important in contributing successfully to the proceedings and their outcome. Establish a good rapport with the lawyer will help in many matters. In the early years of practice, an appearance in the witness box can seem a frightening ordeal. High court judges are to be addressed as "My Lord" or "My Lady". Sessions court judges are to be addressed as "Your Honor". Magistrate court judges are to be addressed as "Sir"/"Madam".

The psychiatrist should remember that his answers to questions are taken down or documented. Answer directly or simply to the questions which is asked. In cross examination, he may be asked to answer a question with a "Yes" or "No" only, but it is the duty of the psychiatrist with the permission of the magistrate/

judge to explain the facts to the court and to request the privilege of modifying the "Yes" or "No", so, that it may entirely represent the facts. In the "Witness Box", sometimes, the other party's lawyer may cross examine. The psychiatrist, sometimes feel that the lawyer's cross examination is threatening, hostile or even offensive. He must be careful, clear, honest and take no offence. The judges usually come for the rescue to protect the experts from unacceptable bullying. In the witness box, the psychiatrist may have his notes and papers in front of him and will be allowed to refer to them. The expert should speak up clearly and audibly. It is best to speak more slowly than one would in normal conversation. It is important for the expert to stick on to his own opinion. As experience is gained, many psychiatrist become increasing expert in giving evidence and as a result, they are a valuable asset to the justice system.

DO'S AS AN EXPERT EVIDENCE

- Try to present himself in a smart, confident, and professional way.
- The psychiatrist must be punctual.
- He must dress appropriately.
- Appear confident (but not arrogant).
- Speak clearly and audibly.
- Keep to the point.
- Evidence should be comprehensible and simple language.
- Keeps sentences short.

DON'TS AS AN EXPERT EVIDENCE

- Do not use jargon.
- Do not use technical expressions not generally understandable by a lay person.
- Do not use words of foreign origin, (e.g. cyclothymia instead of "mood swings").
- Do not use polysyllabic or uncommon words.
- Do not lose your temper even if provoked by the council.
- Do not confront.

THE PSYCHIATRIST AS A DEFENDANT

1. When people get more awareness of their rights they would like to claim compensation for real or imagined wrongful acts by the doctors.
2. In this regard, psychiatrists will have to defend themselves in cases of so called negligence. Hence, maintaining good records or notes will be of much helpful to the doctor.
3. The psychiatrist should be aware of the fact that "Ignorance of the law is not a defence."
4. The doctor should be courteous that when acting in good faith, sometimes they tend to break the provisions of MHA. He should be in a position to tell that the civil procedures for admission were followed.

RIGHTS OF EXPERT WITNESSES

The expert witness has several rights in court (Danner, 1983).

1. If the expert is unclear about how they should answer a question, or whether they must answer the question posed, they may ask the judge.
2. The expert may ask the judge whether the material asked for is privileged.
3. The expert may refuse to answer questions that they do not understand. They may also ask examining counsel to clarify or repeat the question.

CREDIBILITY OF EXPERT WITNESS

The expert witness's style of speech has considerable impact on his or her credibility (Lubet, 1998).

In controlled studies of mock testimony, powerful speech was found to be more convincing and credible than powerless speech (Conley, Obar, and Lind, 1978). Powerless speech tends to make more frequent use of the following (Erickson, et al. 1978);

1. Intensifiers (so, very, surely): I surely did.
2. Hedges (Kind of, I think, I guess).
3. Especially formal grammar.
4. Hesitation forms (uh, well, you know).
5. Gestures (using the hands to point while saying "over there").
6. Questioning forms (rising, question intonation in declarative contexts).
7. Excessive politeness (please, thank you, sir).

ABUSE OF PSYCHIATRIC TESTIMONY

- Needel (1980) identified three possibilities for the potential abuse of psychiatric testimony.
- Experts who offer biased opinions based on either calculated or unconscious prejudices.
- Physicians lacking in psychiatric sophistication who give psychiatric testimony.
- Fully qualified experts who unintentionally or through laziness perform an examination that does not serve as a professionally adequate basis for their conclusions.

THE ETHICAL PROBLEMS FOR PSYCHIATRISTS IN THE COURT

Often the psychiatrist are used as a "Hired Gun" withholding part of the truth to endorse a particular legal position and giving testimony without adequate knowledge. It is wrong to devote too much time to court work, when skilled professional services are in such short supply (Gunn, 1991). Long wrangles in court may be entertaining but often they have little impact on the patients future and they can divert the doctor away from treatment.

THE MYTH AND REALITY OF EXPERT EVIDENCE

Psychiatrist believe that the expert evidence they give in the "Court of Law" is unbiased and unprejudiced and is going to be the most valuable evidence in deciding the case. But, many forensic psychiatrist have had the painful experience of learning that their report is not used (or) expert is to be requested to examine the case (or) that the report is not to be shown to the court fully, but selected aspects will be used to assist in eliciting oral evidence. Psychiatrists must also face cross examination which may tend to place him in a negative and defensive position.

SUGGESTED READING

1. Bhujang PM. Mentally ill and the law. Universal Publishing Corporation, 2003.
2. Blueglass R, Bowden P. Principles and practice of forensic psychiatry, 1990.
3. Nambi S. Legal aspects of psychiatry—Indian perspective. Manashanthi Mental Health Care Pvt Ltd, 2008.
4. Rix KJB. The psychiatrist as expert witness. Part 2: Criminal Cases and the Royal College of Psychiatrists Guidance. Advances in psychiatric treatment, 2008;14:109-14.
5. Somasundaram O. Criminal responsibility—An overview. Indian journal of psychological medicine, 2001.
6. Tasman A, Kay J, Lieberman JA. Psychiatry, volume 1. Advances in Psychiatric Treatment, John Wiley and Sons Ltd, 2008.

24 Chapter

Rights of the Mentally Ill and the Responsibilities of the Caregivers

INTRODUCTION

Right is a power, privilege, demand or claim possessed by a particular person by virtue of law. Every legal right that one person possesses, imposes corresponding legal duties on other persons.

Protection of human rights of persons suffering from mental disorder is the basic responsibility of the caregiver, community, and the Government. Even though, there are many laws and legislations enacted, still there is violation of human rights of persons suffering from mental disorder in many of our houses, public places, and in other situations. First, we have to understand what is meant by right Human Rights.

HUMAN RIGHTS

"The aim of all political association is the conservation of the natural indisputable rights of man".—Loche

"Human Rights are rights which all persons equally have simply so far as they are human".—Gewirth

Human Rights are the rights relating to life, liberty, equality, and dignity of the individual guaranteed by the Constitution or embodied in the International Covenants and enforceable by Courts in India. Section 2(d), Protection of Human Rights Act, 1993.

HUMAN RIGHTS IN INDIA

Refers to:

- Rights relating to life
- Rights relating to liberty
- Rights relating to equality and
- Rights relating to dignity of the individual.

HOW DOES LEGISLATION HELP TO PROTECT THE RIGHTS OF THE MENTALLY ILL

Legislation can assist persons with mental disorders to receive an appropriate care and treatment. It can protect and promote rights and prevent discrimination.

It can also uphold specific rights, such as the right to vote, to property, to freedom of association, to a fair trial, to judicial guarantees and review of detentions, protection in such areas as housing and employment. Criminal Justice Legislation can ensure appropriate treatment and protection of rights of mentally ill offenders.

INTERNATIONAL MOVEMENTS IN PROTECTING THE RIGHTS OF THE MENTALLY ILL

Key International and Regional Human Rights Instruments Related to the Rights of People with Mental Disorders

- International and Regional Human Rights Instruments
- International Bill of Rights
- Other International Convention Related to Mental Disorders.

Major Human Rights Standards Application to Mental Health

- UN principles for the protection of persons with Mental Health
- Standard Rules on the Equalization of Opportunities for Persons with Disabilities (Standard Rules, 1993).

Technical Standards

- Declaration of Caracas (1990)
- Declaration of Madrid (1996)
- WHO Technical Standards
- The Salamanca Statement and Framework for Action on Special Needs Education (1994).

INTERNATIONAL HUMAN RIGHTS DOCUMENTS BROADLY FALL INTO TWO CATEGORIES

1. Those which legally bind states that have ratified such conventions.
2. Those referred to as international human rights "standards", which are considered guidelines for framing laws concerned with upholding human rights of mentally ill persons.

Human Rights of Persons with Mental Disorders in India

- Constitution of India
- Mental Health Act, 1987
- Persons with Disabilities Act, 1975 and National Trust Act, 1999
- Mental Health Care Act, 2010 – Draft
- National and State Human Rights (Human Rights Commission)
- Protection of Human Rights Act, 1999
- Right to Information Act
- Courts Directives and Public Interest Litigation (PILs)

- The Rehabilitation Council of India Act, 1992
- National Trust Act, 1999
- UN Convention on Rights of Persons with Disabilities, 2006.

Six Fundamental Rights

- Right to Equality (Article 14–18)
- Right to Freedom (Article 19–22)
- Right Against Exploitation (Article 23 and 24)
- Right to Freedom of Religion (Article 25–28)
- Cultural and Educational Rights (Article 29 and 30)
- Right to Constitutional Remedies (Article 32)

MENTAL HEALTH ACT, 1987 (PROTECTION OF HUMAN RIGHTS OF MENTALLY ILL PERSONS)

As per Chapter VIII, Section 81.

No mentally ill person shall be subjected during treatment to any indignity (whether physical or mental) or cruelty.

No mentally ill person under treatment shall be used for purposes of research, unless such research is of direct benefit to him for purposes of diagnosis or treatment.

The mentally ill person or his guardian should give informed consent before any research procedure begins.

No letters or other communications sent by or to a mentally ill person under treatment shall be intercepted, detained or destroyed.

Rights of the Disabled Under the Disabilities Act, 1995

Mental illness and mental retardation are two of the six disabilities mentioned in this Act.

The cardinal rights of the disabled which are enshrined in the name of the Act itself are as follows:

1. Rights to equal opportunity with the non-disabled.
2. Right to protection of the legal rights of the disabled.
3. Right to full participation in the affairs of the life at par with those who are nondisabled.
4. The disabled have been statutorily recognized by this Act and the various forms of disability have been given legal definition.
5. The disabled have the right to be taken care of and rehabilitated in the mainstream of life in terms of this Act and the Government and other authorities and establishments covered by this Act have an obligation to fulfill their duties towards the disabled in the light of the provisions contained in this Act.
6. It is the duty of the central and State Governments to take preventive steps so that the occurrence of disabilities is arrested, provide training to

the staff at primary health centers, improve hygiene health and sanitation measures, screen children at least once a year to indentify risky cases, provide for prenatal, perinatal and postnatal care of mother and child and create awareness amongst the people on the causes and measures to be taken to prevent disability.

7. Every child with disability is entitled to free education in appropriate environment upto the age of 18 years and the Government should set up special schools for imparting special education, promote integration of disabled students in normal schools and provide opportunities for vocational training to disabled children.
8. Disabled children having studied upto fifth class can continue their education as part-time students, through open schools or open universities and are entitled to special books and equipments free of cost from the Government.
9. It is the Government's duty to develop new assistive devices, teaching aids and special teaching material so that disabled children may have equal opportunities in education. The Government has to set up teacher training institutions for training children with disabilities and prepare comprehensive education schemes providing for transport facilities to disabled children to attend school, provide books, uniforms, other materials to them, scholarships, restructured curriculam and amanuensis for blind students.
10. There shall be reservation of posts for the disabled upto one precent each for those who have blindness, impaired hearing or cerebral palsy for which posts will be identified by the Government every three years. Vacancies not filled up can be carried forward to the next year.
11. Special employment exchange to provide for the disabled who seek employment has to be set up by the Government.
12. All Government educational institutions and aided institutions shall reserve upto 3% seats for persons with disabilities. Vacancies are to be reserved in poverty alleviation schemes. Incentives are also to be given to employers to ensure that 5% of workforce is composed of disabled persons.
13. Disabled persons will also be entitled to preferential allotment of land at concessional rates for housing and for rehabilitation purposes.
14. There shall be no discrimination of the disabled in transport facilities, traffic signals on the road, or in built environments. Neither shall there be any discrimination of the disabled in matters of government employment.
15. The Government will regulate recognition of institutions for the disabled or for those with severe disability.
16. The chief commissioner and the State Commissioners will look into the complaints with respect to matters relating to deprivation of rights of the disabled.

17. The Government and local authorities shall undertake rehabilitation of the disabled, grant aid to Non-Government Organizations, devise insurance schemes, for the disabled employees and also frame unemployment allowance scheme for the disabled.
18. Those who avail or attempt to avail benefits meant for the disabled in a fraudulent manner are punishable with imprisonment upto two years or with payment of fine upto ₹ 20,000/–.

Mental Heath Care Act, 2010—(Draft)

Provides the following rights for persons with mental illness:

- Right to access Mental Health Care.
- Right to community living.
- Right to protection from cruelty, inhuman, and degrading treatment.
- Right to equality and nondiscrimination.
- Right to information.
- Right to confidentiality.
- Access to medical records.
- Right to personal contacts and communication.
- Right to make complaints about deficiencies in provision of services.

Right to Access Mental Health Care

All mentally ill persons have a right to access mental health care and treatment from Mental Health Services run or funded by the government. The services should be easily accessible, available, affordable and acceptable by the patients and their caregivers. The services provided include outpatient facilities, aide and long-term care, rehabilitation services or services for special population like children and old age. Mental Health Services shall be integrated into General Health Care Services. As far as possible community based treatment in coordination in their families are to be encouraged than long-term hospital-based treatment. The Mental Health Services should be available at a closed reach and not far away. Persons with below poverty line should be entitled for free treatment. There should not be any discrimination in quality of services. Essential drugs enumerated by who shall be available free of cost to all persons. The government shall allot adequate budgetary provisions for Mental Health Care. The progress of the Mental Health Services should be submitted periodically to the parliament by the Central government and to the Assembly by the State (Government).

Right to Community Living

Persons with mental illness have a right to live with their family in the community. Even if they do not have a home, the Government should provide restrictive community based facility including halfway homes, group homes, etc.

Right to Protection from Cruel, Inhuman and Degrading Treatment

- All persons with mental illness have the right to live with dignity.

- No such person shall be subjected to any cruel, inhuman or degrading treatment in a Mental Health Facility, (MHF).
- They should have safe and hygienic environment, adequate sanitary conditions, facilities for recreation, education and religious practices, privacy especially for women.
- Should not be forced to work in a Mental Health Facility; adequate preparation to live in the community, adequate space and food, women should be provided with sanitary napkins, no compulsory tonsuring, uniform should not be made compulsory, protection from all physical, emotional and or sexual abuse.

Right to Equality and Nondiscrimination

Mentally ill persons are to be treated equally with persons with physical illness. No discrimination based on gender, sex, sexual orientation, religion, culture, caste, social or political beliefs or disability. Medical Insurance for mental illness to be provided like physical illness. Emergency services—ambulance services are essential. Living conditions and any other health services provided to physical illness are to be provided for mental illness.

Right to Information

A person with mental illness or his nominated representative shall have the right to know the following:

- The section under which he is admitted in Mental Health Facility.
- Right to apply for review of admission.
- The nature of mental illness and the proposed treatment plan.
- In the language that the person can understand.
- In the event that complete information is to be provided when the person recovers from the illness. His representative has to be provided with the information immediately.

Right to Confidentiality

The mentally ill person has a right to confidentiality in the context of his mental health and mental health care. All information obtained should be kept in confidential with some exceptions. Right to confidentiality also applies to all information stored in electronic and/or digital format.

Access to Medical Records

Mentally ill persons shall have access to their medical records except in certain situations which may harm the patient. If the information in the medical record is withheld from the mentally ill person, the mentally ill person can apply to the District Panel of Mental Health Review Commission.

Right to Personal Contact and Communication

A person admitted in a Mental Health Facility has the right to receive visitors and make phone calls. If visitors or phone calls are restricted due to some reasons, the persons can apply to the District Panel of Mental Health Review Commission. Mentally ill person in Mental Health Facility can send and receive mail and email. The Medical Officer of Mental Health Facility may restrict some mail or calls but shall not do for the mails or calls from the Court, District Panel of MHRC, SMHA, any MP or MLA, nominated representative, lawyer or legal representative of the person.

Rights to Legal Aid

The person with mental illness shall be entitled to receive free legal services to exercise any of his or her rights under the Legal Services Authorities Act, 1987 and provide the contact details of the availability of the services.

Right to Make Complaints about Deficiencies in Provision of Services

Mentally ill persons admitted in Mental Health Facility has the right to complain regarding deficiencies in provision of care and services. The Medical Officer in charge of the facility. If not satisfied with the response, State Mental Health Authority. If not satisfied with the response, District Panel of Mental Health Review Commission. Judicial appeal is different in addition to complaints with District MHRC.

Human Rights Issues

India is a party to the International Covenant on Civil and Political Rights, and the International Covenant on Economic, Social and Cultural Rights, adopted by the General Assembly of the United Nations on 16th December 1966. After a series of meetings and debates, the Human Rights Commission Bill, 1993 was placed in the Lower House of the Indian Parliament on 14th May 1993. The Protection of Human Rights Ordinance, 1993 was promulgated by the President of India on 28th September 1993 and came to be known as the Protection of Human Rights Act, 1993. This Act further strengthened the provisions under Section 81 of the MHA, 1987 and was welcomed by mental health professionals of the country.

At present, there is a National Human Rights Commission (NHRC) at the centre and a Human Rights Commission (HRC) in every state of India. The recent initiative taken by the NHRC for the overall development of mental hospitals in the country is noteworthy, e.g. Quality Assurance in Mental Health Projects (Channabasavanna, personal communication). Similarly, different states HRCs have taken initiatives to upgrade the state mental hospitals. The initiatives and interventions of the HRCs of Assam, Madhya Pradesh and West Bengal are noteworthy. The HRCs also taken a serious view of any maltreatment of the mentally ill (West Bengal HRC, 1998).

Section 3—"The rights relating to life, liberty, equality and dignity of the individual guaranteed by the constitution are embodied in the International Covenant and enforceable in the Courts of India."

THE NATIONAL HUMAN RIGHTS COMMISSION (NHRC)

The Protection of Human Rights Act, 1993 (PHRA)

Provides for the establishment of a:

- National Human Rights Commission
- State Human Rights Commission in States and
- Human Rights Court.

Functions

Inquires suo moto or on a petition presented to it by a victim or any person on his behalf into complaint of violation of human rights or abetment these of negligence in the prevention of such violation by a public servant and others.

NHRC has given guidelines on various issues like postmortem, etc. which includes guidelines relating to administration of polygraphic test (Lie Detector Test) No. 117/8/97-98 NHRC.

Human Rights Commission Report, 2002

- The National Human Rights Commission (NHRC) has conducted a detailed study of government mental hospitals.
- Of the thirty-three facilities the NHRC studied, all had closed/locked wards, nineteen had no open wards, fourteen had a "jail like structure," sixteen had solitary confinement cells, eighteen did not have a clinical psychologist, and eighteen administered electro-convulsive therapy without anesthesia.
- In sum, the NHRC concluded that "the state of mental health care in the country ... is very poor and the living conditions are horrible."

  Supreme Court of India

  17 April 2002 (334/2001)

  August 6, 2001.

Death of 25 chained inmates in asylum fire in Tamil Nadu a 'spark' for many changes in India.

Erwadi Tragedy and the Supreme Court Intervention

- Even though the MHA was enacted in 1987 and the Government ordered its implementation from 1st April 1993, many States in practice were not implementing the MHA .
- Only after the *Erwadi Tragedy* some years back the Supreme Court ordered all the States to implement the MHA in letter and spirits.
- Even in the adverse situation this order comes as a blessing to protect the rights of the mentally ill.

PUBLIC INTEREST LITIGATIONS

- Dramatic changes in Mental Health Care due to PIL and Supreme Court directives.
- Services of PILs since 1982 (Veena Sethi vs State of Bihar) were successful in initiating reforms.
- Revolutionary change of pathetic Shahdara Mental hospital to IHBAS in Delhi (PIL—1983, Kanpur vs Union of India).
- Similar charges in Agra, Gwalior, Tejpur, Pune and Ranchi.
- "No person should be kept in jail purely on grounds of mental illness", Supreme Court Judgement. (PIL—1989, Sheela Barse vs Union of India.)
- "It is preferable to use modified ECT, under proper supervision", Bombay Highcourt Judgement in 1998 on a civil writ petition.

RIGHTS OF THE MENTALLY ILL PRISONERS

In India, there is no uniform mechanism for providing psychiatric care to mentally ill people in prisons. Each state has its own rules, regulations, and provisions. For decades, may mentally ill, both those with criminal record and those with no criminal record have been admitted to jails especially so in the Eastern part of India.

DETENTION OF NON-CRIMINAL MENTALLY ILL IN THE PRISONS

Following a PIL, the Supreme Court in its verdict, July 18, (1993), on the famous Ms Sheela Barse vs Union Government of India Categorically said "The admission of non-criminal mentally ill persons to jails is illegal and unconstitutional." This protects the Human Rights of the Non-Criminal Mentally Ill, who were kept inside the prisons of many States especially the West Bengal.

THE RIGHTS OF THE LESBIANS AND GAY PEOPLE

Lesbians, Gay men and Bi-sexual and Transgender people all over the world suffer persecution and violence simply for being who they are. They are tortured or ill treated. They are attacked in their homes as well as in the communities to punish and intimidate because of their sexual orientation or gender identity. They are targeted because, their real or perceived sexual identity is seen as threatening the social order. The conspiracy of silence about the torture and ill treatment of lesbian, gay and bi-sexual and transgender people as been broken. Human Rights defence have emerged in many countries around the world. Campaigning for an end to violence and discrimination based sexual identity and to ensure equal dignity and rights for all. ("Crimes of hate, conspiracy of silence"—Amnesty International Publication, 2001)

RIGHT TO REFUSE TREATMENT

It is not legally accepted in India. Historically, the right of mentally ill persons to refuse treatment have been limited compared to persons without mental illness.

Along with development of Mental Health Care in the West, the evolution of the informed consent doctrine and public perception about the quality of care delivered in Institutions—all played important roles with regard to the currently recognized right to refuse treatment. (Applebaum, 1994; Winick, 1997).

Reasons for Refusal

- Actual side effects of medication.
- Illness related –
  - Due to denial of their illness.
  - Delusions about treatment.
  - These people "Pose the greatest clinical challenges".
  - Angry and disagreement about the need to be helpless.

HUMAN RIGHTS ISSUE GIVEN IMPORTANCE IN THE ENSUING MENTAL HEALTH CARE BILL, 2012

Compulsory tonsuring—a common practice on patients of mental illnesses, is all set to be banned. When admitted in any mental institute, such patients will wear their personal clothes and not be forced to wear uniforms provided by the establishment. Now, menstrual care of women mental illness patients will be taken care by the institute.

Instead of being dark and dingy, like many such institutes are, the mental homes will need to have facilities for leisure, recreation and religious practices for patients.

A mental health establishment can also not force inmates to undertake work they do not wish to do. Patients will have to be paid an "appropriate remuneration for the work when undertaken". With one in four families likely to have at least one member with a behavioral or mental disorder in the country, the new Mental Health Care Bill includes some patient-friendly provisions.

DUTIES OF THE FAMILY MEMBERS/CAREGIVERS

It is the responsibility of the family members or the caregivers to get Reception Order from the magistrate through an application. So that their mentally ill person who is refusing to take treatment at home can be admitted in a psychiatric hospital as an involuntary patient. If the family members prefer and admit a mentally ill person through a Reception Order, based on their application in a private hospital or nursing home, it is the duty and responsibility of the family members to pay the cost of maintenance of the mentally ill person. The family members are responsible persons to take care of their mentally ill relative. In case, if the court finds that the mentally ill person is cruelly treated and not under proper care and control that will amount to willful negligence and the relatives shall be punishable with fine which may extend to ₹ 2000.

RESPONSIBILITIES OF THE MANAGER/GUARDIAN OF MENTALLY ILL PERSONS

As per MHA (Section 60)

The manager appointed by the Court under MHA 1987, within six months time should submit a detailed financial report of the patient including his immovable property, other assets, debts and liabilities to the court. The manager should submit the accounts of the property of assets periodically within three months to the court.

- The manager under the direction of District Court.
- Can perform contracts of the mentally ill persons.
- Can dispose of the business premises.
- May dispose of leases.
- If the manager does not perform the duties as per the order of the court the Court may take action against him or may remove him from his guardianship or manager.

DUTIES OF GOVERNMENT

Promotion of mental health and preventive programmes. Creating Awareness about mental health and illness and reducing stigma associated with mental illness. Providing adequate human resource and training. Coordination within the government.

CONCLUSION

Protection of the Human rights of the mentally ill is a positive intent, this demands special legislations. Mental illness should not be viewed as either a "Medical" or "Legal" conditions alone, but as a sociological dimension is needed. Justice Venkatachalliah's Landmark Judgement in the Supreme Court (1988) is a welcome step. Exclusive judicial preoccupation with the medical concept of mental illness is not preferable

The protection of human rights of mentally ill has come to a reasonably accepted state in the law in our country. If we are going to fully implement the constitution of India, the persons with disabilities act and the forthcoming MHC Act 2010 which is expected to replace the Mental Health Act, 1987.

SUGGESTED READING

1. A Handbook on the Right of Information Act, 2005 C Sitaraman and Co Pvt Ltd, 2011. Who Resource Book on Mental Health, Human Rights and Legislation, 2005.
2. Amendments Proposed to the Persons with Disabilities Act, 1995. Ministry of Social Justice and Empowerment, Government of India.
3. Dhanda A. Legal Order and Mental Disorder. Sage Publications, New Delhi, 2000.
4. Bhugra D. Handbook of Psychiatry—A South Asian Perspective; Byword Viva Publisher Pvt Ltd, 2005.

5. Mental Health Care Act, 2010, Ministry of Health and Family Welfare, Government of India, New Delhi.
6. Nambi S. Forensic psychiatry: Psychiatry and law, Indian perspective. Manashanthi Mental Health Care Pvt Ltd, 2011.
7. National Project on preventing torture in India. People's Watch, Tamil Nadu, 2006.
8. The Mental Health Act, 1987. Universal Law Publishing Company, New Delhi, 2004.
9. WHO Resource Book on Mental Health, Human Rights and Legislation.
10. Working Draft of the Rights of persons with Disabilities Act, 2010. Centre for Disability Studies, NALSAR, University of Law, Hyderabad, India.

25 Chapter

Medicolegal Implications Where Psychiatrists can be Involved

INTRODUCTION

A Thorough Understanding of the Statutory Regulations of this Country

All practicing psychiatrists should understand the basic fact that legislation forms an essential component of the mental health care delivery. Hence, a good understanding and knowledge of various laws and legislations involved with mental health practice is very essential with practice of psychiatry.

The public awareness about mental illness is increasing. The role of media in propagating various negligence and deficits are gaining momentum. The literary rate is growing gradually in our country. With all the above reasons, more and more public turn out to be litigious. Sometimes, it is inevitable that each person is in a dilemma as to whether the doctor who is treating him is doing so efficiently or may commit some mistake. The other side of the table, the psychiatrist becomes paranoid as to whether the patient will become a litigant. Hence, there is a prevailing suspicious mood in the doctor-patient relationship and the psychiatrist prefers to have a defensive practice. Even though, medicolegal against doctors are increasing day-by-day, the cases against the psychiatrists are only few in our country. That does not mean that psychiatric professional must be indifferent and ignorant towards medicolegal implications and they must be cautious in their day-to-day practice and they should be careful and vigilant in treating each and everyone of their patients. There are several areas to be considered in this aspect:

Duties and Obligations

a. Good understanding of the rules and regulations existing in India relating to mental disorders.
b. **Documentation:** This is the best defense in case of any medicolegal case against the psychiatrists. The documentation must be correct, up-to-date and medical records should be carefully preserved. It is essential that every event of the illness of the person getting treated has to be recorded in a detailed manner.

   There should not be any effort to suppress, alter or manipulate any mishap or failure, which is likely to be found out. If any such thing is done and if it is likely to be found out, it will act as a proof of guilt on the part of the doctor.

It is always prudent to be straight forward and truthful. One should stick to the facts even if there is some mistake, it is better to record the same and later defend one's case. All the investigations, side or adverse effects, the progress of the illness, good or bad outcome, however, minor, it must be recorded in the case record file then and there. If something is done, (e.g. An investigation) and it is not recorded, it is considered not to be done. In good clinical practice, if something is not recorded, that means it is not done.

c. **Importance of medical records:** Medical records are very important documents, which are useful for clinical diagnosis and treatment follow-up cases research, certification, insurance claims, and as documentary evidence in enquires and judicial proceedings.
d. **Certification:** Psychiatrists are to issue certificate about their patient's mental status on different situations of a psychiatrist certifies that a person is suffering from severe mental illness that means that has lot of future complications including civil and criminal responsibility. A certificate should be complete in the sense it should contain the patient's name, age, sex, occupation, date of admission, date of discharge (if he or she is an inpatient) and thorough notes of the complaints history, thorough physical and mental status examination necessary investigation and their results and the psychiatrist's opinion about the diagnosis and future advice—all these have to be mentioned and if something is not clear, it is better to mention the same instead of guesswork.
e. **Expert evidence**: Psychiatrists are required to give evidence as an expert witness in the court of law. The Indian Evidence Act, 1858 (Section 45 and 46) provides, for the opinion of experts who have special skills, training, and experience. Medical professional including psychiatrists are also privileged witnesses under this section Expert witnesses have the following privileges:
   - Permitted to refer to other cases
   - Take assistance of notes, books, etc.
   - Give opinion.

Expert witness may be requested for variety of purposes both in civil and criminal issues. Psychiatrists should not be reluctant to attend course or to give opinion regarding the cases which they treat. It is the duty of every psychiatrist to assist in the process of justice.

Court Attendance

In case of court attendance as an expert witness, the psychiatrist should note the following points:

1. He should accept the summons issued by the court and except on a dire emergency he should present himself in the Court of Law in the specified date and time.
2. He has to prepare himself by going through the mental and the clinical details along with the relevant documents.
3. The psychiatrist must be polite and answer only to the questions in a simple and clear language and he is in a position to tell only the facts and should

not express his emotions. Always, he should remember that he is in the court premises and not in the hospital sittings. He should remember whatever he has conveyed as an expert witness, it is up to the judge to decide about how much he can take up.

Complaints Against Psychiatrist

Complaints against psychiatrist and psychiatric hospital and nursing homes are not uncommon. These complaints can be under different provisions and platforms.

a. **Professional bodies:** In the case of psychiatrist, who is also a medical doctor, a complaint can be lodged in the State or Central Medial Council for any malpractice or misconduct. Similarly, a complaint can be lodged against the psychiatrist in Indian Psychiatrist Society also. These professional bodies will conduct inquiry, and if found guilty, the psychiatrist will be punished accordingly.
b. **Civil:** This involves the following—Tort: Tort is a civil wrong, breach of contract or breach of trust. The purpose of Law of Tort is to compensate these people who have started laws for damage as a consequence of their legal rights being violated. Negligence, nuisance, trespass, are some of the examples of tort. Medical negligence is usually considered on the principles laid down in "Law of Tort."

Contract

When the patient approaches a psychiatrist or psychiatric nursing home/hospital, the relationship between the psychiatrist/hospital and patient is contractual in nature. Breach of contract entitles the suffered parties the remedies, which are specified in the contract itself.

Consumer Protection Act (CPA), 1986

In the recent past, Consumer Protection Act has gained much competence and at times looked upon by the mentally persons as a constant threat. CPA is trying to protect the interest of the consumers (patients and their relatives and providing them means to get quick justice. CPA is applicable where the patients are charged with fees, where no fees are charged, CPA is not applicable.

Statutory

The affairs of the mentally ill were common under the person of Mental Health Act, 1987 till today. Soon, the new Act, Mental Health Care Act is expected to replace Mental Health Act.

Criminal

Normally, the criminal liability of any particular offence or offences is related to an identifiable individual or group of individuals. In some exceptional circumstances, the entity that is hospital may be made responsible. Section 304A.

Indian Penal Code (IPC) causing death by negligence. Whoever causes death of any person by doing any rash Act not admitting to culpable homicide, shall be punished with imprisonment of either description for a term which may extend 22 years or with fine or both.

Section 337 of IPC—Rash or Negligent Act resulting in simple hurt. Section 338 of IPC Rash or Negligence Act resulting in previous hurt. Liability may also arise for violation of other acts.

SUGGESTED READING

1. Bhujang PM. Mentally ill and the law. Universal Publishing Corporation, 2003.
2. Blueglass R, Bowden P. Principles and practice of forensic psychiatry, 1990.
3. Nambi S. Legal aspects of psychiatry—Indian perspective, 2009. Manashanthi Mental Health Care Pvt Ltd, 2008.
4. Rix KJB. The psychiatrist as expert witness. Criminal cases and the royal college of psychiatrists guidance. Advances in Psychiatric Treatment, 2008;14:10-9-14.
5. Somasundaram O. Criminal responsibility—An overview. IJPM, 2001.
6. Tasman A, Kay J, Lieberman JA. Psychiatry. Advances in psychiatric treatment, Volume I. John Wiley & Sons, Ltd; 2008.

26 Chapter

Certification in Psychiatry

INTRODUCTION

Psychiatrists are increasingly requested to provide a report/certificate in connection with the administration, legal process for welfare measures. Many psychiatrists find that issuing a certificate is an integral part of their professional work. The role of the psychiatrist in providing medicolegal opinion on behalf of the patient can be as important as making a diagnosis or providing treatment for the patient. The dictionary meaning of a medical certificate is straightforward—a document stating the result of a satisfactory medical examination. Medical certificate is usually issued regarding the treatment of illness, types of illness, recommendation for leave and fitness for duties. Certification for mental illness may be for different purposes such as certification for admission in a psychiatric hospital. Presently, certificates in psychiatry are issued for many purposes other than for committing a patient for hospitalization.

A certificate may be required in psychiatric practice in the following areas:
- Medical leave
- Fitness to resume duty
- Certificate for invalidation from service.

EMPLOYMENT—MENTAL FITNESS

- Matrimonial matters—from family courts for divorce/separation.
- Civil matters—appointment of guardian/managers.
- Disability certificate—for family person and other welfare measures.
- IT exemption.
- Child custody.
- Sexual matters.
- Admission to psychiatric hospital.
- Criminal responsibility.

THE COMMON CAUSES OF REFERRAL FOR CERTIFICATION/ REPORTING

Civil

- Guardianship
- Family pension

- Divorce/separation
- Child custody
- Sexual tests.

Criminal

- To ascertain the criminal responsibility
- Fitness to stand trial
- Rape.

Who can Certify

As specified in the Medical Council of India (MCI) code of medical ethics, registered practitioners are in certain cases bound by the law, to give certificates, notifications, reports or other documents signed by them in their professional capacity for subsequent use in the courts of law for administrative purposes. Any such certificate, report or document which is untrue, misleading or improper is liable to have the doctor's name erased from the Medical Council Register.

Good and Bad Certificates

The certificates and reports display one aspect of the public face of psychiatry. A well-crafted report demonstrates objectivity, detachment, humanity and professionalism. A carelessly constructed report reveals much about the author, does little for the patient and does less for the credibility and image of the profession of psychiatry.

The Structure of the Written Report/Certificate

Psychiatrists vary greatly in how they prefer to present information in reports. Following are some genreal points:

1. A court report/certificate is not a formulation or case presentation, rather, it is presentation of psychiatric information for a non-psychiatric purpose.
2. Clarity is crucial.
3. Avoidance of over inclusiveness and pursuit of legal relevance should be the aim.
4. Technical terms should be avoided wherever possible. If included, then definition and explanation must also be offered.
5. Only facts and opinions that can be sustained under cross-examination should be included. Always indicated the sources of those facts.
6. The defendant may see the report/certificate during subsequent hospital treatment or legal information about others.
7. Avoid disclosing privileged information about others.
8. Remember that others might use the report/certificate during subsequent hospital treatment or legal information about others.
9. Be specific and avoid general terms.
10. Give reasons for conclusions.

11. Avoid value-laden statements.
12. Exclude psychiatric information not directly relevant to the purpose.
13. Include only limited background information.
14. Try to preserve the confidentiality of the report/certificate.

Certification in Civil Matters

The judicial declaration of liability to manage affairs due to unsoundness of mind differs other investigations of mental incapacity because it determines civil stability. Once a person is declared of unsound mind, she/he cannot participate in any legal transactions, in relations to his or her property, even during a lucid interval, while the certificate remains in force. A finding of incapacity in these proceedings is prima facie evidence of unsoundness of mind in all other legal proceedings. Such certificate can also cause loss of personal autonomy.

PSYCHIATRIC ISSUES IN REPORTS FOR THE CRIMINAL COURTS

- Fitness to plead
- Fitness to stand trial
- Mental state at the time of the alleged offense
- Any psychiatric factors that might assist in understanding or explaining behavior, or have a bearing on forming an intent, or on criminal responsibility
- Mental state at the time of examination
- Recommendations for disposal or treatment
- Prognosis where this seems relevant
- Psychiatric report in a criminal case should contain the following information:
  - Name of defendant and charge
  - Introduction
  - At whose request/documents studied/description of defendant
  - Personal history
  - Family history
  - Previous offending behavior
  - Present offense(s)
  - Findings on clinical examination
  - Information from other sources
  - Investigation
  - Discussion
  - Opinion
  - Certification regarding disability in relation to mental illness.

INDIAN DISABILITY EVALUATION AND ASSESSMENT SCALE (IDEAS)

A scale for measuring and quantifying disability in mental disorders. Best suited for the purpose of measuring and certifying disability for the mentally ill population in India. Patients with the following diagnoses are eligible for disability benefits:

1. Schizophrenia
2. Bipolar disorder
3. Dementia
4. Obsessive compulsive disorder.

Duration of illness = at least 2 years—the number of months the patient was symptomatic in the last 2 years (M124—months of illness) should be determined. Assessment and certification to be done only by the psychiatrists. Recertification to be done once in 2 years.

IDEAS—Items

- Self-care: Includes taking care of body hygiene, grooming, health including bathing, toileting, dressing, eating and taking care of one's health.
- Interpersonal activities (social relationships): Includes initiating and maintaining interactions with others in a contextual and socially appropriate manner.
- Communication and understanding: Includes communication and conversation with others by producing and comprehending spoken/written/nonverbal messages.
- Work: Three areas are employment/housework/education measures anyone aspect.
  - Performing in work/job: Performing in work/employment (paid) employment/self-employment/family concern or otherwise. Measure ability to perform tasks at employment completely and efficiently and in proper time. Includes seeking employment.
  - Performing in housework: Maintaining household including cooking, caring for other people at home, taking care of belongings, etc. Measures ability to take responsibility for and perform household tasks completely and efficiently and in proper time.
  - Performing in school/college: Measures performance in education related tasks.

Scores for Each Item

- 0—No Disability (none, absent, negligible)
- 1—Mild Disability (slight, low)
- 2—Moderate Disability (medium, fair)
- 3—Severe Disability (high, extreme)
- 4—Profound Disability (total, cannot do)

Total score (range: 0–20)

Add scores of the 4 items and obtain a total score.

MI 2Y—Months of illness in the last two years. Interview with informant and case notes if available should be used to determine for how many months in the last two years the patient exhibited symptoms. (Range: 1–4)

MI 2Y	< 6 months	Score is to be added is 1
	7–12 months	fsAdd 2
	13–18 months	Add 3
	> 18 months	Add 4

Global Disability

Total disability score + MI 2Y score = Global disability score (range: 1–20)

Percentages

For the purpose of welfare benefits, 40% will be the cut-off point. The scores above 40% have been categorized as moderate, severe and profound based on the global disability score. This grading will be used to measure change over time.
Score of 0—No disability = 0%
1–7— Mild disability = < 40%
8 and above = > 40%
(8–13 Moderate Disability; 14–19=Severe disability; 20=Profound disability).

DISABILITY ASSESSMENT OF MENTAL RETARDATION

Assess the Intelligent Quotient (IQ)

IQ is to be assessed by using a standardized test like Binet Kamat Test, Alexander's Pass Along Test, Koh's Block Design Test, Draw A Man Test, Sequin form board for children with MR aged above 5 years, Weschlers Intelligence Scale.

Calculate disability as follows:
110-IQ = Disability scoring.
Example : If IQ is 40 the disability is 70% (110-40-70).

ASSESSMENT OF DISABILITY IN PERSONS WITH MENTAL RETARDATION (ADPMR)

Main features of ADPMR:
1. ADPMR is best suited for the purpose of measuring and certifying the level of disability in persons with mental retardation.
2. It is a brief, quick and simple instrument, which can be used, even in busy clinical settings.
3. It comprises five areas namely perceptual-motor, self-care, communication and social, academic and occupational.
4. Basic training is required to use/administer ADPMR.
5. This can be applied either in clinical set-up or even in community based program.

6. Rating/scoring is very simple and is based on direct observation of persons with mental retardation and interview of primary caregiver. Case records can be used as supplementary source of information.
7. Rating can also be done on the basis of information from teachers/guardians of persons with mental retardation.
8. Rating is done on the basis of discrepancies in age appropriate performance.
9. No standardized kit is required for assessment.

Who does the Assessment?

Proper diagnosis and certification can be done jointly by the psychiatrist, clinical psychologist and special educator. However, administration of ADPMR can be done by social worker, rehabilitation personnel, school teachers, nurses and grass root level workers after basic training in its administration and scoring.

Items

- Perceptual-motor: Describes and measures performance in gross motor and fine motor areas in which movement, coordination, balances and postures of the body and its parts are assessed.
- Self-care: Describes and measures performance in eating, toileting, brushing, bathing, dressing, grooming, and maintaining healthy body hygiene and safety.
- Communication and social: Describes and measures performance in receptive and expressive verbal or non-verbal communication and maintaining relationships within community in socially accepted manner.
- Academic: Describes and measures performance in formal and non-formal educational activities. Concepts like body parts, color, shape, size, sex, number, time, money, reading, writing and arithmetic, reasoning and problem solving ability.
- Occupational: Describes and measures performances in domestic, pre-vocational and vocational activities.
  - Domestic: Competencies like cooking, stitching, maintaining cleanliness in house, small repair and maintenance work, taking care of younger siblings and belongings, etc.
  - Prevocational: Visits for vocational placements such as work habits, work-related behaviors, unskilled and semi-skilled, etc. Competency in using simple tools like scissor, hammer, screwdriver, stapler, etc. Has a work habit, able to work under supervision, aware of works hazards.
  - Vocational: Includes performances in work settings, quality and quantity of work, job related behavior and skills.

Scores for each item:

- 0—No disability (none, absent, negligible)
- 1—Mild disability (slight, low)
- 2—Moderate disability (medium, fair)
- 3—Severe disability (high, extreme)
- 4—Profound disability (total, cannot do).

Percentages

For the purpose of welfare benefits, 40% will be the cut-off point. The scores above 40% have been categorized as moderate, severe and profound based on total disability score. This grading will be used to measure change over time.
Score of 0—No disability = 0%
1–7— Mild disability = < 40%
8 and above = > 40%
(8–13-Moderate Disability; 14–19=Severe disability; 20=Profound disability)

MANUAL FOR ADPMR

General instructions: All ratings should be done considering deviation from age appropriate criteria. Information in the five areas is to be obtained by direct observation of the persons with mental retardation, interview of the parents, or primary caregiver with case reports as supplementary source of information. In case of doubts in severity rating, in general the criterion which is fulfilled more frequently should be coded. In selected conditions, intermediate scores like 1.5, 2.5, 3.5 can be used.

Perceptual-Motor

Describes and measures the physical developmental patterns with regard to body balance, coordination of muscles, postures, movement of joints, etc. as per the person's chronological age.

Broadly classified into two areas:

a. *Gross motor*: Neck holding, rolling over, sitting, squatting, kneeling, standing, walking, running, climbing up and down the stairs, etc.
b. *Fine motor*: Holding, screwing/unscrewing, locking/unlocking, cutting with scissors, threading beads/needles, etc.

Guiding observations/questions:

- Does he sit, walk, and run well?
- Does he climb up and down the stairs?
- Does he hold objects (rattle, milk bottle, tumbler using both hands)?
- Does he screw/unscrew jar/bottle lid and take out small objects?
- Does he hold pencil using his three fingers and scribble?

Scoring Disability

0—No disability

Age appropriate performance is observed. Problem in coordination, balance, movement are not present or reported.

1—Mild

Mild impairment in coordination, balance or movement is observed. Performances in activities in gross motor and fine motor areas are mildly delayed. One side of the body may have impaired functioning, but not or little affect on the total movement.

2—Moderate
Functionally independent performance in gross motor and fine motor areas. Clumsiness in walking pattern, moderately in-coordinated movement and balance may be observed.

3—Severe
Marked impairment in coordination, poor balance and restricted movement. Markedly delayed gross motor and fine motor areas. Needs assistance for mobility.

4—Profound
Immobile, very restricted movement of joint or little mobility, requires physical assistance for mobility even in familiar settings, hand functions are severely impaired, no or little balance uncoordinated movement or little coordination may be present.

Self-care

Describes and measures the adaptability in the area of personal care as per the age and social norms.

Broadly classified into two areas:

a. Self-help activities: Such as eating, drinking, toileting, brushing, bathing, dressing and grooming skills, etc.
b. Personal hygiene, physical health and safety. Guiding observations/questions:
    - Does he indicate for toilet needs/independent in toileting?
    - Does he eat independently using hands or spoon?
    - Does he brush self, bath, wear shirts/frock, unbutton/button?
    - Does he wear shoes/slippers correctly and tie laces of shoes?
    - Does he/she apply oil, powder, comb hair, shave, or keep cleanliness during menstrual period?
    - Does he maintain cleanliness and orderliness?
    - Does he take note of danger and hazards, e.g. broken glass, fire, etc.?
    - Does he cross roads independently?

Scoring Disability

0—No disability
Age appropriate independent performances are observed as per the social norms of his immediate environment.

1—Mild
Mild impairment in age appropriate self-care. At times needs intermittent assistance (Cluing/Gestural/Verbal prompts). The person dC3S most of the self-help skills, personal care of the maintain hygiene and cleanliness matching near to the age level (if not exactly). Generally aware of danger and hazards.

2—Moderate

Functionally independent performance in self-care areas. May needs regular and consistent verbal prompting. Fairly aware of danger and hazards. Maintain cleanliness and orderliness with reminder.

3—Severe

Marked impairment in self-help skills areas, needs assistance (physical prompt) for most of the daily living activities.

4—Profound

Totally dependent on others for self-care, maintenance of hygiene and cleanliness. Requires continuous custodial care for self-help activities. Inconsistent/absence of bowel or bladder control.

Communication and Socialization

Describes and measures the ability to follow the commands and instructions and receive messages whether those are verbal, gestures or any other indications. Ability to express their needs at one word level/two word level using phrases sentences or by nonverbal mode such as pointing, using signs gestures, etc. Ability to interact with others in this immediate environment; developing and maintaining relationship with familiar persons and strangers in socially accepted manners.

Broadly classified into three areas:

a. Receptive communication
b. Expressive communication
c. Interpersonal relationships.

Guiding Observations/Questions

- Does he respond to his name?
- Does he say papa, baba, mama, etc.?
- Does he follow one-step simple instructions like "Give me the ball"?
- Does he express his needs using two words phrases/gestures like "Give ball", "Ma come" etc?
- Does he great others or waves hands to say "bye-bye"?
- Does he use sentences or communicates through multiple gestures/signs?
- Does he share possessions with others or play with others?
- Does he express distress or defends self when teased/bullied/exploited by others?
- Does he go about in nearby areas, places/town and come back safely?

Scoring Disability

0—No disability

Communication meets expectation as per his age and socio-cultural context. No difficulty in comprehension and expression. Interactions with others are well-maintained. No problem behaviors observed or reported.

1—Mild
Mild impairment in age appropriate comprehension and expressive verbal or nonverbal language is assessed. Social behaviors are generally accepted by others. However, occasionally problem behavior may be reported in maintaining social interaction.

2—Moderate
A narrow range of verbal and non-verbal expressions is assessed to see if the person is able to follow very simple commands. Has inappropriate social interaction, has frequently reported problem behaviors, quarrelsome, shyness or may have isolation tendency.

3—Severe
There is marked impairment in verbal and non-verbal expressions, limited expressions. There is marked difficulty in following simple commands and may have serious difficulty in interacting with others or maintaining relationships. Problem behavior may be commonly reported.

4—Profound
There is almost nil verbal and non-verbal expressions and is unable to follow simple instructions with total absence of reciprocal social interactions.

Academic

Describes and measures the level of cognitive functioning, concept formation (colors, shapes, sizes, familiar/unfamiliar objects, numbers, etc.) preacademic and academic performances in the areas of reading, writing and arithmetic. Scholastic performances (if attended/attending school) are assessed, recorded and scored accordingly.

Guiding Observations/Questions

- Does he point/name body parts?
- Does he point/name common objects?
- Does he differentiate colors, sizes (big/small), shapes, etc.?
- Does he write 3-letters words, name and address?
- Does he know addition, subtraction?
- Does he do minor purchasing?
- Does he read/write sentences or paragraphs?

Scoring Disability

0—No disability
Average scholastic performances as per his age. If the person is from rural background, he has the concept of reasoning and calculating as per his age.

1—Mild
Mild discrepancies in academic achievements (formal/non-formal). Has basic number concepts. Has basic problem solving ability. Can do simple additions and subtractions. Can read and write small paragraphs. Money exchange present.

2—Moderate

Marked discrepancies in academic achievements (formal/non-formal). Has limited number concepts. Needs help in doing simple addition and subtractions. Functional reading and writing not present like read and write name, address, telephone number. Minimal money exchange present.

3—Severe

Very poor academic performances, appears to be uneducable. May have pre-academic (shape, size, color, etc.) concepts.

4—Profound

Nil or negligible or minimal academic performances, even absence of pre-academic (shape, size, color, etc.) concepts.

Occupational

Describes and measures the performances in occupational activities including household work, prevocational activities, and competencies in work at job site.

Guiding Observations/Questions

a. Does he help mothers/family members/teachers in routine household/classroom activities?
b. Does he perform simple household activities like dusting, cleaning, sweeping, etc.?
c. Does he cook, operate mixer/stone grinder, operate kerosene stove, etc.?
d. Does he fetch milk/water, participates in gardening?
e. Does he do household repair and maintenance work?
f. Does he work in group without disturbing others, follow group norms?
g. Does he maintain standard of work and increase production of items as per demand?

Scoring Disability

0—No disability

Attends regular work at home, at work place as any other persons of his age.

1—Mild

In general, the person is able to do the required work appropriate to his age, sometimes needs supervision or prompting. In general, maintains quality of work. At times quality may not be upto the mark.

2—Moderate

Needs regular and continuous prompting in household or job site activities. Unable to maintain regular work behaviors. Quality of the work is poor.

3—Severe

Requires physical assistance to perform the task. Makes mistakes in simple activities. Cannot be left alone to perform simple tasks. May disrupt others at home or at work place.

4—Profound
Nil or negligible work performances.

Information Checklist for ADPMR

Background Information
Name: ....
Date of Birth: ....
Age: ....
Date of Admission: ....
Education/Class: ....
Informant's Name: ....
Income per Month: ....
Address: ....
....
Date: ....
Registration. No.: ....
Sex: ....
SES: ....
Education: ....
Level of Retardation [10] (Tools Used): ....
Social Maturity [SO]: ....
Associated Conditions: ....
A. Disability (Specify): ....
B. Behavioral Problem (Specify): ....

Scoring Sheet for ADPMR

Items	0	1	2	3	4
I. Perceptual-motor					
II. Self-care					
III. Communication and socialization					
IV. Academics					
V. Occupational					

Total score:
"-"-

Percentage of Disability

- < 40%
- > 40%

Permanent Disability and its Exemption

Income Tax Act Section 80 DDB; Income Tax Rules 11 DD

The specific diseases in psychiatry are:
- Dementia
- Parkinson's diseases

Other disorders

- Motor neuron disease (MND)
- Cancer
- Chorea
- Dystonia musculora deformis
- Hemiballismus
- Aphasia, ataxia.

Certificate is to be done by a Doctor with PG qualification in form 10-1 (The proforma enclosed in the Annexure). They should posses MD, Diploma holders are not eligible to certify.

Income Tax Exemption for Mental Retardation (MR)

Income Tax Act Section 80DD.

80DD deduction in respect of maintenance including medical treatment of handicapped dependant. Where an assessee, who is a resident in India being an individual or a Hindu undivided family has, during the previous 'year: Incurred any expenditure for the medical treatment, training and rehabilitation of a handicapped dependant. The assessee should be allowed a deduction of a sum of ₹ 40,000 in respect of the previous year. "Handicapped dependant means" a person is suffering from a permanent physical disability or is subject to mental retardation; which is to be certified by a psychiatrist in the case of mental retardation; working in Government Hospital (part-time/full-time). The disability should reduce person's capacity for normal work or engaging in a gainful employment or occupation.

The above certificates are to be renewed every year.

To Issue the Proper Certificate—10 Tips

1. Completion
2. Consent
3. Communication
4. Confidentiality
5. Current Medical Research
6. Continued update of knowledge
7. Consult colleagues
8. Cooperation with colleagues
9. Cover (Indemnity Insurance for the Doctor)
10. Confidence.

Issuing Improper (False) Certificate

It is an offense to issue false certificate. It is prudent not to issue any certificate without personally examining the patient and without confirming the identity. A copy should be kept for records. Cases have been reported were recommendations given only on hearsay or just by having a peep at the patient.

Medical Council of India—Code of Medical Ethics

Registered practitioners are in certain cases bound by law, to give certificates, notifications, reports or other documents signed by them in their professional capacity for subsequent use in the courts of justice or for administrative purposes. Any such certificate, report or document which is untrue, misleading or improper is liable to have his name erased from the MC Register. Do not disclose the secrets of a patient that have been learnt in the exercise of your profession; these may be disclosed only in the court of law under orders of the presiding judge. Do not publish photographs or case reports of your patient in any medical or other journal in a manner by which their permission; if the identity is not disclosed his consent is not needed.

CONCLUSION

There is an increasing use of psychiatrist's report/certificate, psychiatric hospitals' record as evidence in the court of law and also for other administrative and welfare measures.

Psychiatrists have several ethical, moral and legal obligations in the performance of their duties. It is very important, therefore, that every psychiatrist should understand the nature of these obligations to the best of their ability.

SUGGESTED READING

1. Aiyar's AN. Indian Tax Laws—2001—Company Law Institute of India Private Ltd, Chennai.
2. Bhujang PM. Mentally ill and the law. Universal Publishing Corporation, 2003. Forensic Psychiatry, Clinical Practice Guidelines. Published by Indian Psychiatric Society, 2009.
3. Blueglass R, et al. Writing reports and giving evidence, Practical forensic psychiatry. Seminars on the Royal College of Psychiatrists, 1995;134-63.
4. Chiswick D, Cop R (ed.). Seminars in practical forensic. The Royal College of Psychiatrists, 1995.
5. Gutheil TG and Appelbaum PS. Clinical Handbook of Psychiatry and the Law. 3rd edition, Lippincott William & Wilkins 2000.
6. IDEAS—Indian Psychiatric Society 2002.
7. Income Tax Rules—Taxmann's, 2001
8. Nambi S. Certification in psychiatric practice in India. The Andhra Pradesh Journal of Psychological Medicine, 2003;7(II):25-30.
9. Persons with Disabilities Act, 1995. Eastern Book Company, 1998.
10. The Mental Health Act, 1987. Bare Act, 2003. New Delhi: Delhi Law House.

27 Chapter

Ensuring Quality Mental Health Care and the Role of the Judiciary and Police Officers

Mental health forms an important component of health. Mental health care delivery in India is gaining a momentum in the recent past. Almost every aspect of life in the modern days is regulated or affected in some way by the Law. All civilization in the world have enacted laws to regulate human behavior so that the weakest can live freely and enjoy all his human rights. There is dynamic relationship between the concept of mental illness, the treatment of the mentally ill and the Law. Legislation is an expression of the society with regard to the way it views and cares for the mentally ill persons. Treatment programs also have a legal component in which they are often controlled by laws on admission and discharge, or on the use of treatment methods or therapeutic drugs; this is likewise the case, where mental health services are a part of social programmes for the sick and the handicapped.

THE RIGHTS OF THE MENTALLY ILL INCLUDE

a. The right to get considerate and competent treatment.
b. The right to be informed about the treatment.
c. The right to give consent.
d. The right for privacy.
e. The same fundamental rights as their citizens, including the right to a decent life as normal as possible.
f. Protection against exploitation and discriminatory, abusive or degrading treatment.
g. Assistance including legal aid to protect their rights.

The freedom of the mentally ill person cannot be ensured by legal formality alone, it requires a "Human" touch.

THE RIGHTS OF THE MENTALLY ILL

Right to demand:

- The same fundamental rights as their fellow citizens including the right to a decent life, as normal and full as possible
- Legal safeguards against abuse appeal
- Necessary treatment in the least restrictive setup and as far as possible, to treatment and care in the community

- Rehabilitation
- Personal autonomy, privacy, freedom of communication
- Special education
- Training
- Economic and social security
- Family and community life employment
- Protection against exploitation and discriminatory, abusive, or degrading treatment
- Assistance, including legal to protect their rights.

In the legal point of view, whenever, we mentioned mental illness, most of the time it indicates only the severe or major mental disorder. Here, the person is unable to control his behavior, his thinking is deranged, he loses his touch with reality and finally he has no insight into his condition (that is not aware that he is suffering from a severe mental illness, which needs treatment). Persons suffering from physical disorders themselves will seek medical help, whereas persons suffering from severe mental illnesses never accept that they are ill and come forward for treatment. Hence, most of the time, it is the possibility of the relatives or the community or the government to take care of these persons.

When we aim at quality mental health care delivery, everybody in the society is responsible, but often in practice, the mental health professionals and the law enforcing agencies are held responsible. It is essential that the judicial officers and the police officials need to be oriented about the various legal provisions related to mentally ill persons.

THE LAWS RELATING TO PSYCHIATRY IN INDIA

Mental Health Legislations

- Mental Health Act, 1987.
- Persons with Disabilities Act, 1995 (PDA).
- Child Care and Protection Act, 2000 (Juvenile Justice Act).
- Rehabilitation Council of India Act, 1992.

Civil Laws Relating to Mentally Ill Persons

- Indian Evidence Act 1925, Section 118.
- Law of Contract Section 6, 11, and 12.
- Right to Vote to Stand for election—Act 326, 102 of the Constitution of India.
- Indian Succession Act, 1925 (Testamentary Capacity) Section 59.
- Marriage and Mental Health Legislation
  - Hindu Marriage Act, 1955 and 1976.
  - Indian Divorce Act, 1869.
  - Parsi Marriage and Divorce Act, 1936.
  - Dissolution of Muslim Marriage Act, 1939.
  - The Special Marriage Act, 1954.
  - The Family Courts Act, 1984.

Criminal Laws Related to Psychiatry

- Provisions as to accused persons of unsound mind (Sections 328–339 CrPc 1973).
- Criminal Responsibility Section 84 IPC, 1860
- Attempt to commit suicide Section 309 IPC
- Right of private defence against an insane person Section 98 IPC
- Unnatural offenses Section 377 IPC (Sexual perversions)
- Affrays (Section 159 in Mania)
- Misconduct in public under intoxication e.g. Alcohol deference section 510 IPC.

Other Special Acts Related to Mental Health

- Narcotic Drugs and Psychotropic Substances Act, 1985. (Amended 1988).
- Domestic Violence Act, 2005.

Legislation assists persons with mentally ill to receive appropriate care and treatment. It protects and promotes rights, and prevents discrimination. Legislations uphold specific rights, such as the right to vote to property, to freedom of association, to a fair and to judicial guarantees. Criminal justice legislation ensures appropriate treatment and protection of the rights of the mentally ill offenders.

THE MENTAL HEALTH ACT, 1987

This is the important Act in India governing all the matters relating to the treatment and care of mentally ill persons. It makes better provision with respect to the property and affairs of the mentally ill.

Admission of Mentally Ill Person in Psychiatric Hospital/Nursing Home (As Per MHA, 1987)

- Admission without reception order—
  - Admission on voluntary basis of any adult (Section 15 of MHA of 1987).
  - Admission of minors by parents or guardian (Involuntary–Section 19 of MHA 1987).
  - Admission of uncooperative, unwilling patients under special circumstances (Involuntary—Section 19 of MHA 1987).
- Admission with reception order (all involuntary).
  - Reception order on application. (Section 20 to 22 of MHA 1987).
  - Reception order for wandering mentally ill and mentally ill person cruelly treated or not under proper care and control. (Section 23 to 25 of MHA 1987).
  - Admission after inquisition by District Court. (Section 26 of MHA 1987).

Admission with Detention Order (All Involuntary—Section 27 of MHA 1987)

- For mentally ill prisoners and army, navy, and air force personnel.
- Admissions in psychiatry hospitals may be of two kinds:
  1. Voluntary
  2. Involuntary
- The involvement of Police and Judiciary comes only in the involuntary admissions.

When involuntary admission is considered?

- Presence of mental illness.
- Immediate physical danger to himself and/or others because of his mental illness.
- Inability to engage in rational decision making regarding the acceptance of mental illness.
- Absence of less restrictive alternative.
- Admission includes a therapeutic purpose.

The Role of Police Personnel in the Care of the Mentally Ill

1. In the case of the wandering dangerous mentally ill—Mental Health Act, 1987.
2. In the case of mentally ill person cruelly treated are not under proper care and control—Section 25 MHA.

   In both these above situations, the police officer incharge of the corresponding police station should take the alleged mentally ill in his custody and to produce before the judicial magistrate or commissioner of police. In case of a city within 24 hours to obtain a reception order, after obtaining reception order from the judicial magistrate or commissioner of police, the alleged mentally ill person should be taken to the psychiatric hospital for the purpose of admission.
3. Accompanying the mentally ill prisoners formally from the prison to the psychiatric hospital or vice versa.
4. To retake into custody of persons, who escaped from the psychiatric hospital, who were admitted through reception order back into the hospital (Section 48 of MHA).
5. To investigate the persons who attempted suicide (IPC Section 309 of MHA).
6. A juvenile in conflict with the law is apprehended by the police (Special juvenile police unit), who can immediately report the matter to a member of the board under juvenile justice act (Section 10 of JJA, 2000).

   The police officer arresting the juvenile shall inform the parent/guardian/probation officer/public servant/social worker. (JJA 2000 Section 32).
7. The inspector general of persons is expected to inspect the mentally ill prisoners along with the visiting committee members once in three months to assess the state of mind of mentally ill prisoners and report (Section 39 of MHA).

Suggestions to Improve the Care of the Mentally Ill for the Police Personnel

- Periodic psychoeducation/sensitization program.
- Developing a positive attitude towards mentally ill. The mentally ill should be treated as a diseased person and not a delinquent person.
- Playing a proactive role.
- Creation of a Mental Health Cell in the City Police limit with the help of Mental Health Professionals/NGO's.

The Role of the Judiciary in the Care of the Mentally Ill

Judiciary and Psychiatry are two important subjects, which are concerned with the behavior of the individual in the society and the welfare of the society. The judiciary has many roles to play in the care of mentally ill as per the MHA, 1987.

Role of Judiciary in the Admission of a Mentally Ill Person in a Psychiatric Hospital/Psychiatric Nursing Home

The judicial intervention in the admission of mentally ill into a psychiatric hospital comes only for the category of involuntary admissions.

- The judicial magistrate are empowered to issue a reception order for a mentally-ill person on application either by the relative of a mentally ill person or by the officer in charge of a psychiatric hospital on a prescribed application with two medical certificates of which one should be from the Government Hospital. (Section 20, 21, 22 of MHA of 1987)
- The judicial magistrate is empowered to issue a reception order for a person alleged to have been suffering from mental illness for wandering and brought by the police officer in charge of the respective police station. (Section 23 and 24 of MHA of 1987)
- Also, the Magistrate is empowered to issue a reception order in case of a mentally ill person, who is cruelly treated or not under proper care and control. (Section 25 of MHA of 1987).

Admission after Judicial Inquisition

- Any District Court holding an inquisition regarding any person, who is found to be mentally ill is of opinion that is necessary, the district court can issue an reception order to admit such person as an inpatient in a psychiatric hospital/ psychiatric nursing home. (Section 26 of MHA of 1987)
- Admission and detention of mentally ill prisoners (Criminals), an order under Section 330 CrPc (under trial prisoners) or Section 335 CrPc (not guilty by the reason of unsoundness of mind), Section 3 of the Prisoners Act, 1900 (3 of 1900). A detention order can also be issued for these mentally-ill prisoners into psychiatric hospital/psychiatric nursing home.

  A detention order can also be issued under: Section 144 of the Air Force Act, 1950 (45 of 1950) or under Section 145 of the Army Act, 1950 (46 of

1950) or under Section 143 or Section 144 of the Navy Act, 1957 (62 of 1957).

- Magistrate can issue an reception order for detention of mentally ill person (For persons who were already issued reception order under section 22, 24 or 25 of MHA). Pending his removal to psychiatric hospital or psychiatric nursing home for a period not exceeding 30 days in any other hospital.
  - In all the above admission procedures, where a reception order is issued by the Magistrate or District Court shall forthwith send a certified copy of the order or medical certificates, three medical officers in charge of the psychiatric hospital.
  - No Magistrate or District Court shall pass a reception order in any psychiatric hospital outside the State in which Magistrate or District Court exercises jurisdiction. (Section 33 of the MHA).
  - The magistrate has the power to appoint substitute person upon whose application the reception order has been made, e.g. after the death of the person, who applied for the admission.

Role of Judiciary as a Member of the Visiting Committee or Board of Visitors

The Judicial Magistrate forms one of the members of the visiting committee or board of visitors for the psychiatric hospital (mainly for the State Mental Hospital) to monitor the admissions, discharges, and other facilities of the hospital. The visiting committee is expected to visit the hospital once a month.

Duty of the Magistrate in Discharge of Person Admitted in Psychiatric Hospital

Any person admit through reception order for treatment of mental illness in a psychiatric hospital for treatment may make an application to the Magistrate along with the certificate from the medical officer of the hospital for discharge. If the Magistrate can pass an order of discharge if he is fit or dismiss his application if he is not fit. (Section 43 and 44 of MHA)

Grant Leave of Absence for Persons Admitted in Psychiatric Hospital Through Reception Order

The Magistrate may issue an order for granting leave of absence (temporary discharge) on application by a relative or guardian. (Section 46 of MHA)

The Responsibilities of the District Court in the Case of the Mentally Ill

Any person aggrieved by any order of the magistrate can appeal against that order through the District Court within 60 days from the date of the order and the decision of the District Court on such appeal will be final. (Section 49 of MHA)

Judicial Inquisition Regarding Alleged Mentally Ill Person Possessing Property, Custody, Office Person, and Management of his Property

An application for holding an inquisition into the mental condition of a person may be made either:

- By any of his relative.
- A public curator.
- By the Advocate General of the State.
- The District Court can serve a notice to the alleged mentally ill person or the person having the custody of that person to produce before the court for examination for the purpose of holding the inquisition.
- The District Court may issue order for the manager to perform contracts, to dispose of business premises, to dispose of leases, to dissolve and disposal of property of partnership, power to transfer of stocks, securities, or shares belonging to mentally ill. (Section 64 to 74 of MHA), where the District court has the reason to believe that any person who is found to be mentally ill after inquisition has ceased to be mentally ill, it may direct any court subordinate to it to enquire whether is ceased to be mentally ill and if so, shall order all actions taken in respect of the mentally ill person under this Act to be set aside (Section 73 of MHA). The District Court can order the relative or the guardian for payment of cost of maintenance out of the State of mentally ill person or from a person regularly bound to maintain him.

  (Section 79 of MHA), where a mentally ill person is not represented by a legal partner, the District Court, or Magistrate, shall assign a legal partner to represent him at the expense of the State, if he is poor, otherwise, the fees should be changed from the property of such person.

Measures to Improve the Quality of Services by Legal and Judiciary with Regard to the Care of the Mentally Ill

- Legal aspects of psychiatry with specific relevance to Indian scenario should be emphasized as a special branch for the students of law.
- Periodic orientation programmes to be conducted for the legal professionals and the judiciary.
- Regular lectures in Forensic Psychiatry and field visits to the psychiatric hospitals are to be included in the curriculum of Judicial Academy.

SUGGESTED READING

1. Dalal PK, Pargaokar A, Kala AK. Mental health legislation in India—shortcomings and solutions. International Conference of SAARC Psychiatric Federation in Agra, 2005.
2. Indian Psychiatric Society—Recommendation of Mental Health Legislation, 2002.
3. Mental Health: New understanding, new hope, WHO—The World Health Report, 2011.
4. Mental Health Act, 1987.

5. Nambi S. Legal Aspects of Psychiatry—Indian Perspective. Manashanthi Mental Health Care Publications, 2008.
6. Nambi S. Mental Health Act, 1987—an evolution, presented in the Indian Psychiatric Society South Zone Conference, Mangalore, 1994.
7. Nambi S. Private Psychiatric Practice and Mental Health Legislation in India, Paper presented at the First Annual Conference of IAPP, New Delhi, 2000.
8. The Mental Health Act, 1987 (14 of 1987), New Delhi. Universal Law Publishing Company (private), 2004.
9. Verma VK, Verma SK. Mental Health Legislation in Ten Asian Developing Countries – the practical need for change, international Digest of Health Legislation, 1984;35(2).

28 Chapter

Forensic Psychiatry: Its Relevance in Postgraduate Training

Forensic psychiatry is a clinical subspecialty within the medical speciality—psychiatry. The subject is concerned with area where psychiatry and the law meet. It overlaps interfaces and interacts with psychiatry and law in all aspects. Law is the sanctioning discipline and psychiatry is the therapeutic discipline.

Forensic psychiatry is firmly rooted in the medical science of psychiatry, but also requires some knowledge of criminology, the law, criminal justice, and public policy, institutional dynamics, ethics and organization of services for mentally disorders offenders. Due to various reasons, forensic psychiatry was reared as Cinderella, much neglected, ignored, misinterpreted and misunderstood.

BASIC KNOWLEDGE AND SKILLS IN FORENSIC PSYCHIATRY FOR POSTGRADUATES

Assessment

- Assessment of behavioral abnormalities.
- Assessment of risk and dangerousness.
- Writing reports for courts and mental health review tribunals.

Knowledge

- Mental health legislation and relevant criminal and civil law
- The range of services for mentally-disordered offenders
- How to use them
- Ability to give evidence in court.

Therapeutic Skills

- Understanding and using security as a means of control and treatment.
- The treatment of chronic disorders, especially where behavioral problems are exhibited, such as severe psychoses and personality disorders.
- Skills in psychological treatments for behavior disorder (particularly psychotherapy).

SYLLABUS IN FORENSIC PSYCHIATRY FOR MD PSYCHIATRY COURSE

The syllabus can be covered under the following six headings:
- Psychocriminology
- Laws relating to psychiatry in India
- Civil and criminal responsibility
- Confidentiality, competence, Consent and certification in psychiatry
- Forensic issues in special population
- Rights of the mentally ill.

Psychocriminology

This chapter deals with the following concepts:
- Psychiatric causes of aggression and violence.
- Characteristic of murder by mentally ill person—homicides by people with mental illness, myth and reality.
- Crime and psychiatric disorder
  - Crime and schizophrenia
  - Crime and epilepsy
  - Crime and substances use disorders
  - Crime and affective disorders
  - Crime and personality disorders
  - Crime and mental retardation.

Laws Relating to Psychiatry in India

- The care and treatment legislation (Mental health legislations)
- Criminal responsibility formulation (Criminal laws)
- Civil status provisions (Civil laws).

Mental Health Related Legislation

A thorough knowledge about the various aspects of Mental Health Act, 1987 and detailed account of Mental Health Care Act, 2010 (DRAFT).
- Persons with Disability Acts, 1996.
- Rehabilitation Council of India Act, 1992.
- Consumer Protection Act, 1986.
- Juvenile Justice (Care and Protection of Children) Act, 2000.

Civil Laws Related to Mentally Ill Persons

Marriage and mental health registration:
- Hindu Marriage Act, 1955 and 1976.
- The Special Marriage Act, 1954.
- Dissolution of Muslim Marriage Act, 1939.
- Indian Divorce Act, 1869.
- Parsi Marriage Plus Divorce Act, 1936.

- The Family Courts Act, 1984.
- The Evidence Act, 1925, Section 118.
- Law of Contract Section 6, 11 and 12.
- Right of Vote and Stand for Election Act 326, 102 of the Constitution of India.
- Testamentary capacity—Indian Succession Act, 1925, Section 59.

Criminal Laws Related to Psychiatry

Provisions as to accrues persons of unsound mind sections 328–339, CrPc 1973–criminal responsibility section 84 IPC 1860—Attempt to commit suicide section 309 IPC—Right private defence against an insane person section 98 IPC (Sexual Perversions)—misconduct in public under intoxication. (For example: Alcohol intoxication section 510 IPC).

Other Special Acts Related to Mental Health

- Narcotic Drugs and Psychotropic Substances Act, 1985 (Amended 1988).
- Domestic Violence Act, 2005.

Criminal Responsibility

This area deals with the criminal responsibility.

Criminal responsibility is covered under section 84 of Indian Penal Code. This Act deals with the relieving of the crime committed by a mentally ill person who as committed the crime under the influence of mentally illness. This section is based on the famous McNaughton Act. Knowledge about the various criteria for a prisoner with mental illness who is fit to stand "Trial".

Ethical Issues in Psychiatry—Confidentiality, Competence, Consent and Certification in Psychiatry

This chapter deals with the importance of maintaining confidentiality and also guidelines for seclusion and restraint of mentally ill persons.

- Negligence in psychiatric practice.
- Informed consent in psychiatric practice.
  - Competency
  - Information to be provided
  - Voluntaries
  - Alternatives.

Certification in Psychiatry Practice

The preparation structure and content of good certificate in psychiatry practice.

- Certification for criminal cases.
- Certification in civil matters.
- Disability assessment certification certificate for mental illness and mental retardation.
- Certificate for various concession and government benefits.

Forensic Issues in Special Population

- Forensic issues in child psychiatry.
- Forensic issues in women.

- Forensic issues in elderly.
- Sexual disorders—forensic issues.

Rights of Persons with Mentally Illness

- Rights to access mental health care.
- Right to community living.
- Right to protection from cruel inhuman and degrading treatment.
- Right to equality and non-discrimination.
- Right to information.
- Right to confidentiality.
- Access to mental records.
- Right to personal contacts and communication.
- Right to legal aid.
- Right to make complaints about deficiencies in provision of services.

FORENSIC PSYCHIATRY TRAINING FOR POSTGRADUATE IN INDIA

The number of PG center in psychiatry has tremendously increased the recent past. Hence, it is necessary to chat out the syllabus and the training which should be uniform to all the centers in India. The MD post graduate in psychiatry should have minimum:

- One month posting in a forensic psychiatry unit of a recognized psychiatry hospital.
- Minimum 30 hours of theory in forensic psychiatry.
- This can be reduced to 20 days clinical training and 20 hours of theory for Diploma Students (DPM).
- In the university examination theory papers, one of the papers there should be questions for minimum 25% in MD, and minimum 15% for DPM in essential.

All the MD psychiatry postgraduates whether undergo they training in private or government medical colleges. This clinical training for one month should be compulsory. If the PG centers disorder not have a forensic psychiatry unit there should be attached to the forensic psychiatry unit of the one of the 37 psychiatry hospitals who has psychiatry units.

It has long been known that there is dynamic relationship between the concepts of mental illness, the treatment of the mentally ill and the law. Legislation forms and integral and essential component of the mental health care delivery system. With nearly three crores of the population in India suffers from severe mental illness there is a strong need to have a special training in forensic psychiatry.

For this purpose we need to have psychiatrist who are specially qualified in forensic psychiatry. Therefore, it is high time that the Indian Psychiatric Society should come forward to represent the government and the MCI to have higher speciality courses like Diploma or Fellowship or DM in Forensic Psychiatry.

SUGGESTED READING

1. Agarwal AK. Ethics in psychiatry. Indian Journal of Psychiatry, 1994;36:1-5-11.
2. Agarwal AK, Gupta SC. Ethical issues in psychiatry. Souvenir of the Annual Conference of Indian Psychiatric Society and World Psychiatric Association held at Jaipur (1993, 1998).
3. Appelbaum PS. A health information infrastructure and the threat to confidentiality of health records. Psychiatric Serv, 1998;49:27-28, 33.
4. Appelbaum PS. Privacy in psychiatric treatment: Threats and responses. Am J Psychiatry 2002;159:1809-18.
5. Bhugra D (ed). Handbook of Psychiatry, 2005.
6. Gutheil TG. Paranoia and progress notes: A guide to forensically informed psychiatric record keeping. Hosp Community Psychiatry,1980;31:479-82s.
7. Nambi S. Legal aspects of psychiatry—Indian perspective, 2008. Manashanthi Mental Health Care Pvt Ltd.
8. Oyebode F. Clinical errors and medical negligence. Advances in Psychiatric Treatment, 2006;2:22-7.

29 Chapter

Starting Career in Practice—Handling Legal Issues

Abstract
Young Psychiatrists who start their practice should be familiar with the legal provisions governing the psychiatric practice in India. Many of the comprehensive legislations in relation to psychiatry can be referred, whenever there is a need. But some basic knowledge about the law which interferes with day-to-day practice is very much essential. Most of the text books in psychiatry which our young psychiatrists are very much familiar during their postgraduate days, are mostly western. The legal aspects of psychiatry should be based on Indian laws to practice in India. This article will give a bird's eye view regarding various legal aspects of psychiatry in India. This is not a complete reference. Young psychiatrists are requested to refer comprehensive text book of forensic psychiatry with Indian Perspective for the holistic knowledge.

INTRODUCTION

The young psychiatrists should know some basic administrative, ethical and legal provisions in India related to psychiatric practice. It is very essential to understand that legislation forms an integral component in the implementation of mental health care. Legislation is an expression of society with regard to the way it views and cares for mentally ill individuals. It has long been known that there is a dynamic relationship between the concept of mental illness, the treatment of the mentally ill, and the law.

Every civilization has its own rules and regulations in controlling and modifying the human behavior. In India, also, we have multiple rules, regulations, and laws related to psychiatric disorders. Every young psychiatrist should have some basic understanding of the legal provisions existing in India.

MENTAL HEALTH CARE LEGISLATIONS

Mental Health Act,1987

This Act governs the matters to treatment and care of the mentally ill and also have provisions with respect to the safety of the properties and affairs and also take care of their rights.

A thorough knowledge about the various aspects of this Act is essential:

- Mental Health Care Act, 2010, (Draft).
- Persons with Disabilities Act, 1996.
- Juvenile Justice (Care and Protection of Children) Act, 2000.

Civil Laws Related to Mentally Ill Persons

- Marriage and Mental Health Legislation: Various laws related to marriage and divorce existing in India and Family Court Act, 1984.
  - The Evidence Act 1925 Section 118.
  - Law of Contract Section 6, 11, and 12.
  - Right to Vote and Stand for Election Act 326,102 of the Constitution of India.
  - Testamentary Capacity—Indian Succession Act 1925, Section 59.

Criminal Laws of Mentally Ill Criminals Related to Psychiatry

Mentally ill persons who commit a crime are dealt in:

- Sections 328–339, CrPc 1973.
- Criminal responsibility—Section 84 IPC 1860.
- Attempt to commit suicide—Section 309 IPC.
- Right to private defence against an insane person—Section 98 IPC.
- Misconduct in public under intoxication, e.g. alcohol intoxication section 510 IPC.

Other Special Acts Related to Mental Health

- Narcotic Drugs and Psychotropic Substances Act, 1985 (Amended 1988).
- Domestic Violence Act, 2005.

Mental Health Care Legislation

The young psychiatrists who start this practice either in government service or in the private sector should understand that the psychiatric practice in India is governed by MHA, 1987 and its rules (Both Central and State Government Rules) framed thereafter. Psychiatrists who take up teaching and research have minimal regulations to follow like admission of a mentally ill person in a teaching or general hospital psychiatric ward (mostly voluntary in nature). Psychiatrists who are in the research should adhere to the protection of the rights of the mentally ill when they do research and in no way there should be any violation of human rights at any stage of their research. They should also have a working knowledge about the guidelines framed by the Indian Council of Medical Research (ICMR) in conducting research in clinical settings. Those who are involving in private practice should understand the rules and regulations laid down by MHA, 1987 and MHCA, 2010 in establishing and maintaining private psychiatric hospitals.

It is mandatory to get licence from the State Mental Health Authority to establish and maintain a private psychiatric hospital. As per the Act, the private psychiatric hospital should constitute visitors committee as required by MHA. There should be provisions for various modalities of treatment and other psychological methods of therapies.

The young psychiatrist should be aware of the provisions laid down in the draft of the MHCA 2010, which will be enacted soon for regular implementation. The new Act MHCA, 2010 is giving much importance to the rights of the mentally ill instead of the Central and State Mental Health Authorities of MHA, 1987. The new Act proposes to have mental health review commission in the Central and State level.

The persons with Disabilities Act (equal opportunity, protection of rights, and full participation Act (1996) is an Act which protects the rights and provides equal opportunities of the disabled persons, mental retardation and mental illness are included as disabilities in this Act. This Act provides the mentally-disabled individuals to live a full life and making full contribution each in accordance with his or her ability. There should not be any discrimination just because they are mentally ill.

ETHICAL ISSUES IN PSYCHIATRIC PRACTICE

Ethics is the science of norms of behavior for any group; a code of conduct decided by a group of person in a particular society. It provides a framework to gain one's own behavior in a particular setting.

Some Selected Ethical Principles for Psychiatrists

a. Confidentiality.
b. Restraint in release of information to third parties. It is very important in psychiatric practice to keep many informations provided by the patient or by their relatives to keep as confidential and need not be disclosed to any persons.
c. Informed consent: The voluntary and continuing permission of the patient to receive a particular treatment based on an adequate knowledge of the purpose, nature, likely effects and risks of the treatment including the likelihood of its success and any alternatives to it. Informed consent should be obtained for the following conditions in psychiatric practice:
   - Admission of a person to a psychiatric hospital on a voluntary basis.
   - Procedures like ECT, psychosurgery and other invasive investigatory procedures like lumbar puncture, spheoidal EEG, etc.
   - Penthathol analysis (narco-analysis).
   - Drug treatments like disulfiram therapy and clozapine therapy.
   - Administration of any research drugs (Drug trials).
d. Competency: Legally, only competent persons may give informed consent. The following four standards for determining incompetence were suggested:
   - Communication of choice
   - Understanding of relevant information provided
   - Appreciation of available options and consequence
   - Rational decision-making.

A valid consent can be either expressed (oral or in writing) or implied from the patient's action.

e. Guidelines for seclusion and restraint of mentally ill persons:
   The mentally ill persons:
   - Is likely to commit self-harm or suicide.
   - The mentally ill person poses a threat to the community because of his dangerousness due to mental illness.
   - The mentally ill person presents a specific threat to innocent third parties.

   Hence, it is necessary in psychiatric practice, occasionally, not often, we have to seclude and restrain the mentally-ill persons.

Indications for Seclusion and Restraint

- Behavior or threats that create or imply danger to the patient or others.
- Safe and uncontrolled access for medical procedures.
- Involuntary evaluation or treatment of incompetent.

The Indian Psychiatric Society Guidelines on Ethical Issues,1989

To maintain a high-level of ethical conduct, the psychiatrists are expected to follow the following principles:

- Responsibility
- Competence
- Benevolence
- Moral standards
- Patient's welfare
- Confidentiality.

LEGAL IMPLICATIONS

The relationship between the mentally ill person and psychiatrist is complex, sensitive, and vital. Hence, it is always better to be careful and vigilant.

1. To have some basic knowledge about all the statutory regulations of our country like Mental Health Act and others.
2. *Documentations*: The best defense in case of complaints against psychiatrist is correct up-to-date and clear medical records.

   The young psychiatrists should know whenever he attends to a patient's either as outpatient or inpatient. The comprehensive history, the investigation results, the physical and mental status examination with a provisional or final diagnosis should be documented. Every important information has to be recorded in good clinical practice. "If something is not documented, that means it is not done".
3. *Medical records:* Medical records are vital documents that are to be kept in safe custody for years together, since, they are documentary evidence in inquiries and judicial proceedings. The psychiatrist would have seen a case

and after that there may not be any follow-up after three or four years. Later also the court may summon the doctor to give evidence regarding the mental status of the patient.

4. *Certifications*: The psychiatrists are oblidged to issue certificates for various purposes. It is very essential that he or she should know that issuing improper or false certificate is not only unethical but also an offence. While issuing certificate the psychiatrist should ensure:
   - To take complete history
   - Thorough examination
   - If necessary to admit and observe
   - Carry out necessary investigations
   - Take other experts' opinion whenever necessary
   - To give opinion on only those issues, in which one is certain
   - If something is not clear better to mention the same. No need to guess or imagine
   - Not to issue the certificate for a person whom he has not personally examined or examined long time back.
5. *Expert evidence*: Psychiatrists are required to give evidence as expert as witnesses as per section 45, 46 of Indian Evidence Act. The psychiatrists have the following privileges:
   - Permitted to refer other cases
   - Take assistance of notes, books, etc.
   - Give opinion (Hence also known as Opinion Witness).
6. *Response of doctors to court summon:* It is the duty of every psychiatrist to assist in the process of Justice. Hence, psychiatrists are advised not to ignore the court summons unless it is dire emergency.
7. *Do's and Don'ts as expert evidence:*

   Do's
   - The psychiatrist must be punctual.
   - He must dress appropriately.
   - Appear confident (but not arrogant).
   - Speak clearly and audibly.
   - Keep to the point.
   - Evidence should be comprehensible and simple language.
   - Keep sentences short.

   Don'ts
   - Do not use jargon.
   - Do not use technical expressions not generally understandable by a lay person.
   - Do not use words of foreign origin, e.g. cyclothymia instead of 'mood swings'.
   - Do not use polysyllabic or uncommon words.
   - Do not lose your temper even if provoked by the Council.

Replies to questions, although, put by the advocate, will be addressed to the Judge and Head of Jury. The conventional appellation to the judge is "Your Honour" in the lower courts and "Your Lordship" in High Courts. Most often, the council and judges are courteous and considerate towards the expert witness, but their questions will be probing in nature.

In all cases, it is advisable to go over the case files and documents briefly before and to refresh the memory. In criminal cases, it may be helpful to see the accused again before the proceedings start. This is particularly important where the issue is fitness to plead.

The performance in the witness box and the impressions that the witness makes on the court are obviously important in contributing successfully to the proceedings and their outcome.

CRIMINAL AND CIVIL ISSUES (RESPONSIBILITIES) IN PSYCHIATRY

Criminal Responsibility

Persons suffering from severe mental illness will be acquitted of their crime if they have committed the crime because of the reason of his unsoundness of mind. This is based on the famous "The McNaughton Rules", the relevant section of IPC 84, says "Nothing is an offence which is done by a person who, at the time of doing it, by reason of unsoundness of mind, is incapable of knowing the nature of the act, or that he is doing what is either wrong of contrary to law".

Legal insanity is different from medical insanity, the person is considered to be suffering from insanity only when he is not knowing what he is doing is right or wrong or not knowing what he is doing is against law or not knowing the consequences of the act.

Fitness to Stand Trial

When a mentally ill prisoner who committed a crime is observed by the court that he is not fit to stand trial, he will be sent for psychiatric treatment. After the treatment is over, it is the duty of the treating psychiatrist to ascertain his fitness to plead based on the following principles:

- Is oriented to place, person and time.
- Understands the questions asked.
- Understands the nature of the charge.
- Understands the difference between guilty and not guilty.
- Is able to instruct his advocate.
- Is able to follow the evidence presented in the court.
- Is able to challenge the selection of jurors.

A person may be suffering from severe mental disorder, but still be fit to stand trial.

Civil Responsibility

Before the Court of Law, all persons are considered to be sane, (normal). Otherwise, it is to be proved. A person has no responsibility in the full conditions, if he is proved to be an insane person.

Testamentary Capacity

As per Section 59 of the Indian Succession Act, 1925, "Every person of sound mind, not being a minor, may dispose of his property by will".

A Will can be declared invalid if it is proved that at the time of making the will, the testator:

- Was of unsound mind.
- Did not have the mental capacity to understand the consequences of the act.

Witness

Under the Indian Evidence Act, 1872 (section 118), a lunatic is incompetent to give evidence in a Court of Law, if he is unable to understand the questions asked or to give rational answers to them by virtue of lunacy.

Contract

Under the Indian Contract Act, 1872 (section 11) every person to be competent to contract, must be a major and sound of mind, i.e. he is capable of understanding the contract and of forming a rational judgment as to its effect upon his interests.

Transfer of Property

Under the Transfer of Property Act, 1882 (section 7) only persons competent to contract, are authorized to transfer of property.

The Right to Vote and the Right to Stand for Election

No person of unsound mind can contest an election or exercise the franchise of voting.

Marriage

Marriage is a legal contract between an adult male and an adult female of sound mind. Marriage can be declared null and void or the person is incapable of getting married because of severe mental illness. Secondly, because of the continuous presence of some major mental disorders divorce can be granted for the aggrieved person.

<table>
<tr><th colspan="2">An unsoundness of mind as affecting the capacity to marry</th></tr>
<tr><td>Hindu Marriage Act, 1955 (HMA)
• A Hindu Marriage is voidable if either party
• Is incapable of giving a valid consent as a consequence of unsoundness of mind, or
• Though capable of giving a valid consent as a consequence of unsoundness of mind, or Though capable of giving a valid consent has been suffering from mental disorder of such a kind or to such an extent as to be unfit for marriage and the procreation of children.
• Has been subject to recurrent attacks of insanity.</td><td>Indian Divorce Act, 1869
A Christian marriage is voidable if either party was a lunatic or idiot.</td></tr>
<tr><td rowspan="2">The Special Marriage Act 1954 (SMA)
Applicable to persons from any religion undergoing a civil marriage. Has provisions similar to the HMA except that a marriage under the SMA is void.</td><td>Parsi Marriage and Divorce Act, 1936
Unsoundness of mind is not ground for annulment.</td></tr>
<tr><td>Muslim Law
A person of unsound mind cannot contract a marriage and such a marriage if contracted is void. However, if the guardian of the person of unsound mind considers such marriage to be in his interest and in the interest of society and is willing to take up all the monetary obligations of the marriage then such a marriage can be performed.</td></tr>
</table>

<table>
<tr><th colspan="2">Unsoundness of mind as a ground for divorce</th></tr>
<tr><td rowspan="2">Hindu Marriage Act, Special Marriage Act and Parsi Marriage and Divorce Act
Respondent has been incurably of sound mind or has been suffering continuous or intermittently from mental disorder of such a kind and to such an extent that the petitioner cannot reasonably be expected to live with him.</td><td>Dissolution of Muslim Marriage Act, 1939
A Muslim woman can seek divorce on the ground that her husband has been insane for period of two years.</td></tr>
<tr><td>Indian Divorce Act, 1869 Amendment 2001 (for Chrisitians)
Unsoundness of mind is a ground of divorce on two conditions that is it must be incurable and it must be at least for two years immediately before the filing of the petition.</td></tr>
</table>

Consumer Protection Act, (1986)

Medical profession has come under the purview of the Consumer Protection Act as per the Supreme Court judgment in 1995, which has created an anxiety among medical professionals. The Law is trying to protect the interest of the consumers (patients and/or caregivers) and providing them means to get quick justice. The service rendered to a patient by a doctor would fall within the "Ambit of Service", only when a fee is charged for the service. If there is no fee, the Consumer Protection Act (1986) is not applicable.

Objectives of Consumer Protection Act

- The rights of the consumer to seek redressal against unscrupulous exploitation.
- Right to consumer education and others.

The second objective is very relevant to the practice of Psychiatry, which includes the informed consent. The three levels of implementing Consumer Protection Act are:

- District forum with jurisdiction up to 5 lakhs claim.
- State forum with jurisdiction up to 20 lakhs claim.
- National forum far beyond 20 lakhs.

Even though psychiatrists have a fear whether any of their patients turn out to be a litigant and go to the consumer forum, most of the time, it is not happening so. The incidents of claim against Psychiatrists still remain much lower than that of claims against other medical specialists (less than 3%).

Steps for prevention:

- A good doctor-patient relationship.
- Psychoeducation.
- Proper record keeping.
- Obtaining informed consents wherever necessary, above all.
- A good ethical psychiatric practice.

Witness

Under the Evidence Act, 1872 (section 118), a lunatic is incompetent to give evidence in the Court of Law, if he is unable to understand the questions asked or to give rational answers to them by "Virtue of Lunacy".

Right to Vote and Right to Stand for Election

Under Article 326 of the Constitution of India, no person declared to be of "Unsound Mind" could vote. Under Article 102 of Constitution of India, a person is disqualified from being chosen as or for being a member of either House of Parliament, if he is of unsound mind and stands so declared by the Competent Court.

This is true for practically all official and responsible positions.

Driving

Anyone applying for a Driving License or who holds the license must declare whether he has suffered from any mental disorder. A person who is suffering from severe mental disorder, that includes severe learning disability, dementia, etc. are not entitled to have a valid driving license as per the Road Traffic Act and Driving License Act of India.

MEDICAL INSANITY VERSUS LEGAL INSANITY

When civil or criminal issues related to the mentally ill come to the Court of Law, the concept of mental illness viewed in the court is different from medical concept. In the Court of Law, a person is considered to be insane or of unsound mind, only when a person is:

- Incapable of knowing the nature of the act he is doing.
- Not knowing what he is doing is right or wrong or what he is doing is contrary to law.
- Not knowing the consequences of the act.

CONCLUSION

A working knowledge of the law that regulates the practice of Psychiatry, assist young psychiatrists to provide good care to their patients and avoid unnecessary and counter-productive defensive practices. Psychiatrists cannot be expected to be as knowledgeable of the Law as Lawyers, but they do need to understand how the Law and Psychiatry interact in various common clinical situations. Good Psychiatry and Law are complementary.

SUGGESTED READING

1. Bhujang PM. Mentally Ill and the Law, Mumbai. Universal Publishing Corporation, 2003.
2. Mental Health Care Act. Ministry of Health and Family Welfare, Government of India, New Delhi, 2010.
3. Nambi S. Forensic Psychiatry, (Psychiatry and Law) Indian Perspective. Manashanthi Mental Health Care Pvt Ltd, 2011.
4. Nambi S. Legal Aspects of Psychiatry. Indian Journal of Psychological Medicine, 2000.
5. Nambi S. Marriage, Mental Health and Indian Legislation, Presidential Address at the 57th Annual Conference of the Indian Psychiatric Society, 2005.
6. Rosner R. Principles of practice of forensic psychiatry. Arnold Publications, 2003.
7. The Mental Health Act, 1987, (Bare Act, 2003), Delhi Law House with Mental Health Authority Rules, 1990 along with State Mental Health Rules, 1990.
8. The Persons with Disabilities (Equal Opportunities, Protection of Rights and Full Participation) Act, 1995 along with the Person with Disabilities (Equal Opportunities, Protection of Rights and Full Participation) Rules, 1996.

30 Chapter

Special Investigations in Forensic Psychiatry—Merits and Demerits

Merits and Demerits: For a long time, investigators in criminal law and psychiatrists believe that they could get the truth or the fact from a person, who is an offender and who is not willing to come out with regular methods used by the police during investigation, since they wanted more scientific literary and dependable method of bringing out the truth. Hence, methods like hypnosis, abreaction using pentothal sodium analyzing the variation in the neurophysiology during lying by using polygraphy and some more methods were started gaining importance in the investigations of the criminal justice system.

Evaluation of amnesia in a forensic psychiatry setting is a very difficult task. There is a lack of clinical studies of amnesia in forensic psychiatry settings and as a result, the incidents of organic amnesia and psychogenic amnesia (dissociative amnesia) are not clear. Malingered amnesia is also seen frequently in forensic settings as well as being the arguably most common manifestations of all malingering. The true incidents of amnesia in forensic settings in specific clinical situations, such as homicide and in many other instances is poorly understood or there is insufficient research available.

THE AMYTAL INTERVIEW: (THE PENTOTHAL ANALYSIS) ABREACTION

This was introduced in the 1930s as a treatment for patients suffering from psychosis. The Amytal interview has been used in non-psychotic persons and has been mostly used as a diagnostic tool in catatonia, hysterical states, usually with muteness and various stupors. It is also used in abreactions to recover memory in dissociative amnesia and fugue states, the later being the most controversial application.

In 1940, Sargent and Slater, reported the rapid recovery of memory with amytal in troupes acutely distressed by battle conditions. In fact, they claim it to be more effective than hypnosis. In another study, Sargent and Slater (1941) described one-third of a group hospitalized patients with psychogenic amnesia in World War II as malingering. In over 200 patients, Lambert and Rees, (1944) found that amytal interview was the best method of recovering memory when compared with suggestions and hypnosis.

A double blind, placebo controlled study on Amytal was completed by Dysken, et al. (1979). Though, these authors had some reservations on the use of and the effectiveness of the procedure, they feel that occasionally in catatonia they can reduce negative symptoms.

Rand (1997) conducted a study of serial Amytal intervals in a variety of clinical conditions and concluded that it was the useful clinical and therapeutic tool. A recent literature review by Kavirajan (1999), which detailed seven controlled Amytal studies against placebo refer to only one study that was superior to placebo in promoting verbalization and alertness.

The use of Amytal as an adjunct to psychotherapy is known as narcotherapy and there are four basic techniques.

1. *Simple Abreaction:* The recall of suppressed memories with relief of associated negative affect.
2 *Narco Suggestion:* It is the treatment with the use of suggestion while the patient is under the influence of Amytal.
3. *Narco analysis:* Abreaction accompanied by posthypnotic suggestion.
4. *Narco synthesis:* Requested repressed material and abreaction forming part of a more comprehensive psychotherapeutic approach, where the repressed memories obtained in the Amytal interview are integrated in the ongoing psychotherapeutic sessions. Narcoanalysis using many courts have refused to admit any testimony established by narcoanalysis.

METHODOLOGY OF PENTATHOL ANALYSIS

The usual procedure is to have the patient in a slightly darkened quite room on a couch or chair that allows him or her to recline. Informed consent should be obtained. A butterfly needle or narrow bore-scalp vein needle is inserted into a superficial vein, usually on the hand and a solution of 5% pentathol (500 mg pentathol in 10 mL of sterile water) is injected at a rate of 0.5 mental/minute or 25 mg/minute. Normally, a dose of between 150–350 mg of pentathol is required to achieve this optimum state. The interview itself has no specialized technique, except that a degree of suggestion of relaxation is maintained.

Hypnosis

Hypnosis has had a long but checkered career in the courtroom, repeatedly being either overvalued or undervalued as the cause of crime and instrument of truth telling or a contaminant of testimony. Original debates whether or not hypnotic suggestion would be considered expiratory incriminal defence. This point of view is no longer taken seriously. More recently, hypnosis has been used as a means of refreshing the memories of witnesses and victims resulting in considerable medical/psychological, legal debate about the velocity of hypnotically refreshed testimony.

Now a days, hypnosis is also occasionally being used as a diagnostic tool in assessing the criminal responsibility of defendants with dissociative disorders.

Hypnosis is not especially helpful in simply adding details in routine situations, especially in view of the challenges to the credibility of a witness with whom it is used. The laboratory literature on hypnosis in memory enhancement suggest that while a hypnotized witness may provide more correct information and he or she also provides more incorrect information and is not good at detecting his or her poor accuracy.

In summary, both the advantages and dangers of hypnosis has been oversold.

There are situations in which it can help to provide additional information and there are risks of testimony that may occur. Our current ability to measure hypnotic responsiveness increases the empirical basis for evaluating the role and usefulness of hypnosis in the forensic setting.

Hypnosis can assist in managing trauma related problems and can intensify social influence on witnesses and victims. It deserves a measured and carefully evaluated place in a legal process.

The New Jersy State Supreme Court offered the following guidelines to safeguard the integrity and accuracy of the recovered information.

- The interview be conducted by a trained psychologist
- The qualified individual be independent and not responsible to be the prosecutor, investigators, or defense
- Written information from law enforcement personnel be reviewed
- Prior to the hypnosis, a written account of the alleged events be obtained
- All contact with the individual be recorded (preferably with audio and video) and
- Only the hypnotist and subject should be in the room during the interview.

The accuracy of information obtained during hypnotic states has three main potential limitations:

- It is easily possible to lie while under the effects of barbiturates.
- Hypnotics are well-known to increase an individual's suggestibility.
- The cognitive effects of the drug are such that information obtained while under the effects of the drug is likely distorted and therefore inherently unreliable (Piper, 1993).

PENTATHOL INTERVIEW, HYPNOSIS, AND POLYGRAPHY

- The combination of hypnosis and pentathol are known as narco-analysis.
- Pentathol interviewing has been consistently described as a useful technique although expectations of outcome from the subject with regard to the drug being used are the expertise of the interviewer are important predictors of success. In order to study amnesia, in a forensic setting, polygraphy or lie detection technique was used to evaluate alcohol and drug-induced amnesia.

Polygraphic Technique

- Polygraphic technique is usually referred as the Lie Detector and also in the same context it is also known as Lie Detection Technique.

- There are two schools of thought as to the reliability of the polygraph in detecting deception. The history of the modern polygraphs dates back to 1895, where a mission was used to record blood pressure and pulse in order to detect deception in criminals. Records, pulse, blood pressure, heart rate, and muscle movements. The sesnors are attached to the person.
- The machine was called a hydrosphygmograph, later, monitoring respiratory rate and skin conduction study also were included.
- One school sees it as a reliable technique and reports that studies have shown it to be about 90% reliable in detecting deception. The other school sees the polygraph as unreliable and based on assumptions that are flawed scientifically. The polygraph today is used widely by the Law Enforcement agencies in the United States.

The test procedure consists of three phases:
Phase I: The pre-test interview
Phase II: Chart recording.
Phase III: Diagnosis.

A set of questions prepared and reactions are measured. Baseline is established by asking questions whose answers investigator knows, lying is associated with perceptible physiological and behavioral changes and wave patterns in the graph.

Deviation from the baseline, it is like diagnosing a syndrome not even a disease by just taking notes of body temperature.

Perpetrators

Perpetrator has details in brain. According to Lawrence A Farewell (1995), words, pictures, flash, mermer, and the four stages include the following:

1. Crime scene evidence collection.
2. Brain evidence collection.
3. Computer evidence analysis.
4. Scientific research.

The three main components include:

1. Target
2. Irrelevance
3. Probes.

In India, polygraph is used at merely one or two places in the investigatory proceedings but most of the judiciary maintain that polygraphy is inadmissible in any criminal trial. It is not also legal to force a person to undergo polygraphy. The polygraph works on the principle that deceptive subjects in physiological and emotional energy to lie. The scientific validity of polygraph testing is questionable. There is some evidence for the validity of polygraph testing in criminal investigations, but there is very little scientific support for its validity in screening situations of any type. The most significant criticism of the validity of the polygraphic technique relates to a lack of any scientific basis of the technique itself. There is a lack of standardization in the procedure.

When I was 11-years-old, I went along with a friend to convey a message to his uncle who worked in a police station. In the courtyard, police were beating a hard-core pickpocket who already had enough beating marks on his body. A very old and thin looking policeman who was going off duty, stopped on seeing this, went to the senior in the beating team and requested with folded hands, "*Huzoor*, if you permit, can I also give him a slap?" Permission was given with a nod and the slap delivered.

I remembered the incident some months back while watching news on TV, which was showing narcoanalysis being performed on scamster Telgi. The man was lying down, semi-sedated, mumbling some words when prodded by light slaps on the cheeks by the psychologist who was holding a questionnaire. There were other people around, all in white coats. The TV clip itself went on for 20 minutes. The whole procedure must have lasted much longer. The mental health professional in the interrogating team reminded me of the old policeman. Both had no logical or scientific reason to do what they did. And it was certainly unethical to make it degrading by doing it on television. Remember, even if Saddam's death sentence was right, his death video was not and it shocked the conscience of the world. Sometimes, when you talk of ethics in such contexts, the question is asked, "Did he think of ethics while killing innocent people?" Answer to that is, that this is the difference between him and the civilized society.

The turning point of narco analysis in India came in 2002. In June 2002, 3 months after the burning of a train bogie by a crowd at Godhra in Gujarat and the subsequent massacre of Muslims, seven persons accused of burning the train were brought to the Sree Sayaji General (SSG) Hospital in Vadodara. They were interrogated and doctors from the medical college department of anesthesia, surgery and psychiatry carried out a narcoanalysis. Since then it has been used very frequently in high profile criminal cases with a lot of pre and post-test publicity in print and electronic media. In some cases, videos of the narco-analysis actually being conducted were shown on television. Results of narco-analysis, however, are not admitted as evidence in any country in the world, including India.

SUGGESTED READING

1. Agarwal AK. A review of Indian psychiatry research and ethics. Indian J Psychiatry 2010;52(7):297-305.
2. Kala AK. Of ethically compromising positions and blatant lies about 'Truth Serum', Indian J Psychiatry, 2007;49(1):6-9.
3. Rosner R. Principles and Practice of Forensic Psychiatry, 2nd edn, 2003.

31 Chapter

Forensic Articles in Indian Journal of Psychiatry—Revised

Abstract

Articles related to Forensic Psychiatry published in the Indian Journal of Psychiatry and Neurology and Indian Journal of Psychiatry during the last 60 years revisited. During these years, around 50 articles have been published in this subject. Psycho-criminology is the theme dealt with in most of the articles. Highlights of some of the important articles are mentioned.

Key words: Forensic Psychiatry, Mental Health Legislation, Psychocriminology

INTRODUCTION

It is a great opportunity to review the articles related to forensic psychiatry, which were published in the Indian Journal of Psychiatry (IJP) during last 60 years.[1]

In the modern days, almost every aspect of life is regulated or affected in some way by Law. All civilizations in the world have enacted laws to regulate human behavior, so that, even the weakest can live freely and enjoy all the Human Rights. Legislations form the important component in the implementation of Mental Health Care. There is a dynamic relationship between the concept of Mental Illness, the treatment of the Mentally ill, and the law.

"Forensic Psychiatry is a poorly defined specialty with little organized training in most countries." (WHO working group) Working knowledge of the Law that regulates the practice of psychiatry assists clinicians in providing good care to patients. Psychiatrists cannot be expected to be as knowledgeable of the Law as lawyers, but they do need to understand how the Law and Psychiatry interact in various common clinical situations.[2]

In reviewing the forensic-related articles published in the Indian Journal of Psychiatry (IJP) during last 50 years, it is noted that there are only around 50 articles cited. If we were to classify these articles, they would fall under the following three heading:

1. Psycho-criminology related articles—there are around 38 articles.
2. Mental health legislation articles—numbered around 5
3. The others are around eight.

There is one letter to the Editor and Book Review for the book titled "Psychiatry and Law" by JC Marfatia in 1972. These are other interesting findings in analyzing these articles. There are totally eight articles related to forensic psychiatry during the past 50 years of IJP, which include one invited editorial. They are:

1. Indian Journal of Neurology and Psychiatry of October 1949, the editorial titled "Indian Lunacy act" (author unknown).
2. BB Sethi "Cult of Violence" in 1984.
3. BB Sethi "Need for Growth of Forensic Psychiatry" in 1984.
4. SM Channabasavanna "Dialogue with Judiciary" in 1985.
5. AK Aggarwal "Mental Health and the Law" in 1992.
6. TSS Rao "Psychiatrist and the Science of Criminality" in 2007.
7. TSS Rao "Criminal Behavior—A dispassionate look at parented disciplining practices" in 2007.
8. AK Kala invited Editorial titled of "Ethical Compromising Positions and Blatant Lies about Truth Serum" in 2007.

These are two articles of Murthy Rao oration delivered by RC Kapoor in 1994 tilted "Violence in India—A Psychological Perspective" and LP Shah in 1999 titled "Forensic Psychiatry in India—Current Status and Future Development".[3]

It is heartening to note that the two presidential addresses are in Forensic Psychiatry, the first one by O. Somasundaram 1987 on "The Indian lunacy Act —1912"[4] the historic background; and the second one by S Nambi on "Marriage, Mental Health and Indian Legislation" in 2005. It is to be noted here that the Presidential Address by JK Trivedi in 2004 on "Terrorism and Mental Health" is also to be taken into account. Incidentally, both these presidents are from Chennai, South India. At this juncture, it is to be noted that majority of the forensic psychiatry articles in the last 50 years, around 20 are from the South and many of them are from Chennai centre. The Central zone (Lucknow) followed by North and West zone represent the second, third, and fourth in the descending order in this category. Even though, the East zone members have done some pioneering work in forensic psychiatry, only a few articles have been published. It is to be noted here that there are three forensic psychiatry articles authored by foreign authors and one by military (Navy) psychiatrists. Apart from the two presidential addresses specifically in forensic psychiatry, Vidysagar's Presidential Address in 1973 and VSP Basyam's Presidential Address in 1997 have some important points mentioned about Forensic Psychiatry and Mental Health Legislation.

When we review the forensic psychiatry articles in the IJP articles, we cannot miss one name, i.e. O somasundaram of Chennai. Among all the articles on Forensic psychiatry published by the IJP, the contribution by O Somasundaram is nearly one-fourth. His articles include following:

1. Guilty but insane-some aspects of psychiatric crime—1960
2. Insanity vs criminal responsibility—1964
3. Psychiatrically 11/under trail patients—1969
4. Men who kill their wives—1970
5. Crimes of persons with epilepsy—1972
6. The mothers who kills their children—1973
7. Crimes of persons with schizophrenia—1974

8. Crimes of persons with affective disorder—1977
9. Murder in Tamil Nadu—a study of murder trial—1980
10. A study of delinquent
11. The Indian Lunacy Act—1912 the historic background: The Presidential Address.
12. The Psychiatry of Assailants of Tamil Nadu Chief Ministers—1992.

In his Presidential Address on "The Indian Lunacy Act, 1912, the historic background, he traced the evaluation of legislation of various countries with a special mention on British Legislations. At that time, he mentioned that the Indian Lunacy Act was out modeled and should be replaced and that there is a need to change the Act for a more comprehensive Mental Health Act.

Nambi, in his Presidential Address in 2005, mentioned the changing concepts of marriages in India with special emphasis on the increased rate of divorce. He narrated the relation between marriage and various mental health problems. The important aspect of his article in "Marriage, Mental Health, and Indian Legislation" is the various legal procedures outlined by different personal laws in this country. He also mentioned as to how the unsoundness of mind affects the capacity to marry and form a ground for divorce, based on these personal laws prevailing in India.[5]

It is worthy to mention here, two important articles: One by BB Sethi in his editorial in 1984 and the other by LP Shah in his DLN Murthi Rao Oration in 1999. To quote BB Sethi[6] "Majority of patients who require the expertise of a Psychiatrist are those who may harm themselves or the society, are not able to look after the welfare of their family or property and may turn out to be dangerous if allowed to act out of their thinking. Their management quite often requires taking away their basic civil rights, involving freedom, activities and residence. According to existing laws in force, such restraints can be imposed only through a due process and thus it is imperative that the psychiatrists be familiar with these." To quote LP Shah ,[3] "a large number of mental health, legal and Law enforcement professionals are ignorant of Mental Health Related Laws. This is indeed a very shocking state of affairs and there is an urgent need to correct the situations. To quote LP Shah again, "There is hardly any literature in India, clarifying the topics like negligence, informed consent, confidentiality, certification, seclusion, suicide, homicide and the complication of various therapies." He also recommended that the level of teaching and research in the area of Forensic Psychiatry be upgraded and the in-service programmes for the medical and psychiatric personnel. The judiciary and the Law Enforcement Bodies as well as Social Welfare Organization to protect the Human Rights of the Mentally ill be enhanced.

CONCLUSION

Forensic Psychiatry is a clinical subspecialty of psychiatry. The subject is concerned with an area where Psychiatry and Law meet. It overlaps interfaces and interacts with psychiatry is the therapeutic discipline. Due to various reasons, Forensic Psychiatry is reared as Cinderella in our country, which, is much neglected, ignored, misinterpreted and misunderstood. It is very essential that more and more articles based on the modern concept of Forensic Psychiatry and the practical implementation and difficulties of various laws relating to mental health should be published periodically in the IJP. Of course, there are a few psychiatrists in the country with interest in Forensic Psychiatry, who carry out some work in this area, but the main problem of our authors of this article have presented and published more than 50 articles in various souvenirs, regional journals and in the national and international conferences and CMEs, but, hardly only one or two of these have been published. We have to understand that the scientific work which is carried out should be documented or published; if not documented it means it is not done.

REFERENCES

1. Indian Journal of Psychiatry, E-Journal, 2009. Accessible at archives section, www.indianjpsychiatry.org.
2. Nambi S. Legal aspects of psychiatry—Indian perspective. Manashanti Publications, 2008.
3. Shah LP. Forensic psychiatry in India current status and future developments. Indian J Psychiatry, 1999;41:179-85.
4. Somasundaram O. The Indian Lunacy Act, 1912: The Historic Background. Indian J Psychiatry, 1985;29:3-14.
5. Nambi S. Marriage, mental health and the Indian legislation. Indian Journal of Psychiatry, 2005;47:3-14.
6. Sethi BB. Need for growth of forensic psychiatry. Indian Journal of Psychiatry, 1984;26:1-2.

Annexure—1

The Mental Health Care Bill, 2012

CLAUSE

Part I—Preliminary

1—Short title.
2—Objects and purposes of the Act.
3—Interpretation.

Part II—Access to Mental Health Care

4—Cost, accessibility, etc. of health care.
5—Quality of health care.
6—Responsibility of national and county governments.
7—Counselling and aftercare services.
8—Promotion of community mental health care.
9—Mental health interventions in primary care.
10—Access to medication and psychosocial interventions.
11—Access to medical insurance.

Part III—Determination of Mental Illness

12—Determination of mental illness.
13—Principles for determination of mental illness.
14—Determination by medical practitioner.

Part IV—Rights of Persons with Mental Illness and Duties of Mental Health Care Providers

15—Right to mental health care.
16—Protection from discrimination.
17—Legal capacity.
18—Consent to treatment.
19—Access to information.
20—Confidentiality of information.
21—Disclosure of confidential information.
22—Conditions at mental health care facilities.

23—Persons not to be subjected to forced labour.
24—Protection against abuse and cruel and degrading treatment.
25—Person to be informed of rights.
26—Rights of families and carers of persons with mental illness.
27—Best practices.
28—Right to representation.
29—Right to participate in treatment planning.

Part V—Provisions on Admission and Treatment

30—Voluntary admission.
31—Informed consent.
32—Involuntary admission.
33—Emergency admission and treatment.
34—Considerations for emergency cases.
35—Duration of emergency treatment.

Part VI—Mentally Ill Offenders

36—Facilities for mentally ill offenders.

Part VII—Seclusion and Restraint

37—Seclusion or restraint to be in accordance with the law.
38—Conditions for restraint or seclusion.

Part VIII—Review, Appeals, Discharge and Transfer of Person with Mental Illness

39—Review of mental health status.
40—Appeals.
41—Discharge of person with mental illness.
42—Transfer of person with mental illness.

Part IX—Care and Administration of Property of Persons with Mental Illness

43—Application for administration.
44—Receipt of evidence.
45—Order for administration.
46—Duties of a manager.
47—Inventory of property.
48—Penalty.
49—Removal of manager.

Part X—Mental Health Care Board

50—Establishment of the Board.
51—Functions of the Board.

The Mental Health Care Bill, 2012

A Bill for an Act of Parliament to provide for the care, treatment and rehabilitation of persons with mental illness; to provide for the procedures for admission, treatment and general management of persons with mental illness; to provide for the establishment of the Mental Health Care Board and for connected purposes. Enacted by the Parliament of Kenya, as follows:

Part I—Preliminary	
1. This Act may be cited as the Mental Health Care Act, 2012.	Short title.
2. (a) The objects and purposes of this Act are to—promote the mental health and well being of all, including reducing the incidences of mental illness; (b) co-ordinate the prevention of mental illness, access to mental health care, treatment and rehabilitation services to persons with mental illness; (c) reduce the impact of mental illness, including the effects of stigma on individuals, family and the community; (d) promote recovery from mental illnesses and enhance rehabilitation and integration of person with mental illness into the community; (e) ensure that the rights of a person with mental illness are protected and safeguarded.	Objects and purposes of the Act
3. In this Act, unless the context otherwise requires— • "Board" means the Mental Health Care Board established under section 50 of this Act; • "Cabinet Secretary" means the Cabinet Secretary of the Ministry for the time being responsible for matters relating to health; • "care treatment and rehabilitation" includes preventive and after care services such as counselling psychotherapy and vocational care; • "court" means the magistrate's court; • "health care provider" means a person or institution duly licensed and accredited under the written law for the time being in force to provide health care services; • "least restrictive alternative" means health care environment involving minimum emotional, physical and social restraint during home, community or institutional-based care; • "medical practitioner" means a person registered under the Medical Practitioners and Dentists Act as a medical practitioner; • "mental health care facility" means an institution, whether private or public, duly licensed to provide mental health care services; • "mental health" means a state of well-being in which the individual realizes his or her own abilities, can cope with the normal stresses of life, can work productively and fruitfully and is able to make a contribution to his or her community; • "mental illness" includes any disorder, impairment, disability or handicap of the mind, including mental impairment as a result of alcohol, drugs or substance abuse; • "person with mental illness" means a person diagnosed as suffering from a mental illness; • "psychosocial interventions" include counselling, aftercare services and integration; and • "representative" means spouse, next of kin, partner, parent or guardian of the person with mental illness having legal capacity to make decisions on behalf of the person with mental illness.	Interpretation Cap 253

Part II—Access to Mental Health Care	
4. (a) Mental health care shall be affordable, equitable and accessible to all. (b) The national and county governments shall ensure that there is adequate funding for mental health care services to meet requirements for staffing, facilities, medication and equipment to ensure the highest attainable quality in provision of mental health care services as required under this Act. (c) A person with mental illness shall be entitled to receive funds from the National Development Fund for Persons with Disabilities established under the Persons with Disabilities Act, 2003 or such other fund as may be established under any written law for the time being in force to cater for persons with disabilities.	Cost, accessibility, etc. of health care No. 14 of 2003.
5. Mental health care shall be of the highest quality possible and shall be provided in a manner that— (a) preserves the dignity of the person with mental illness; (b) takes into consideration and allows for treatment options which helps a person with mental illness to cope by himself or herself with the mental health illness affecting him or her; (c) provide relevant clinical and non-clinical care aimed at reducing the impact of the mental illness and improving the quality of life of the person with mental illness.	Quality of health care
6. The national and county governments shall determine and co-ordinate the implementation of their health policies and measures in a manner that— (a) ensures the provision of mental health care and treatment at health establishments at the community, primary, secondary and tertiary levels; (b) promotes the provision of community-based care and treatment; (c) ensures that adequate funding is allocated to mental health care; (d) promotes the rights and best interests of persons with mental illness; and (e) promotes and improves the mental health status of the people. In the provision of mental health care, priority shall be granted to community health and primary mental health care and treatment as opposed to institutionalization of the person with mental illness, having regard to the mental health condition of the person with mental illness, economic and social status of the community. Where a person with mental illness has been discharged from a mental health care facility, efforts shall be made towards re-integration of the person into the community and specialized and personalized after-care services required to enable the person with mental illness live a decent and dignified life outside the facility.	Responsibility of national and county governments

7. A person with mental illness has the right to appropriate physical and mental medical care and treatment, as well as, to the widest extent possible, counselling, rehabilitation and after care support necessary to help the person with mental illness recover from the illness.	Counseling and aftercare services
8. The national and county governments shall ensure that community mental health is promoted by— (a) providing appropriate resources, facilities, services, personnel and programs to allow persons with mental illness to be attended to at the community level; and (b) ensuring that there exists a supportive environment that facilitates access to care and treatment and other necessary after care and supportive services. Community mental health services shall undertake the provision of— (a) outpatient services to persons with mental illness clinics in health centres and general hospitals; (b) rehabilitation and aftercare services for persons with mental illness after discharge from a mental health facility; (c) supervised homecare and support for persons with mental illness; and (d) services for the promotion of mental health.	Promotion of community mental health care
9. Mental health interventions in primary care shall— (a) be comprehensive, ranging from prevention to early intervention through treatment and continuing care and prevention of relapse; (b) target the populations that are at different levels of risk including children, women, youth, elderly persons, refugees and those affected by catastrophic incidences and emergencies. (c) include education, awareness and training on mental health promotion and interventions. The families and carers of persons with mental illness shall be accorded support necessary to reduce their exposure to mental illnesses caused by catastrophic incidences and emergencies, and interaction with the person with mental illness.	Mental health interventions in primary care
10. A mental health care facility shall have access to the same level of resources as any other health establishment, and in particular— (a) qualified medical practitioners, including psychiatrists, psychologists, psychiatric nurses, counsellors, psychotherapists and other qualified professional staff in sufficient numbers, and with adequate space to provide each person with mental illness with privacy and a programme of appropriate therapy; (b) diagnostic and therapeutic equipment; (c) adequate, regular and comprehensive treatment, including supplies of medication; and (d) appropriate professional care. The national government shall ensure that all medication required in the treatment of persons with mental illness is included in the essential drug list.	Access to medication and psychosocial interventions

The Board shall liaise with the Cabinet Secretary responsible for education to integrate into the syllabus instructions relating to mental health, including instructions on prevention, treatment, rehabilitation and other general information on mental health and related illnesses.	
11. Every person is entitled, if the person so wishes, to medical insurance covering treatment to a person suffering from mental illness and no insurance company shall make any insurance policy providing insurance against sickness which excludes or restricts the treatment of persons suffering from mental illness. A person with mental illness shall not be discriminated against or subject to unfair treatment in obtaining adequate health insurance for the care and treatment of physical and mental health problems from public and private health insurance providers. Any person or insurance company that contravenes the provisions of this section commits an offence and shall be liable, on conviction, to a fine not exceeding five hundred thousand shillings, or to imprisonment for a term not exceeding three years, or both.	Access to medical insurance.
Part III—Determination of Mental Illness	
12. A determination that a person has a mental illness shall be made in accordance with the provisions of this Act and the regulations made under the Act.	Determination of mental illness
13. (a) A determination of mental illness shall not be made on the basis of political, economic or social status or membership in a cultural, racial or religious group, or for any other reason not directly relevant to the mental health status of a person. (b) A family or professional conflict, or non-conformity with moral, social, cultural or political values or religious beliefs prevailing in a person's community, shall not be a determining factor in the diagnosis of mental illness. (c) A background of past treatment or hospitalization as a person with mental illness shall not of itself justify any present or future determination of mental illness.	Principles for determination of mental illness
14. A determination as to whether a person is suffering from mental illness shall be made by at least two accredited health practitioners with at least three years experience on matters related to mental health.	Determination by medical practitioner
Part IV—Rights of Persons with Mental Illness and Duties of Mental Health Care Providers	
15. (a) Every person has the right to the highest attainable mental health care. (b) A person with mental illness shall be treated in a humane and dignified manner, and shall have his or her privacy respected. (c) A person with mental illness has the right to protection from physical, economic, social, sexual and other forms of exploitation, abuse and degrading treatment.	Right to mental health care

16. (a) A person shall not be discriminated against on the ground that he or she is suffering from mental illness. (b) Every person with mental illness shall have the right to exercise all civil, political, economic, social and cultural rights accorded to every person by the Constitution and any other written law in force in Kenya.	Protection from discrimination
17. (a) Where a person is, by reason of his or her mental illness, deemed by law not to have legal capacity, such person shall be entitled to the appointment of a personal representative to manage or conduct his or her affairs. (b) Where a court or other competent body finds that a person with mental illness is unable to manage his or her own affairs, measures shall be taken, so far as is necessary and appropriate to that person's condition, to ensure the protection of his or her best interests.	Legal capacity
18 (a) Every health care provider shall, where the person with mental illness is capable of making an informed decision on the need for treatment, inform the person with mental illness of his or her right to choose an appropriate treatment of his or her own choice, and obtain written consent prior to administering any treatment. (b) Where a person with mental illness is incapable of making an informed decision on the need for treatment, such consent must be sought and obtained from the personal representative as appointed under this Act, unless the treatment is provided under section 33 (emergency admission and treatment).	Consent to treatment
19. (a) Every person with mental illness is entitled to access to full information regarding his or her mental and other health status, clinical records and other related information maintained by mental health care facilities and service providers in accordance with Article 35 of the Constitution, subject to restrictions necessary to prevent serious harm to the health of the person with mental illness or to the public. (b) Any information withheld under section 20 (1) shall be accessible to the personal representative of a person with mental illness duly appointed under this Act. (c) Whenever information is withheld from a person with mental illness or his or her representative, the person with mental illness or his or her representative shall receive notice of such withholding and the reasons for it and such decision shall be subject to a review by the Board and further judicial review. (d) Any representations made by a person with mental illness or his or her representative shall, on request, form part of that person's records. (e) The Cabinet Secretary shall make regulations generally on access to information under this section, and without prejudice to the generality of the foregoing, such regulations may provide for—	Access to information

• the procedure for making an application for access to information; • the person or persons eligible to apply for access to the information; • the duration within which the mental health care facility shall make such records available upon receipt of the application; • exceptional circumstances where such information may be withheld.	
20. (a) All information obtained in the context of care and treatment of a person with mental illness is confidential and such confidentiality shall be maintained by those in possession of such information. (b) A person or a mental health care facility may not disclose any confidential information, except under circumstances enumerated under section 21.	Confidentiality of information
21. A person or mental health care facility may disclose confidential information relating to a person with mental illness where such disclosure— (a) is required by law or ordered by a court; (b) is in the public interest; (c) is necessary to prevent the likelihood of serious harm to the person with mental illness or to others; (d) is necessary for purposes of treating the person with mental illness and in the best interest of the person with mental illness.	Disclosure of confidential information
22. The environment and living conditions at a mental health care facility shall be as close as possible to those of the normal life of persons of similar age as those housed in the facility and in particular shall include— (a) facilities for recreation and leisure activities; (b) facilities for education and religious practice; (c) facilities for communication; (d) facilities suited to the social and cultural background of a person with mental illness, and for appropriate vocational rehabilitation measures to promote reintegration of the person in the community, including vocational guidance, counselling and placement; (e) facilities necessary to ensure that the privacy and dignity of a person with mental illness is protected as required by this Act. Every mental health care facility shall be inspected by the Board at least once every six months to ensure that the conditions, treatment and care of persons with mental illness comply with the provisions of this Act and any other relevant written law.	Conditions at mental health care facilities
23. (a) A person with mental illness shall not be subjected to forced labor, whether within or outside a mental health care facility. (b) Every person with mental illness in a mental health care facility has the right to receive remuneration for any work done, similar to that payable to a person without mental illness.	Persons not to be subjected to forced labor

24. Every person, body, organization or mental health care facility providing care and treatment to a person with mental illness shall take steps to ensure that— (a) persons with mental illness are protected from exploitation, abuse, or any cruel and degrading treatment; (b) persons with mental illness are not subjected to any forced labor; and (c) care and treatment services are not used as punishment or for the convenience of other people. A person who witnesses any form of abuse against a person with mental illness shall report the incident immediately to the police, the Board or any other competent authority.	Protection against abuse and cruel and degrading treatment
25. (a) A person with mental illness shall be informed of his or her rights under the law by the mental health care provider attending to him or her, in a form and language which the person understands, which information shall include an explanation of those rights and how to exercise them. (b) Where the person with mental illness does not understand such information or does not have mental capacity for such understanding, the rights shall be communicated to the representative of that person.	Person to be informed of rights
26. The families and carers of persons with mental illness have the right to— (a) access information regarding the medical status and treatment plans of a person with mental illness; (b) receive support and services from the relevant government agencies in taking care of person with mental illness; (c) be involved in the formulation of mental health policy, legislation and plans; (d) be involved in the legal processes including decision-making, reviews and appeals relating to a person with mental illness.	Rights of families and carers of persons with mental illness
27. (a) In making a decision under this Act concerning the care or treatment of a person with mental illness, including a decision to make an admission order in relation to a person, the best interests of that person shall be the principal consideration with due regard being given to the interests of other persons who may be at risk of serious harm. (b) Where it is proposed to make a recommendation or an admission order in respect of a person with mental illness, or to administer treatment to such person under this Act, the person shall, so far as is reasonably practicable, be notified of the proposal and be entitled to make representations in relation to it, either in person or through a representative, and before deciding the matter, due consideration shall be given to any representations duly made under this subsection. (c) In making a decision under this Act concerning the care or treatment of a person with mental illness, including a decision to make an admission order, due regard shall be given to the need to respect the right of the person to dignity, integrity and privacy.	Best practices

28. (a) A person with mental illness is entitled to choose and appoint a representative of his or her own choice, to represent him or her in any manner, including in any complaint procedure or appeal. (b) A person with mental illness is entitled to, where necessary, the services of an interpreter who shall be made available free of charge. (c) A person with mental illness or his or her representative has the right to produce at any hearing independent medical reports or any other oral or written reports or any other evidence that is relevant to his or her mental health status. (d) A person with mental illness or his or her representative has the right to attend, participate and be heard in any hearing.	Right to representation
29. (a) A person with mental illness has a right to participate in the formulation of his or her treatment plans. (b) Where a person with mental illness is incapable of exercising the right under subsection (1) due to his or her mental illness, his or her representative, spouse, next of kin, partner, associate, parent or guardian shall be entitled to participate in the formulation of treatment plans.	Right to participate in treatment planning
Part V—Provisions on Admission and Treatment	
30. A person who presents himself or herself voluntarily to a mental health care facility for treatment or admission shall be entitled to receive appropriate care and treatment or to be referred to an appropriate mental health care facility.	Voluntary admission
31. (a) No mental health care, treatment or admission shall be accorded to a person with mental illness without the person's informed consent or that of his or her representative. (b) In order for consent to be valid under this section, it shall satisfy the following conditions— • the person with mental illness or his or her representative shall be competent to give the consent; • consent shall be given freely without threats or improper inducements; • there shall be appropriate and adequate disclosure of all relevant information relating to treatment, including information on the kind, purpose, likely duration and expected benefits of the treatment; • choices, where available, shall be given to the person with mental illness in accordance with prescribed clinical practice; • consent shall be documented in the person's records.	Informed consent

32. A person may be admitted involuntarily to a mental health care facility as a person with mental illness, or, having been admitted voluntarily as a person with mental illness, be retained involuntarily as a person with mental illness in the mental health care facility, if a qualified mental health care medical practitioner determines, in accordance with this Act, that the person has a mental illness or disorder and considers that— (a) because of mental illness or disorder, there is a serious likelihood of immediate or imminent harm to that person or to other persons; or (b) in the case a person whose mental illness or disorder is severe and whose judgment is impaired, failure to admit or retain the person is likely to lead to a serious deterioration in his or her condition, or will prevent the giving of appropriate treatment that can only be given by admission to a mental health facility in accordance with the principle of the least restrictive alternative. A mental health care facility may receive an involuntarily admitted person with mental illness, only if the facility has been designated to do so by law and only for the duration necessary to stabilize the person with mental illness, and provide mental health care services to him or her. The following factors shall be considered in cases of involuntary admission— (a) there is evidence of a mental illness of a specified severity; (b) there is likelihood of immediate or imminent harm to the person with mental illness or others, and a deterioration of the person's condition if treatment or admission or both are not given; (c) the treatment can only be given by way of admission to the health facility.	Involuntary admission
33. An emergency admission or treatment of a person with mental illness shall be administered where there is immediate and imminent danger to the health and safety of the person with mental illness or other people, and the nature of such immediate and imminent danger is such that there need to be urgent care and treatment to stabilize the person with mental illness.	Emergency admission and treatment
34. (a) For any case to be considered an emergency, there shall first be shown that the time required to comply with substantive procedures would cause delay and lead to harm to the person with mental illness or to other people. (b) Where the requirements in subsection (1) have been satisfied, the person with mental illness may be admitted to the health facility or be given treatment based on the assessment carried out by a qualified medical practitioner or other accredited mental health practitioner.	Considerations for emergency cases

35. (a) Emergency admission or treatment shall not be prolonged for duration longer than necessary to stabilize the person with mental illness and in any case, shall not be prolonged beyond a period of seventy-two hours, and shall be allowed only to the extent that it is necessary to treat the person with mental illness. (b) Emergency treatment shall not include— • depot neuroleptics; • electroconvulsive therapy; • sterilization; • psychosurgery or other irreversible treatment. (c) Procedures for emergency treatment or admission or both may be initiated immediately by a spouse, next of kin, partner, parent or guardian and authorized by a qualified medical practitioner if it is assessed that the person with mental illness is likely to require care beyond the stipulated time limit for emergency treatment. (d) The family of the person with mental illness or their representative shall be immediately informed of the emergency procedures undertaken. (e) A person with mental illness, his or her family or representative have the right to appeal against emergency admission or treatment to the Board. (f) The Cabinet Secretary may, on the recommendations of the Board, make regulations on emergency treatment and admission.	Duration of emergency treatment
Part VI—Mentally Ill Offenders	
36. (a) Whenever a medical practitioner is of the opinion that a prisoner or a remandee is of unsound mind, the practitioner may, by order under his or her hand in the form prescribed, direct that such prisoner be removed to a mental health facility within the prison or outside the prison and be treated while under detention. (b) Where a prisoner or remandee transferred to a mental health facility pursuant to subsection (1) is, in the opinion of the person in charge of such mental health facility, no longer mentally ill, the person in charge of the mental health facility shall inform the officer in charge of the prison from which the prisoner was removed, and the prisoner shall then be delivered into the custody of the officer of that prison if still liable to be confined in prison, and if not so liable, shall be released. (c) The period during which the prisoner has been detined in the mental health facility under this section shall be recorded as part of the prisoner's term of imprisonment. (d) Mentally ill offenders shall be entitled to have their criminal cases expedited and given priority over other cases. (e) The Director of Public Prosecutions and other state officers shall expedite the process of granting mentally ill offenders within the criminal justice system the necessary authorizations and examinations and at no cost.	Facilities for mentally ill offenders

(f) Mentally ill offenders shall be provided mental health care and treatment by the government. (g) There shall be special cells for mentally ill prisoners within which they shall be held separately from the rest of the prisoners or other persons with mental illness, and receive mental health care and treatment of the same quality and with the same frequency as other person with mental illness. (h) Mentally ill prisoners with severe mental illness may be thansferred to a mental health care facility where they can receive appropriate treatment and care.	
Part VII—Seclusion and Restraint	
37. (a) A person with mental illness shall not be physically restrained or secluded except in accordance with the law and the set procedures and upon authorization by a qualified mental health care practitioner. (b) Physical restraint or seclusion shall only be used where it is the only means available to prevent immediate or imminent harm to the person with mental illness or other people. (c) Physical restraint or seclusion shall not be prolonged beyond the period which is strictly necessary to administer treatment to the person with mental illness necessary to allow him or her to co-habit peacefully with other users within the facility, his or her family or with members of the community. (d) All instances of physical restraint or seclusion, their reasons, nature and extent shall be recorded in the person's medical records. (e) A person with mental illness who is restrained or secluded shall be kept under humane conditions and shall be under the care and regular supervision of a qualified mental health care practitioner within the facility. (f) A representative of the person with mental illness shall be given prompt notice of the restraint or seclusion of the person with mental illness. (g) The review of the mental health status of a person with mental illness under seclusion or restraint shall be done in accordance with Part VIII of this Act.	Seclusion or restraint to be in accordance with the law
38. Where a person with mental illness is physically restrained or secluded, a mental health care practitioner shall— (a) ensure that it is in the best interests of that person; (b) the mental health care facility has adequate facilities to ensure the safety of that person; (c) ensure the restraint or seclusion is not used as a punishment to the person with mental illness or for the convenience of the staff of the health facility. Restraint and seclusion shall be implemented alongside other forms of treatment only as a last resort and when other forms of treatment fail.	Conditions for restraint or seclusion

Part VIII—Review, Appeals, Discharge and Transfer of Person with Mental Illness	
39. The mental health status of a person with mental illness shall be reviewed periodically by a mental health care practitioner, and such review shall include a review of— (a) the nature of the illness; (b) the need for care and treatment; (c) the type of care and treatment provided; (d) the need for referral, transfer or discharge; and (e) any other matters related to the mental health status of the person with mental illness. The review of the mental health status of a person with mental illness may be initiated by— (a) the person with mental illness; (b) the mental health care practitioner in charge of managing the person with mental illness; (c) a representative of the person with mental illness; (d) the mental health care practitioner in charge of the facility; (e) any other person upon proof of the nature of their interest; or (f) the Board. The procedure for review shall be as prescribed under this Act.	Review of mental health status.
40. Any decision made under review shall be subject to appeal in the first instance to the mental health care practitioner in charge of the facility, and further to the Board. A person with mental illness or his or her representative who is not satisfied with the decision of the Board on appeal may appeal further to the High Court.	Appeals
41. A person with mental illness shall be discharged where— (a) the mental health care practitioner in charge of managing the person makes a decision to discharge the person as a result of a review; (b) the person can no longer receive any other or further treatment from a mental health care facility and appropriate efforts are being made towards re-integration of the person into the community, and for specialized and personalized aftercare service.	Discharge of person with mental illness
42. Where a mental health care practitioner is of the opinion that it would be for the benefit of a person with mental illness admitted in a mental health care facility, or that it is necessary for the purpose of obtaining special treatment for such person, the person may be transferred to another mental health care facility after obtaining consent from— (a) the person with mental illness; or (b) the representative of the person with mental illness; or (c) the other mental health care facility where the person with mental illness is being transferred to. A person with mental illness in a health facility other than a mental health care facility may be transferred from the health facility to a mental health care facility.	Transfer of person with mental illness

Part IX—Care and Administration of Property of Persons with Mental Illness	
43. An application for an order for the management and administration of the estate of a person with mental illness may be made to the court by a parent, spouse or child who has attained the age of eighteen years, friend, relative or any interested person under whose care or charge the person with mental illness is. an application under subsection (1) shall be accompanied by an affidavit setting out the grounds upon which it is made and shall give full particulars as to the property and relatives of the person to whom it relates. Where the application relates to a person duly admitted as a person with mental illness, the application shall be accompanied by a certified true copy of the appropriate admission or treatment and particulars in respect of that person. The notice of the application shall, unless the court considers its service impracticable, inexpedient or would be ineffectual, be served upon the person in respect of whom the application is made in such manner as the court may direct. The court may direct that a copy of such notice be served upon any relative of the person with a mental illness or upon any other person to whom in the opinion of the court notice of the application should be given. The court may require the person in relation to whom an application is made to attend at a place and time as it may appoint for the purpose of being personally examined by the court, or by a registered medical practitioner or any other person as the court may desire in order to have a report of the mental capacity and condition of such person.	Application for administration
44. The court shall receive evidence on affidavit or otherwise and consider any report submitted to it under the provisions of this Act as to the mental capacity of the person to whom the application relates as may be produced before it. The court may, in any proceedings under this Act, make inquiries into the properties belonging to a person alleged to be suffering from a mental illness.	Receipt of evidence
45. The court may make such order as it finds necessary for the administration and management of the estate of any person with mental illness, for the purpose of making provision for the person's maintenance and that of members of his immediate family who are dependent upon him or her, and for the payment of his or her debts. The court may appoint a fit and proper person to be the manager of the estate of a person with mental illness for the purposes of safeguarding the property of that person. The court shall, by notice in the Gazette, inform the public of the appointment of a person as the manager of the estate of a person who is suffering from mental illness and may allow any person to lodge an objection to the appointment.	Order for administration

A manager appointed under subsection (3) shall act in accordance with the directions of the court, and shall exercise powers for the management of the estate as may be expressly conferred upon him or her, either specifically or generally, by any order or direction of the court or any other relevant written law. A manager shall not, without express permission of the court, mortgage, charge, or transfer any immovable property or lease that property for a term exceeding three years.	
46. Where a manager is appointed under this Part, the court may order that the manager shall have such general or special powers for the management of the estate as the court considers necessary, and proper regard being had to the nature of the property whether movable or immovable of which the estate may consist. Notwithstanding subsection (1), a manager shall not, without special permission of the court— (a) mortgage, charge or transfer by sale, gift, surrender or exchange any immovable property of which the estate may consist; (b) lease any such property for a term exceeding five years; or (c) invest in any securities other than those authorized under the Trustee Act. A manager shall not invest any funds or property belonging to the estate of which he or she is a manager, in any company or undertaking in which he or she has an interest, nor on the purchase of immovable property under the authority of section 4(1) (d) of the Trustee Act without prior consent of the court. A manager shall perform his or her duties responsibly taking into account the best interests of the estate of the person who is suffering from mental illness. Every conveyance or other instrument made in pursuant to an order of the court shall be valid and have effect as if it were made by the person, being of sound mind and in respect of whose estate the order is made.	Duties of a manager Cap 167 Cap 167
47. Every person appointed to be a manager of the estate of a person with mental illness under this Part shall, within six months of the date of his or her appointment, deliver to the court and to the Public Trustee an inventory of the property belonging to the person in respect of whose estate he or she has been appointed manager and all sums of money, goods and effects as he or she receives on account of the estate, together with a statement of debts owed by or due to such person, in the prescribed form. The representative or any person having capacity to act as the representative of a person with mental illness may, upon payment of such fee as may be prescribed, inspect and obtain a copy of any inventory, statement or account delivered to the court and to the Public Trustee pursuant to subsection (1).	Inventory of property

An interested person who does not fall in the category of persons mentioned in subsection (2) above may, on payment of such fee as may be prescribed, make an application to the court to inspect and obtain a copy of any such inventory, statement or account delivered to the court and to the Public Trustee pursuant to subsection (1). The Public Trustee shall report annually to the Cabinet Secretary and the Board on all accounts delivered to him or her under subsection (1). Where any person, by petition to the court, impugns the accuracy of any inventory or statement or of any annual account made under this section, the court may summon the manager and inquire summarily into the matter, and make such order as it considers proper, or may refer the petition to a magistrate having jurisdiction in the place where the property belonging to the estate concerned is situated, for inquiry and report, and upon receipt of the magistrate's report, the court may make such order as it considers necessary.	
48. A manager who contravenes the provisions of this Part shall be liable, upon conviction, to imprisonment for a term not exceeding three years or a fine not exceeding five hundred thousand Kenya shillings, or to both. Any property of a person who is mentally which is lost due to maladministration of his or her estate shall be a civil debt recoverable summarily.	Penalty
49. The court may, on its own motion or upon application, for any sufficient cause, remove any manager or guardian appointed by it under this Part, and may appoint any other fit person in his or her place, and may make such order as it considers necessary to ensure that the person removed transfers the property under his or her care, and of which he or she was manager, to his or her successor, and accounts to the successor for all money received or disbursed by him or her in connection with the property.	Removal of manager
Part X—Mental Health Care Board	
50. There is established a board to be known as the Mental Health Care Board. The Board is a body corporate with perpetual succession and a common seal and shall, in its corporate name, be capable of— (a) suing and being sued; (b) taking, purchasing or otherwise acquiring, holding, charging or disposing of movable and immovable property; (c) borrowing money or making investments; (d) entering into contracts; and (e) doing or performing all other acts or things for the proper performance of its functions under this Act which may lawfully be done or performed by a body corporate.	Establishment of the Board

The Board shall be the successor to the Board known as the Kenya Board of Mental Heath existing immediately before the commencement of this Act, and subject to this Act, all rights, obligations, assets and liabilities of that Board existing at the commencement of this Act shall be automatically and fully transferred to the Board and any reference to the Kenya Board of Mental Heath in any contract or document shall, for all purposes, be deemed to be a reference to the Board established under subsection (1). The provisions of the First Schedule shall apply upon the commencement of this Act.	
51. The functions of the Board shall be to— (a) co-ordinate the mental health care activities in Kenya; (b) advise and make recommendations to the Government on the state of mental health and mental health care facilities; (c) approve the establishment of mental health facilities; (d) inspect mental health facilities to ensure that they meet the prescribed standards; (e) assist, where necessary, in the administration of mental health facilities; (f) receive and investigate any matter referred to it by a person with mental illness or relative or any representative of a person with mental illness concerning the treatment of the person with mental illness at a mental health facility and where necessary to take, or recommend to the Cabinet Secretary, any remedial action; (g) initiate and organize community or family-based programmes aimed at promoting mental health and prevent incidences of mental illness; (h) perform such other functions as may be conferred upon it this Act or any other written law or may be necessary in the carrying out of the Board's functions.	Functions of the Board Functions of the Board
52. The Board shall consist of— (a) the Director of Mental Health; (b) the Director of Medical Services; (c) three medical practitioners with specialization and experience on mental health care nominated by each of the following bodies and appointed by the Cabinet Secretary— • representative body of psychiatrists; • representative body of psychologists; • representative body of counsellors; (d) one person representing caregivers of persons who are mentally ill appointed by the Cabinet Secretary; (e) one person appointed by the Cabinet Secretary having sufficient levels of experience in advocating for the rights of mentally ill persons; (f) the Chief Executive Officer. In appointing the members of the Board under subsection (1)(c), (d) and (e), the Cabinet Secretary shall take into consideration gender balance and diversity in qualifications of persons being appointed.	Membership of the Board

The members of the Board shall, at their first meeting, elect a chairperson from amongst the members of the Board appointed under subsection (1)(c), (d) and (e). A person shall not be appointed as a member of the Board if such person— (a) has been convicted of an offence by a court of competent jurisdiction and sentenced to imprisonment for a term of six months or more; (b) is adjudged bankrupt or has entered into a composition, scheme or arrangement with his or her creditors; (c) is disqualified under the provisions of any other written law from appointment as such. A member of the Board other than an ex-officio member shall hold office for a period of three years, but shall be eligible for re-appointment for a further and final term of three years. A member of the Board, other than an ex-officio member, may— (a) at any time resign from office by notice in writing to the chairperson; (b) be removed from office if the member— • has been absent from three consecutive meetings of the Board without the permission of the chairperson; • is adjudged bankrupt or enters into a composition scheme or arrangement with his or her creditors; • is convicted of an offence involving dishonesty or fraud; • is convicted of a criminal offence and sentenced to imprisonment for a term exceeding six months or to a fine exceeding ten thousand shillings; • is incapacitated by prolonged physical or mental illness or is deemed otherwise unfit to discharge his or her duties as a member of the Board.	
53. The Board shall have all powers necessary for the proper performance of its functions under this Act and in particular, but without prejudice to the generality of the foregoing, the Board shall have power to— (a) enter into contracts; (b) manage, control and administer its assets in such manner and for such purposes as best promote the purpose for which it is established; (c) determine the provisions to be made for capital and recurrent expenditure and for the reserves of the Board; (d) receive any grants, gifts, donations or endowments and make legitimate disbursements therefrom; (e) enter into association with such other bodies or organizations within or outside Kenya as it may consider desirable or appropriate and in furtherance of the purposes for which it is established; (f) open such banking accounts for its funds as may be necessary; (g) invest any of its funds not immediately required for its purposes; (h) undertake any activity necessary for the fulfilment of any of its functions.	Powers of the Board

54. The conduct and regulation of the business and affairs of the Board shall be as provided in the Second Schedule. Except as provided in the Second Schedule, the Board may regulate its own procedure.	Conduct of business and affairs of the Board
55. The Board may, by resolution either generally or in any particular case, delegate to any committee or to any member, officer, employee or agent of the Board, the exercise of any of the powers or the performance of any of its functions or duties under this Act or under any other written law.	Delegation by the Board
56. The remuneration payable to members of the Board shall be determined by the Salaries and Remuneration Commission.	Remuneration of members of the Board
57. There shall be a Chief Executive of the Board who shall be appointed by the Board through a competitive process. The Chief Executive Officer shall hold office for a term of five years, on such terms and conditions of employment as the Board may determine, and shall be eligible for re-appointment. The Chief Executive Officer shall be an ex-officio member of the Board but shall have no right to vote at any meeting of the Board. The Chief Executive Officer shall— (a) subject to the direction of the Board, be responsible for the day to day management of the Board; (b) in consultation with the Board, be responsible for the direction of the affairs and transactions of the Board, the exercise, discharge and performance of its objectives, functions and duties, and the general administration of the Board; (c) be the secretary of the Board.	Chief Executive Officer
58. The Board may appoint such officers, agents and other staff as are necessary for the proper and efficient discharge of its functions under this Act, upon such terms and conditions of service as the Board may determine.	Staff
59 The common seal of the Board shall be kept in the custody of the Chief Executive Officer or of such other person as the Board may direct, and shall not be used except upon the order of the Board. The common seal of the Board, when affixed to a document and duly authenticated, shall be judicially and officially noticed, and unless the contrary is proved, any necessary order or authorization by the Board under this section shall be presumed to have been duly given. The common seal of the Board shall be authenticated by the signature of the chairperson of the Board and the Chief Executive Officer. The Board shall, in the absence of either the chairperson or the Chief Executive Officer, in any particular matter, nominate one member of the Board to authenticate the seal of the Board on behalf of either the chairperson or the Chief Executive Officer.	The common seal of the Board

60. No matter or thing done by a member of the Board or by any officer, member of staff, or agent of the Board shall, if the matter or thing is done bonafide for executing the functions, powers or duties of the Board under this Act, render the member, officer, employee or agent or any person acting on their directions personally liable to any action, claim or demand whatsoever. Any expenses incurred by any person in any suit or prosecution brought against him or her in any court, in respect of any act which is done or purported to be done by him or her under the direction of the Board, shall, if the court holds that such act was done bonafide, be paid out of the general funds of the Board, unless such expenses are recovered by him in such suit or prosecution.	Protection from personal liability
61. The provisions of section 60 shall not relieve the Board of the liability to pay compensation or damages to any person for any injury to him or her, his or her property or any of his or her interests caused by the exercise of any power conferred by this Act or any other written law or by the failure, wholly or partially, of any works.	Liability for damages
Part XI—Financial Provisions	
62. The funds of the Board shall consist of— (a) donations, grants, loans or gifts made to the Board and approved by the Cabinet Secretary and the Cabinet Secretary for the time being responsible for matters relating to finance; and (b) such fees, monies or assets as may accrue to or vest in the Board in the course of the exercise of its powers or the performance of its functions under this Act or under any written law. There shall be paid out of the funds of the Board any expenditure incurred by the Board in the exercise of its powers or the performance of its functions under this Act.	
63. The financial year of the Board shall be the period of twelve months ending on the thirtieth June in each year.	Financial year
64. At least three months before the commencement of each financial year, the Board shall cause to be prepared estimates of its revenue and expenditure for that year. The annual estimates shall make provision for all estimated expenditure of the Board for the financial year and in particular, the estimates shall provide for the— (a) payment of the salaries, allowances and other charges in respect of members and staff of the Board; (b) payment of pensions, gratuities and other charges in respect of members and staff of the Board; (c) proper maintenance of the buildings and grounds of the Board; (d) maintenance, repair and replacement of the equipment and other property of the Board; and	Annual estimates

(e) creation of such reserve funds to meet future or contingent liabilities in respect of retirement benefits, insurance or replacement of buildings or equipment, or in respect of such other matter as the Board may deem appropriate. The annual estimates shall be approved by the Board before the commencement of the financial year to which they relate and, once approved, the sum provided in the estimates shall be submitted to the Cabinet Secretary for approval. No expenditure shall be incurred for the purposes of the Board except in accordance with the annual estimates approved under subsection (3), or in pursuance of an authorization of the Board given with prior written approval of the Cabinet Secretary.	
65. The Board shall cause to be kept proper books and records of accounts of its income, expenditure and assets. Within a period of three months after the end of each financial year, the Board shall submit to the Auditor-General, its accounts together with— (a) a statement of the income and expenditure of the Board during that year; and (b) a balance sheet of the Board on the last day of that year. The accounts of the Board shall be audited and reported upon in accordance with the provisions of the Public Audit Act, 2003.	Accounts and audit No.12 of 2003
66. The Board may invest any of its funds in securities in which for the time being trustees may by law invest trust funds, or in any other securities or banks which the Treasury may, from time to time, approve for that purpose. The Board may place on deposit, with such bank or banks as it may determine, any moneys not immediately required for its purposes, as it may determine.	Investment of funds
Part XII—Miscellaneous Provisions	
67. A person who commits an offence under this Act for which no penalty is prescribed shall be liable, on conviction, to imprisonment for a term not exceeding five years or a fine not exceeding five hundred thousand shillings, or both.	General penalty
68. The Mental Health Act is repealed.	Repeal Cap 248
69. The Cabinet Secretary may, on the recommendation of the Board, make regulations generally for the better carrying into effect the provisions of this Act. Without prejudice to the generality of the foregoing, regulations made under subsection (1) may— (a) prescribe anything required by this Act to be prescribed; (b) provide for the setting of quality standards and norms for care, treatment and rehabilitation of person with mental illness; (c) provide for matters related to the rights and responsibilities of person with mental illness in mental health facilities; (d) prescribe the forms to be used under this Act;	Regulations

(e) prescribe the forms and procedures to be used in the authorization and licensing of mental health institutions and the conditions to be attached under such authorization or licence; (f) provide for accreditation of mental health practitioners as well as mental health facilities.	
First Schedule Transitional Provisions	
1. In this Schedule— • "appointed day" means the day on which this Act comes into force; • "assets" include all property movable or immovable and all estates, easements and rights whether equitable or legal in, over or out of property, choses-in-action, money or goodwill of the former institutions whether situated in Kenya or elsewhere; • "former Board" means the Board known as the Kenya Board of Mental Heath existing immediately before the commencement of this Act.; • "liabilities" means liabilities, debts, charges, duties and obligations of every description, whether present or future, actual or contingent, and whether to be observed or performed in Kenya or elsewhere; and • "rights" means all rights, powers, privileges and immunities whether actual, contingent or prospective, whether observed or performed in Kenya or elsewhere.	Interpretation
2. (a) On the appointed day, all the funds, assets and other property, both movable and immovable, which immediately before such day were vested in the former Board shall, by virtue of this paragraph, vest in the Board. (b) On the appointed day, all rights, powers and liabilities, which immediately before such day were vested in, imposed on or enforceable against the former Board shall, by virtue of this paragraph, be vested in, imposed on or enforceable against the Board. (c) If, on the appointed day, any suit, appeal, arbitration or other proceedings of whatever nature and wheresoever instituted in relation to the business of the former Board which is, by virtue of this paragraph, transferred to the Board, shall not abate, be discontinued or be in any way prejudicially affected by reason of such transfer of the business of the former Board or of anything contained in this Act, and any suit, appeal arbitration or other proceedings shall be continued, and enforced by or against the Board. (d) In the case of assets and liabilities arising under any loans which vest in the Board on the appointed day, the Board may enter into such arrangements or agreements over such rights and liabilities with the Government or any other third party.	Assets and liabilities

3. Any reference in any written law or in any document or instrument to the former Board shall, on and after the appointed day, be construed to be a reference to the Board.	Reference to former Board
4. Any proceedings pending immediately before the appointed day to which the former Board was a party shall be continued as if the Board was a party thereto in lieu of the former Board.	Proceedings
5. Every agreement, deed, bond or other instrument to which the former Board was a party or which affected the former Board and whether or not of such a nature that the rights, liabilities and obligations thereunder could be assigned, shall have effect as if the Board were a party thereto or affected thereby instead of the former Board and as if for every reference (whether express or implied) therein to the former Board there were substituted in respect of anything to be done on or after the appointed day.	Agreements, deeds, etc
6. The administrative decisions made by the former Board or by the Cabinet Secretary which are in force immediately before the appointed day shall, on or after such day, have force as if they were directions made by the Board or the Cabinet Secretary under this Act.	Administrative decisions
7. (a) Any person who, at the commencement of this Act, is a member of staff of the former Board shall, on the appointed day, become a member of staff of the Board on the same or improved terms and conditions of service as may be specified by the Cabinet Secretary. (b) Notwithstanding subparagraph (1), a member of staff of the former Board may retire on the basis of abolition of office in accordance with the existing regulations.	Staff
8. Where on the appointed day— (a) any disciplinary proceedings against any member of staff of the former Board are in the course of being heard or instituted, or have been heard or investigated by the former Board but no order or decision has been made thereon; (b) any such member of staff is interdicted or suspended, The Board shall— (a) in the case of paragraph (a), carry on and complete the hearing or investigation and make an order or render a decision, as the case may be; and (b) in the case of paragraph (b), deal with such member of staff in such manner as it deems appropriate having regard to the offence committed by him or her, including the completion of disciplinary proceedings that have been commenced against that member of staff.	Disciplinary proceedings
Where on the appointed day, any penalty, other than dismissal, has been imposed on any member of staff of the former Board pursuant to disciplinary proceedings against him or her and the penalty has not been, or remains to be, serviced by such member of staff, he or she shall, on his or her transfer to the Board, serve or continue to serve such penalty to its full as if it had been imposed by the Board.	Pension

(a) A member of staff of the former Board who becomes a member of staff of the Board shall continue to be governed by the existing Government pension scheme. (b) Where any person whose services are transferred to the Board is, on the appointed day, a member of any statutory voluntary pension scheme or provident fund, the person shall for the purpose of this Act, continue to be governed by the same regulations under those schemes or funds, as if he or she had not been so transferred, and for purposes of the regulations governing those schemes or funds, service with the Board shall be deemed to be service in the former Board.	
Second Schedule	
Provisions as to the Conduct of Business and Affairs of the Board	
1. The Board shall meet not less than four times in every financial year and not more than four months shall elapse between the date of one meeting and the date of the next meeting. Notwithstanding the provisions of subparagraph (1), the chairperson may, and upon requisition in writing by at least five members shall, convene a special meeting of the Board at any time for the transaction of the business of the Board. Unless three quarters of the total members of the Board otherwise agree, at least fourteen days' written notice of every meeting of the Board shall be given to every member of the Board. The quorum for the conduct of the business of the Board shall be five members including the chairperson or the person presiding. The chairperson shall preside at every meeting of the Board at which he is present but, in his absence, the members present shall elect one of their numbers to preside, who shall, with respect to that meeting and the business transacted thereat, have all the powers of the chairperson. Unless a unanimous decision is reached, a decision on any matter before the Board shall be by a majority of votes of the members present and voting and, in the case of an equality of votes, the chairperson or the person presiding shall have a casting vote. Subject to subparagraph (4), no proceedings of the Board shall be invalid by reason only of a vacancy among the members thereof.	Meetings
2. If a member is directly or indirectly interested in any contract, proposed contract or other matter before the Board and is present at a meeting of the Board at which the contract, proposed contract or other matter is the subject of consideration, that member shall, at the meeting and as soon as practicable after the commencement thereof, disclose the fact and shall not take part in the consideration or discussion of, or vote on, any questions with respect to the contract or other matter, or be counted in the quorum of the meeting during consideration of the matter.	Disclosure of interest by Board members

Notwithstanding subparagraph (1), if the majority of members of the Board present in a meeting are of the opinion that the experience or expertise of a member referred to in subparagraph (1) is vital to the deliberations of the meeting, the Board may permit the member to participate in the deliberations subject to such restrictions as it may impose but such member shall not have the right to vote on the matter in question. (3) A disclosure of interest made under this paragraph shall be recorded in the minutes of the meeting at which it is made. A member of the Board who contravenes subparagraph (1) commits an offence and is liable to imprisonment for a term not exceeding six months, or to a fine not exceeding one hundred thousand shillings, or both.	
Any contract or instrument which, if entered into or executed by a person not being a body corporate, would not require to be under seal, may be entered into or executed on behalf of the Board by any person generally or specially authorized by the Board for that purpose.	Execution of instruments
The Board shall cause minutes of all resolutions and proceedings of meetings of the Board to be entered in books kept for that purpose.	Minutes
Memorandum of Objects and Reasons	
The objective of this Bill is to provide a legal framework for the care, treatment and rehabilitation of persons with mental illness. It seeks to establish procedures for admission, treatment and overall management of persons with mental illness. **Part I** contains preliminary provisions. **Part II** contains provisions relating to access to mental health care. It among other things require that such care be affordable, equitable and accessible to all. Similarly, it spells out the responsibilities of the national and county governments regarding provision of mental health care. **Part III** contains provisions on the determination of mental illness, and lays down the principles to be followed in making that determination. **Part IV** contains provisions relating to the rights of persons with mental illness, and the duties of mental health care provides. The objective of this Part is to ensure that persons with mental illness are treated with dignity and respect due to them as human beings, and that mental health care providers carry out their duties in a manner consistent with the objectives sought to be achieved by this Bill. **Part V** contains provisions relating to the admission and treatment of persons with mental illness. **Part VI** provides for mentally ill offenders and stipulates how they should be dealt with under the criminal justice system. **Part VII** contains provisions on the seclusion and restraint of persons with mental illness. **Part VIII** provides for the review, appeal, discharge and transfer of persons with mental illness. **Part IX** provides for the care and administration of the property of persons with mental illness. This is intended to ensure that such property does not go to waste on account of the illness of such person.	

Part X contains provisions on the establishment, powers and functions of the Mental Health Care Board as the body responsible for the co-ordination of mental health care activities in Kenya. **Part XI** contains financial provisions relating to the Board. **Part XII** contains miscellaneous provisions. The enactment of this Bill shall not occasion additional expenditure of public funds. Dated the 24th July, 2012.	**Joseph Lekuton** *Member of Parliament*

Annexure—2

IDEAS—
Indian Disability Evaluation and Assessment Scale, 2002

A Scale for Measuring and Quantifying Disability in Mental Disorders

INDIAN PSYCHIATRIC SOCIETY

2002

CONTENTS

PREAMBLE

The development of the Indian Disability Evaluation and Assessment Scale (IDEAS) signifies a major milestone in the care and rehabilitation of the mentally ill persons in this country. Ever since the enactment of the comprehensive Persons with Disabilities Act (PDA, 1995), with the mentally ill persons in its ambit, paucity of a suitable scale for evaluation of the psychiatric disabilities has been perceived as a major stumbling block for its implementation by the administrators and distressing the mental health professionals. This distress and the concern for the patients lead the Executive Council of the IPS commit to develop an official IPS scale for psychiatric disabilities and get it announced in the Presidential Address at the ANCIPS, 2001 (Pune). The task was taken up in right earnest by the Rehabilitation Specialty section of IPS. The release of this official IPS disability scale is the culmination of that effort and the fulfillment of the commitment made by us at the ANCIPS, 2001. It also signifies the initiative of the IPS to take up and complete socially relevant and professionally significant projects year-bound and, if needing publication, to release them during a prime time joint session at the next ANCIPS.

While acknowledging the excellent work done by the Rehabilitation Specialty Section headed by Dr R Thara and Dr T Murali in this project, it is our fond hope that, with the follow-up efforts by the IPS, IDEAS would gain acceptance by Government of India and State Governments and break the impasse in the implementation of the Disabilities Act and lessen the sorrow and suffering of the mentally ill persons and their unfortunate families in our country.

Dr S Nambi
Honorary General Secretary

Dr KA Kumar
President

and

Executive Council
Indian Psychiatric Society

ANCIPS-2002
Kolkata

PREFACE

As in many walks of life, it was a prolonged and arduous struggle for recognition and status for psychiatric disability among other disabilities. Despite opposition from outside the mental health fraternity and skepticism from within it, disability caused by mental disorders has at last come to stay. The "seventh disability" as it is called now was first included in the Persons with Disabilities Act passed by the Indian Parliament in 1995. The Amendment Committee formed soon after, also examined the status of psychiatric disability in great detail and from various perspectives before concluding that it must be retained in the Act.

It was however like a child without a name. Most policy planners were struck by the lack of comparability with other disabilities mainly because there were no guidelines on its measurement. Although a few tools are available for this purpose, they did not seem quite appropriate for the purpose of certifying disability and quantifying it. In 2000, I therefore suggested that the IPS should take upon itself this task of providing the necessary tool for its quantification and in the capacity of Chairperson, Rehab Committee offered to do it. The Council agreed immediately and even formed a Task Force, which met once in Chennai and discussed this in great detail.

Our experiences and researches with several disability tools for over two decades and the discussions I had with several colleagues familiar with disability led me to evolve a simple instrument consisting only of 4 items. The field trial of International Classification of Functioning (formerly ICIDH 2) has also helped us immensely in this process. The fact that it had to be used widely, rated by people with different backgrounds and in busy clinical settings determined its brevity and simplicity.

The next stage was to field test this. This was done in 8 centers and the cumulative data was then analyzed at SCARF. The field centers also provided valuable feedback on the basis of which some changes were made. The validity of the instrument has been established and some reliability determined. The details of this process can be seen in the ensuing pages.

This has been envisaged to be used primarily for measuring disability for certification and according some benefits for those mentally disabled. It is likely that for research purposes, a more detailed instrument may be required.

I hope this will be accepted by the psychiatric fraternity and used extensively for measuring this disability.

No instrument can be regarded as perfect in all its dimensions. I would appreciate inputs and feedback from many of you, which will help us refine and better IDEAS.

ACKNOWLEDGMENTS

I wish to thank and acknowledge the contribution of the following persons:

- Prof KA Kumar, President and Dr S Nambi, Secretary, IPS.
- Dr T Murali, Convenor, Rehabilitation Committee of IPS
- Investigators and staff of the Field Centers:

Bengaluru	:	Dr Kalyansundaram
Kolkata	:	Dr KL Narayanan
Chennai	:	Dr S Nakkeerar
Lucknow	:	Dr JK Trivedi
Thrissur	:	Dr KS Shaji
Thiruvananthapuram	:	Dr VS Mani
Vellore	:	Dr KS Jacob

- My colleagues Dr S Padmavati and TN Srinivasan for periodic inputs and help in analysis of data Dr Mubeen and Ms Anuradha in data collection and Mr Albert Joseph for data entry and analysis.

Dr R Thara

DESCRIPTION OF "IDEAS"

General guidelines:
- IDEAS is suited best for the purpose of measuring and certifying Disability.
- It is therefore a brief and simple instrument, which can be used, even in busy clinical settings.
- Some training is required in the use of IDEAS.
- This is to be used only on outpatients and those living in the community. Not appropriate for inpatients.
- Rating should be done only based on interviews of the primary caregivers. Case records and patient interviews can be used to supplement information.
- Only in rare instances when no primary caregiver is available should the rating be based only on patient interview. This should then be documented.
- The gender specification "he" has been used for convenience and refers to both genders.
- Probe questions help to guide one through the interview and to help identify dysfunction in one or more activities.

Diagnostic Categories

Patients with only the following diagnoses as per ICD or DSM criteria are eligible for disability benefits:
- Schizophrenia
- Bipolar Disorder
- Dementia
- Obsessive Compulsive Disorder

Duration of Illness

The total duration of illness should be at least 2 years. For the purpose of scoring, the number of months the patient was symptomatic in the last 2 years (MI 2Y-months of illness in the last 2 years) should be determined.

Who does the Assessment?

Diagnosis and certification can be done only by the Psychiatrist. Administration of IDEAS can be done by trained social workers, psychologists, or occupational therapists.

Frequency of Re-certification

Psychiatric Disability will be reassessed every 2 years and re-certified.

The feasibility of doing this in the rural areas will however have to be examined.

Items

Selfcare: Includes taking care of body hygiene, grooming, health including bathing, toileting, dressing, eating and taking care of one's health.

Interpersonal activities (Social relationships): Includes initiating and maintaining interactions with others in a contextual and socially appropriate manner.

Communication and understanding: Includes communication and conversation with others by producing and comprehending spoken/written/ nonverbal messages.

Work: Three areas are employment/housework/education measures anyone aspect.

- ***Performing in work/job:*** Performing in work/employment (paid) employment/self employment/family concern or otherwise. Measure ability to perform tasks at employment completely and efficiently and in proper time. Includes seeking employment.
- ***Performing in housework:*** Maintaining household including cooking, caring for other people at home, taking care of belongings, etc. Measures ability to take responsibility for and perform household tasks completely and efficiently and in proper time.
- ***Performing in school/college***: Measures performance in education related tasks.

Scores for Each Item

0–No	Disability (None, absent, negligible)
1–Mild	Disability (Slight, low)
2–Moderate	Disability (Medium, fair)
3–Severe	Disability (High, extreme)
4–Profound	Disability (Total, cannot do)

Total Score (Range: 0–20)

Add scores of the 4 items and obtain a total score.

MI 2Y- Months of illness in the last 2 years. Interview with informant and case notes if available should be used to determine for how many months in the last 2 years the patient exhibited symptoms. (Range: 1–4)

MI2Y:	< 6 months	: Score to be added is 1
	7–12 months	: Add 2
	13–18 months	: Add 3
	> 18 months	: Add 4

GLOBAL DISABILITY

Total Disability score + MI2Y score = Global Disability score (Range: 1–20).

Percentages

For the purpose of welfare benefits, 40% will be the cut-off point. The scores above 40% have been categorized as Moderate, Severe and Profound based on the Global disability score. This grading will be used to measure change over time.

Score of
0–No Disability = 0%
1–7: Mild Disability = < 40 %
8 and above = > 40 %
(8–13-Moderate Disability; 14–19 = Severe Disability; 20 = Profound disability)

MANUAL FOR "IDEAS"

In order to score this instrument, information from all possible sources should be obtained. This will include interview of patient, the caregiver and case notes when available.

Selfcare

This should be regarded as activity guided by social norms and conventions.
The broad areas covered are:

- Maintenance of personal hygiene and physical health
- Eating habits
- Maintenance of personal belongings and living space.

Guiding Questions

a. Does he look after himself, wash his clothes regularly, take a bath and brush his teeth?
b. Does he have regular meals?
c. Does he take food of right quality and quantity?
d. Does he dress appropriately (weather conditions, over dressing)?
e. Does he take care of his personal belongings with reasonable standard of cleanliness and orderliness?
f. Does he seek treatment for health conditions and comply with advice?

Scoring of Disability

0 = No disability
Patient's level and pattern of selfcare are normal, within the sociocultural and economic context.

1= Mild
Mild deterioration in selfcare and appearance (not bathing, shaving, changing clothes for the occasion as expected). Does not have adverse consequences, such as hazards to his health. No embarrassment to family.

2 = Moderate
Lack of concern for selfcare should be clearly established, such as deterioration of physical health, obesity, tooth decay and body odors.

3 = Severe
Decline in selfcare should be marked in all areas. Patient wearing torn clothes, would only wash if made to and would only eat if told. Evidence of serious hazards to physical health. (Malnutrition, infection, patient unacceptable in public).

4 = Profound
Total or near total lack of selfcare (Example: risk to physical survival, needs feeding, washing, putting on clothes, etc. Constant supervision necessary)

Interpersonal Activities

Includes patient's ability to form and maintain social relationships. This would be applicable to family, friends, colleagues and society at large. Ability for emotional response, such as showing tolerance, responding to criticism or praise, and love and affection. Activities of engaging in physical intimacy. Ability to interact in a socially appropriate manner (reduction or excess).

Guiding Questions

- What is his behavior with others?
- Do you think his behavior in social situations (at work, social gatherings) is appropriate?
- What is the nature of his relationship with other family members?
- Is he able to regulate verbal and physical aggression?
- Is he able to initiate social interactions on his own?
- How does he behave with strangers?
- Is he able to maintain friendship?
- Does he show physical expression of affection and desire?

Scoring

0 = No
Patient gets along reasonably well with people. No friction in interpersonal relationships.
1 = Mild
Some difficulty in initiating and maintaining social interaction. Friction on isolated occasions. However, his social behavior is generally acceptable to others.
2 = Moderate
Definite difficulty in social interaction and interaction considered unhealthy/ inappropriate. May be seen on more than few occasions. Could isolate himself from others and avoid company.
3 = Severe
Serious difficulty in initiating and maintaining social interaction. Behavior in social situations is undesirable and generalized. Causes serious problems in daily living/or work. Patient is socially isolated.
4 = Profound
No attempts at engaging in any kind of social interaction. Family afraid of potential consequences.

Communication and Understanding

- Understanding spoken messages as well as written and non-verbal messages.
- Ability to produce meaningful messages in order to communicate with others.
- Ability to converse in groups, such as chatting and discussing.
- Use of communication devices, such as telephone, email, internet, etc.
- Any reduction/excess of these behaviors should be considered.
- All modes of communication should be considered.

Questions

a. Does he avoid talking to people/talk excessively at times?
b. Is he able to start, maintain and end a conversation?
c. Does he indulge in reading, writing and other communication devices, such as telephone, e-mail, etc?
d. Is he able to comprehend verbal/non-verbal communication?
f. Are others able to comprehend his communication ?
g. Do you need to encourage him to be more communicative?

Scoring

0 = No disability
Patient communicates with people as much as can be expected in his socio-cultural context. No difficulty in comprehension.
1 = Mild
Patient described as uncommunicative. Communication inappropriate (as in excitement). No active avoidance, but speaks only when spoken to. Could have some difficulty in comprehension.
2 = Moderate
A narrow range of communication. Communication can be too brief/in excess, incomplete or incomprehensible.
3 = Severe
Evidence of more generalized, active avoidance of any kind of communication. Serious difficulty in comprehension.
4 = Profound
All communication is nil or a bare minimum. Communication totally incomprehensible.

Work

This includes employment, housework and educational performance. Score only one category in case of an overlap.

Guiding Questions

a. Is he/she employed/unemployed/housewife/student?
b. If employed, does he go to work regularly?
c. Does he like his job and is he coping well with it?
d. How is his competence at work?

Scoring

0 = No disability
Patient goes to work regularly and his output and quality of work performance are within acceptable levels for the job.
1 = Mild
Noticeable decline in patient's ability to work, to cope with it and meet the demands of work. May threaten to quit.
2 = Moderate
Declining work performance, frequent absences, lack of concern about all this. Financial difficulties foreseen.
3 = Severe
Marked decline in work performance, disruptive at work, unwilling to adhere to disciplines of work. Threat of losing his job.
4 = Profound
Has been largely absent from work, termination imminent. Unemployed, and making no efforts to find jobs.
Housewives
In similar ways, housewives should be rated on the amount, regularity and efficiency in which tasks in the following areas are completed. Consider the amount of help required completing these.

Acquiring daily necessities, making, storing and serving of food, cleaning the house, working with those helping with domestic duties, such as maids, cooks, etc. looking after possessions and valuable in the house.
Students
Assess the score on performance in school/college, regularity, discipline, interest in future studies, behavior at the educational institution. Those who had to discontinue education on account of mental disability and unable to continue further should be given a score of 4.

IDEAS
(Indian Disability Evaluation and Assessment Scale)

Scoring Sheet

Items	*0*	*1*	*2*	*3*	*4*
I. Selfcare					
II. Interpersonal activities					
III. Communication and understanding					
IV. Work					

A. Total score (I + II + III + IV) (Range 0–16)
B. MI2Y score (Range 1–4)
Global score (A + B) (Range 1–20)
Percentage of disability (< 40% or > 40%)

RESULTS OF FIELD STUDIES

The sample was drawn from 8 centers all over the country. They were a good mix of patients attending mental hospitals, outpatient clinics of psychiatry in general hospitals and rehabilitation centers. The four diagnostic groups were also included.

Total number of cases included in the field study = 1078

Centerwise Distribution:

- Bengaluru (RFS) = 03
- Kolkata (Antara) = 110
- Chennai:
  - IMH = 160
  - SCARF = 260
- Lucknow (KGM) = 100
- Thrissur (GH) = 135
- Thiruvananthapuram (GGH) = 100
- Vellore (CMC) = 110

Gender and Age Distribution

- Males = 665 (61.6%)
- Females = 413
- Mean age of patients + 37.4 ± 11.53
- Mean duration of illness = 8.61 ± 6.55 years.
- This was the total duration of illness and not MI2Y.

Diagnostic Break-up

- Schizophrenia = 560
- Schizoaffective = 13

Mood disorders

- * Depression = 97
- * Mania = 116
- Bipolar disorder = 198
- Dementia = 21
- OCD = 59
- Others = 14

Table 2.1: Mean scores of items (N = 1078)

Items	*Mean Scores*	*Range*
Selfcare	0.97 ± 1.13	0-4
Interpersonal activities	1.54 ± 1.15	0-4
Communication and understanding	1.46 ± 1.18	0-4
Work	2.11 ± 1.42	0-4

A. Total score (Range 0–16)	Mean = 6.05 ± 4.13
B. Total duration (Range 1–4)*	Mean = 2.88 ± 1.07 years
Global score (A + B) (Range 1–20)	Mean = 8.93 ± 4.39

* Please note that experience during field trails showed that it was rather difficult to compute total duration of illness in certain episodic illnesses. It was also felt that equating the duration of episodic disorders and chronic disorders would not be the right thing to do. Hence, this has now been changed to months of illness during the last 2 years (MI2Y).

Ideas Means Score

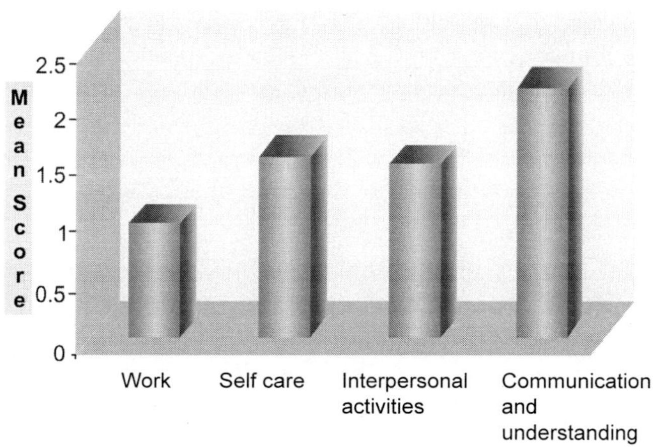

IDEAS

Reliability

Due to logistic reasons, it was not possible to conduct intracenter reliability exercises. Intracentre reliability was done in a few centers between two raters. The kappa value was 0.76 revealing the need for some training in the use of IDEAS.

Internal consistency was calculated. The alpha value was 0.8682 indicating good internal consistency between the items.

Validity

Face validity: The draft instrument was circulated among a team of mental health and disability professionals. Their opinions were sought as to whether at face value, the instrument appeared to be measuring the desired qualities. There was a general consensus on the 4 items of the instrument.

Content validity: During the work of some Indian centers on the ICIDH, several focus group discussions were held. More were held in SCARF for the purpose of this study. The group members consisting of patients, families, and professionals also felt that the items of the schedule were critical in the measurement of this disability.

Criterion validity was established by comparing IDEAS with SAPD (Schedule for the Assessment of Psychiatric Disability), which has been standardized in India. Both these instruments were administered on 223 caregivers at SCARF and also scored independently by two raters. Correlation for all the 4 items was good.

CONCLUSION

We now have a simple, but comprehensive instrument developed and standardized in India. It is primarily meant for measuring disability for the purpose of certification and therefore produces values, which can be converted into percentages similar to what is practiced for other disabilities. It can be used on the field and in busy clinical settings. It is largely dependent on the information provided by the primary caregiver. Since it is on a 5-point scale, any changes occurring during re-assessments can be picked up.

Annexure—3

Specimen Certificates

- *Courtesy:* Dr S Haque Nizamie
- Paper presented at IPS National Midterm CME
- "Legal Aspects of Psychiatry, Indian Perspective", Chennai, 2008

FORM OF CERTIFICATE RECOMMENDED FOR LEAVE OR EXTENSION OR COMMUTATION OF LEAVE (MCI – 2002)

Signature of patient or thumb impression ______________________________
To be filled in by the applicant in the presence of the Government Medical Attendant, or Medical Practitioner.
Identification marks:
1. ____________
2. ____________

I, Dr ____________________________________ after careful examination of the case certify hereby that _____________ whose signature is given above is suffering from _______________ and I consider that a period of absence from duty of___________________ with effect from ______________________________ is absolutely necessary for the restoration of his health.

Place_______________ Signature of Medical attendant __________________.

Date ________________ Registration No. _____________________
(Medical Council of India/State Medical Council of ______________State)

Note: The nature and probable duration of the illness should also be specified. This certificate must be accompanied by a brief resume of the case giving the nature of the illness, its symptoms, causes and duration.

FORMAT OF THE TREATMENT CERTIFICATE PROVIDED AT THE "CENTRAL INSTITUTE OF PSYCHIATRY", WHICH USES SOME SPECIFICATIONS WHICH ARE PERTINENT TO ITS ISSUE, AS MENTIONED ABOVE:

No.:__________ Date:_________

TREATMENT CERTIFICATE

This is to certify that Shri/Smt/Kum ___________________________ with registration no. _________ dated ______ has consulted this hospital as an outpatient.

He/She has been under treatment from ______________ to _______________

He/She has last attended OPD in the following dates
ii. _________________ iii. ___________________________

Date of admission (if applicable) __________ Date of Discharge ___________

Note: This certificate acknowledges only that the above named patient has been under treatment at this hospital without opining the nature, type, duration, severity clarification if any, may be sought from the hospital.

Chief Medical Officer

FORM OF CERTIFICATE RECOMMENDED FOR FITNESS (MCI – 2002)

Signature of patient or thumb impression ______________________________
To be filled in by the applicant in the presence of the Government Medical Attendant or Medical Practitioner.
Identification marks:
1. ____________
2. ____________

I, Dr ____________________ after careful examination of the case certify hereby that ____________________ on restoration of health is now fit to join service.

Place______________ Signature of Medical attendant _________________

Date ______________ Registration No.____________________

(Medical Council of India/State Medical Council of ______________State)
FORMAT OF THE TREATMENT CERTIFICATE PROVIDED AT THE "CENTRAL INSTITUTE OF PSYCHIATRY", WHICH USES SOME SPECIFICATIONS WHICH ARE PERTINENT TO ITS ISSUE, AS MENTIONED ABOVE:

No.:_________ Date:_________

TREATMENT CERTIFICATE

This is to certify that Shri/Smt/Kum________________________with registration no. ______________ dated ______________ has consulted this hospital as an outpatient.

He/She has been under treatment from ______________ to ______________

He/ She has last attended OPD in the following dates
ii.__________________________ iii.__________________________

Date of admission (if applicable)____________Date of Discharge__________

Note: This certificate acknowledges only that the above named patient has been under treatment at this hospital without opining the nature, type, duration, severity clarification if any, may be sought from the hospital.

Chief Medical Officer

CERTIFICATE FOR PERSONS WITH DISABILITY DUE TO MENTAL ILLNESS

No: _____________ Dated:_____________

This is to certify that_______________________CRF No__________________

S/D/W of ______ years old M/F, is mentally disabled and was assessed on Indian Disability Evaluation and Assessment Scale (IDEAS) approved by the Government of India, Ministry of Social Justice and Empowerment, for assessment of disability due to mental illness, vide letter no. 16-8/97-NI-I dated 18th February 2002 and published in the Gazette of India).

In the opinion of the medical board, He/She has more than 40% disability.

Board Members:

1.___________________________ 2. ___________________________

3.___________________________ 4. ___________________________

Director: __________________________

CERTIFICATE OF MENTAL RETARDATION FOR GOVERNMENT BENEFITS

This is to certify that Shri/Smt/Kum ______________________________son/ daughter of ____________________of town/city ____________________ with particulars given below:

a. Age: _______________

b. Sex: _______________

c. Signature/Thumb impression: _________________________

Categorization of Mental Retardation
Mild/Moderate/Severe/Profound
Validity of the Certificate: Permanent

Signature of the Government
Doctor/Hospital with seal
Chairperson Mental Retardation
Certification Board

Recent Attested Photograph
Showing the disability affixed here

Dated:____________________

Place:______________________

FOR MENTALLY RETARDED PERSONS

Appendix—Form for the purpose of rail concession to mentally retarded person to be used by the Government Doctor.

Paste Passport Size Photograph Duly Signed and Stamped by the Issuing Doctor/Person

This is to certify that Km/Shri/Smt. ______________________________, whose particulars are furnished below, is a bonafide mentally retarded person and *cannot travel without an escort.*

Particulars of the mentally retarded persons:
Address:______________________________
Fathers'/Husbands' name:______________________________
Age: ______________________________
Sex: ______________________________

Signature or thumb impression
Mentally Retarded person:__________________
Date: __________________
Place: __________________

(Signature of Government Doctor)
Clear seal of Government
Hospital/clinic seal containing full name and Registration no. of doctor

Note: *Certificate should be issued only to those mentally retarded persons Who Cannot Travel Without an Escort. The photo must be signed and stamped in such a way that Doctor's signature in the stamp appears partly on the photo and partly on the certificate.*

The certificate is valid for five years from the date of issue. After expiry of the period of validity of the certificate, the person is required to obtain a fresh certificate. A Photostat copy of thes certificate is accepted for the purpose of grant of concession. The original certificate will have to be performed an inspection at the time of purchase of concessional ticket and during the journey if demanded. No alteration in the form is permitted.

Form No. 10-1 [See Rule II DD]

CERTIFICATE OF PRESCRIBED AUTHORITY FOR THE PURPOSES OF INCOME TAX DEDUCTION UNDER SECTION 80 DDB

1. Name of the patient: ______________________
2. Address: ______________________
3. Father's name: ______________________
4. Name and address of the person on whom the patient is dependent and his relationship with the patient: ______________________
5. Name of the disease or ailment: ______________________
6. For disease or ailments mentioned in item (i) of Clause (a) of sub-rule (1) whether the disability is 40% or more (Please specify the extent)

   Name, address, registration number and qualification of the specialist issuing the certificate, along with the name and address of the Government hospital:

   ____

   ____

   ____

Verification

This is to verify that I, Dr ______________ S/o (W/o) Shri ______________ in the case of the patient Shri/Smt/ Ms ______________ after considering the entire history of illness, with careful examination and appropriate investigatsion, am of the opinion that the patient is suffering from ______________ disease/ ailment during the previous year ending on March ______________.

I certify that the information furnished above is true to the best of my knowledge.

Signature
(Name and Address)

INFORMED CONSENT FOR ELECTROCONVULSIVE THERAPY

I hereby consent to the administration of a course of electroconvulsive therapy to myself/my _____________ (Relation) _____________________________ (Name of the patient) by Dr _____________ (or any other suitably trained doctor disputized by him).

I also consent to the use of an anesthetic and/or a relaxant or sedative for this purpose, at the discretion of the doctors.

I have been explained the nature and the purpose of the treatments, and I have opted for this treatment.

As regards possible side effects and complications, I understand that headache and confusion, immediately after treatment, are common, but short-lasting.

Memory deficit, lasting for a few weeks, is common but there is no scientific evidence of permanent brain damage.

I also understand that, like in other medical and surgical treatments despite all precautions, risk to life cannot be ruled out. Rarely, fractures may occur.

I authorize the doctors concerned to administer emergency treatment for all such complications, shift the patient to other hospital, and/or seek help of other specialists if necessary. I also undertake to bear the financial.

I confirm that I have explained to the patient/relative the nature, purpose and likely effects of this treatment.

Shri/Smt______________________________was the nearest relation available.

Date/Time/Place **Signature of Doctor**

Relative's Approval: (Wherever Relevant)

I _______________________________________(Name) _____________(The closest available relative) of ________________________________(Patient's name) confirm that an explanation of the nature, purpose and likely effects of ECT has been given to me by Dr __________________________________and that I approve of the treatment being given to the patient __________________.

Date/Time/Place **Signature of Relative**

Annexure—4

Madrid Declaration on Ethical Standards for Psychiatric Practice

Approved by the World Psychiatric Association (WPA) General Assembly on August 25, 1996 and amended by the General Assembly in Yokohama, Japan, in August 2002.

DECLARATION OF MADRID

In 1977, the World Psychiatric Association approved the Declaration of Hawaii, setting out ethical guidelines for the practice of psychiatry. The Declaration was subsequently updated in Vienna in 1983. To reflect the impact of changing social attitudes and new medical developments on the psychiatric profession, the World Psychiatric Association has once again examined and revised some of these ethical standards.

Medicine is both a healing art and a science. The dynamics of this combination are best reflected in psychiatry, the branch of medicine that specializes in the care and protection of those who are ill and infirm, because of a mental disorder or impairment. Although there may be cultural, social, and national differences, the need for ethical conduct and continual review of ethical standards is universal.

As practitioners of medicine, psychiatrists must be aware of the ethical implications of being a physician and of the specific ethical demands of the specialty of psychiatry. As members of society, psychiatrists must advocate for fair and equal treatment of the mentally ill, for social justice and equity for all.

Ethical behavior is based on the psychiatrist's individual sense of responsibility towards the patient and their judgment in determining what is correct and appropriate conduct. External standards and influences, such as professional codes of conduct, the study of ethics, or the rule of law by themselves will not guarantee the ethical practice of medicine.

Psychiatrists should at all times keep in mind the boundaries of the psychiatrist-patient relationship, and be guided primarily by the respect for patients and concern for their welfare and integrity.

It is in this spirit that the World Psychiatric Association approved at the General Assembly on 25th August, 1996, the following ethical standards that should govern the conduct of psychiatrists worldwide.

1. Psychiatry is a medical discipline concerned with the provision of the best treatment for mental disorders, with the rehabilitation of individuals suffering from mental illness and with the promotion of mental health. Psychiatrists serve patients by providing the best therapy available consistent with accepted scientific knowledge and ethical principles. Psychiatrists should devise

therapeutic interventions that are least restrictive to the freedom of the patient and seek advice in areas of their work, about which they do not have primary expertise. While doing so, psychiatrists should be aware of and concerned with the equitable allocation of health resources.
2. It is the duty of psychiatrists to keep abreast scientific developments of the specialty and to convey updated knowledge to others. Psychiatrists trained in research should seek to advance the scientific frontiers of psychiatry.
3. The patient should be accepted as a partner by right in the therapeutic process. The psychiatrist-patient relationship must be based on mutual trust and respect to allow the patient to make free and informed decisions. It is the duty of psychiatrists to provide the patient with relevant information so as to empower the patient to come to a rational decision according to personal values and preferences.
4. When the patient is incapacitated and/or unable to exercise proper judgment because of a mental disorder, or gravely disabled or incompetent, the psychiatrists should consult with the family and, if appropriate, seek legal counsel, to safeguard the human dignity and the legal rights of the patient. No treatment should be provided against the patient's will, unless withholding treatment would endanger the life of the patient and/or those who surround him or her. Treatment must always be in the best interest of the patient.
5. When psychiatrists are requested to assess a person, it is their duty first to inform and advise the person being assessed about the purpose of the intervention, the use of the findings, and the possible repercussions of the assessment. This is particularly important when the psychiatrists are involved in third party situations.
6. Information obtained in the therapeutic relationship should be kept in confidence and used, only and exclusively, for the purpose of improving the mental health of the patient. Psychiatrists are prohibited from making use of such information for personal reasons, or financial or academic benefits. Breach of confidentiality may only be appropriate when serious physical or mental harm to the patient or to a third person would ensue if confidentiality were maintained; as in case of child abuse in these circumstances, psychiatrists, should whenever possible, first advise the patient about the action to be taken.
7. Research that is not conducted in accordance with the canons of science is unethical. Research activities should be approved by an appropriately constituted ethical committee. Psychiatrists should follow national and international rules for the conduct of research. Only individuals properly trained for research should undertake or direct it. Because psychiatric patients are particularly vulnerable research subjects, extra caution should be taken to safeguard their autonomy as well as their mental and physical integrity. Ethical standards should also be applied in the selection of population groups, in all types of research including epidemiological and sociological studies and in collaborative research involving; other disciplines or several investigating centers.

Guidelines Concerning Specific Situations

The World Psychiatric Association Ethics Committee recognizes the need to develop a number of specific guidelines on a number of specific situations. The first five were approved by the General Assembly in Madrid, Spain, on 25th August, 1996 and the last two by the General Assembly in Hamburg, Germany, on 8th August, 1999.

- *Euthanasia*: A physician's duty, first and foremost, is the promotion of health, the reduction of suffering, and the protection of life. The psychiatrist, among whose patients are some who are severely incapacitated and incompetent to reach an informal decision, should be particularly careful of actions that could lead to the death of those who cannot protect themselves because of their disability. The psychiatrist should be aware that the views of a patient may be distorted by mental illness such as depression. In such situations, the psychiatrist's role is to treat the illness.
- *Torture*: Psychiatrists shall not take part in any process of mental or physical torture, even when authorities attempt to force their involvement in such acts.
- *Death penalty*: Under no circumstances should psychiatrists participate in legally authorized executions nor participate in assessments of competency to be executed.
- *Selection of sex*: Under no circumstances should a psychiatrist participate in decisions to terminate pregnancy for the purpose of sex selection.
- *Organ transplantation*: The role of the psychiatrist is to clarify the issues surrounding organ donations and to advise on religious, cultural, social and family factors to ensure that informed and proper decisions be made by all concerned. The psychiatrists should neither act as a proxy decision maker for patients nor use psychotherapeutic skills to influence the decision of a patient in these matters. Psychiatrists should seek to protect their patients and help them exercise self-determination to the fullest extent possible in situations of organ transplantation.
- *Psychiatrists addressing the media*: The media has a key role in shaping the attitudes of the community. In all contacts with the media, psychiatrists shall ensure that people with mental illness are presented in a manner, which preserves their dignity and pride, and which reduces stigma and discrimination against them. An important role of psychiatrists is to advocate for those people who suffer from mental disorders. As the public perception of psychiatrists and psychiatry reflects on patients, psychiatrists shall ensure that in their contact with the media they represent the profession of psychiatry with dignity. Psychiatrists shall not make announcements to the media about presumed psychopathology on any individuals. In presenting research findings to the media, psychiatrists shall ensure the scientific integrity of the information given and be mindful of the potential impact of their statements on the public perception of mental illness and on the welfare of people with mental disorders.
- *Psychiatrists and discrimination on ethnic or cultural grounds:* Discrimination by psychiatrists on the basis of ethnicity or culture, whether directly or by aiding others is unethical. Psychiatrists shall never be involved or endorse, directly or indirectly, any activity related to ethnic cleansing.
- *Psychiatrists and genetic research and counseling:* Research on the genetic bases of mental disorders is rapidly increasing and more people suffering from mental illness are participating in such research. Psychiatrists involved in

genetic research or counseling shall be mindful of the fact that the implication of genetic information are not limited to the individual from whom it was obtained and that its disclosure can have negative and disruptive effects on the families and communities of the individuals concerned. Psychiatrist shall therefore ensure that:

- People and families who participate in genetic research do so with a fully informed consent;
- Any genetic information in their possession is adequately protected against unauthorized access, misinterpretation or misuse;
- Care is taken in communication with patients and families to make clear that current genetic knowledge is incomplete and may be altered by future findings;
- Psychiatrists shall only refer people to facilities for diagnostic genetic testing if that facility has:
- Demonstrated satisfactory quality assurance, procedures for such testing;
- Adequate and easily accessible resources for genetic counseling. Genetic counseling with regard to family planning or abortion shall be respectful of the patients' value system, while providing sufficient medical and psychiatric information to aid patients make decisions they consider best for them.

Four Additional Specific Ethical Guidelines

a. Ethics of psychotherapy in medicine

Medical treatments of any nature should be administered under the provisions of good practice guidelines regarding their indications, effectiveness, safety, and quality control. Psychotherapy, in its broadest sense, is an accepted component of many medical interactions. In a more specific and restricted sense, psychotherapy utilizes techniques involving verbal and non-verbal communication and interaction to achieve specified treatment goals in the care of specific disorders. Psychiatrists providing specific forms of psychotherapy must have appropriate training in such techniques. The general guidelines that apply to any medical treatment also apply to specific forms of psychotherapy in regard to its indications and outcomes, positive or negative. The effectiveness of psychotherapy and its place in a treatment plan are important subjects for both researchers and clinicians. Psychotherapy by psychiatrists is a form of treatment for mental and other illnesses and emotional problems. The treatment approach utilized is determined in concert by the doctor and patient and/or the patient's family and/or guardians following a careful history and examination employing all relevant clinical and laboratory studies. The approach employee should be specific to the disease and patient's needs and sensitive to personal, familial, religious and cultural factors. It should be based on sound research and clinical wisdom and have the purpose of removing, modifying or retarding symptoms or disturbed patterns of behavior. It should promote positive adaptations including personal growth and development.

Psychiatrists and other clinicians responsible for a patient have to ensure that these guidelines are fully applied. Therefore, the psychiatrist or other delegated qualified clinician, should determine the indications for psychotherapy and follow its development. In this context the essential notion is that the treatment is the consequence of a diagnosis and both are medical acts performed to take care of an ill person. These two levels of decisions, interventions and responsibilities are similar to other situations in clinical medicine, however this does not exclude other interventions, such as rehabilitation, which can be administered by non-medical personnel.

- Like any other treatment in medicine, the prescription of psychotherapy should follow accepted guidelines for obtaining informed consent prior to the initiation of treatment as well as updating it in the course of treatment if goals and objectives of treatment are modified in a significant way.
- If clinical wisdom, long standing and well-established practice patterns (this takes into consideration cultural and religious issues) and scientific evidence suggest potential clinical benefits to combining medication treatment with psychotherapy this should be brought to the patient's attention and fully discussed.
- Psychotherapy explores intimate thoughts, emotions and fantasies, and as such may engender intense transference and counter-transference. In a psychotherapy relationship the power is unequally shared between the therapist and patient, and under no circumstances shall the psychotherapist use this relationship to personal advantage or transgress the boundaries established by the professional relationship.
- At the initiation of psychotherapy, the patient shall be advised that information shared and health records will be kept in confidence except where the patient gives specific informed consent for release of information to third parties, or where a court order may require the production of records. The other exception is where there is a legal requirement to report certain information as in the case of child abuse.

b. Conflict of interest in relationship with industry

Although most organizations and institutions, including the WPA, have rules and regulations governing their relationship with industry and donors, individual physicians are often involved in interactions with the pharmaceutical industry, or other granting agencies that could lead to ethical conflict in these situations psychiatrists should be mindful of and apply the following guidelines:

- The practitioner must diligently guard against accepting gifts that could have an undue influence on professional work.
- Psychiatrists conducting clinical trials are under and obligation to disclose to the Ethics Review Board and their research subjects their financial and contractual obligations and benefits related to the sponsor of the study. Every effort should be made to set up review boards composed of researchers, ethicists and community representatives to assure the rights of research subjects are protected.
- Psychiatrists conducting clinical trials have to ensure that their patients have understood all aspects of the informed consent from the substitute decision maker. Psychiatrists must be cognizant that covert commercial influence on the trial design, promotion of drugs' trials without scientific value, breach of confidentiality, and restrictive contractual clauses regarding publication of results may reach in different ways encroach upon the freedom of science and scientific information.

c. Conflicts Arising with Third Party Payers

The obligations of organizations toward shareholders or the administrator regarding maximization of profits and minimization of costs can be in conflict with the principles of good practice. Psychiatrists working in such potentially conflicting environments, should uphold the rights of the patients to receive the best treatment possible.

- In agreement with the UN Resolution 46/119 of the "Principles for the Protection of Persons with Mental Illness, psychiatrists should oppose discriminatory practices, which limit their benefits and entitlement, deny parity curb the scope of treatment, or limit their access to proper medications for patients with a mental disorder."
- Professional independence to apply best practice guidelines and clinical wisdom in upholding the welfare of the patient should be the primary considerations for the psychiatrist. It is also the duty of the psychiatrist to protect the patient privacy and confidentiality as part of preserving the sanctity and healing potential of the doctor-patient relationship.

d. Violating the Clinical Boundaries and Trust between Psychiatrists and Patients

The psychiatrist-patient relationship may be the only relationship that permits an exploration of the deeply personal and emotional space, as granted by the patient. Within this relationship, the psychiatrist's respect for the humanity and dignity of the patient builds a foundation of trust that is essential for a comprehensive treatment plan. The relationship encourages the patient to explore deeply held strengths, weaknesses, fears, and desires, and many of these might be related to sexuality. Knowledge of these characteristics of the patient places the psychiatrist in a position of advantage that the patient allows on the expectation of trust and respect. Taking advantage of that knowledge by manipulating the patient's sexual fears and desires in order to obtain sexual access is a breach of the trust, regardless of consent. In the therapeutic relationship, consent on the part if the patient is considered vitiated by the knowledge the psychiatrists possesses about the patient and by the power differential that vests the psychiatrist with special authority over the patient. Consent under these circumstances will be tantamount to exploitation of the patient.

The latent sexual dynamics inherent in all relationships can become manifest in the course of the therapeutic relationship and if they are not properly handled by the therapist can produce anguish to the patient. This anguish is likely to become more pronounced if seductive statements and inappropriate non-verbal behavior are used by the therapist. Under no circumstances, therefore, should a psychiatrist get involved with a patient in any form of sexual behavior, irrespective of whether this behavior is initiated by the patient or the therapist.

Annexure—5

Universal Declaration of Human Rights, 1948

PREAMBLE

- Whereas recognition of the inherent dignity and of the equal and inalienable rights of all members of the human family is the foundation of freedom, justice and peace in the world,
- Whereas disregard and contempt for human rights have resulted in barbarous acts which have outraged the conscience of mankind, and the advent of a world in which human beings shall enjoy freedom of speech and belief and freedom from fear and want has been proclaimed as the highest aspiration of the common people,
- Whereas it is essential, if man is not to be compelled to have recourse, as a last resort, to rebellion against tyranny and oppression, that human rights should be protected by the rule of law,
- Whereas it is essential to promote the development of friendly relations between nations,
- Whereas the peoples of the United Nations have in the Charter reaffirmed their faith in human rights, in the dignity and worth of the human person and in the equal rights of men and women and have determined to promote social progress and better standards of life in larger freedom,
- Whereas Member States have pledged themselves to achieve, in cooperation with the United Nations, the promotion of universal respect for and observance of human rights and freedoms,
- Whereas common understanding of these rights and freedoms is of the greatest importance for the full realization of this pledge.

Now therefore

The General Assembly,

Proclaims this Universal Declaration of Human Rights as a common standard of achievements for all peoples and all nations, to the end that every individual and every organ of society, keeping this Declaration constantly in mind, shall strive by teaching and education to promote respect for these rights and freedoms and by progressive measures, national and international, to secure their universal and effective recognition and observance, both among the peoples of member States themselves and among the peoples of territories under their jurisdiction.

Article 1

All human beings are born free and equal in dignity and rights. They are endowed with reason and conscience and should act towards one another in a spirit of brotherhood.

Article 2

Everyone is entitled to all the rights and freedoms set forth in this Declaration, without distinction of any kind, such as race, color, sex, language, religion, political or other opinion, national or social origin, property, birth or other status. Furthermore, no distinction shall be made on the basis of the political, jurisdictional or, international status of the country or territory to which a person belongs, whether it be independent, trust, non-self-governing or under any other limitation of sovereignty.

Article 3

Everyone has the right to life, liberty and security of person.

Article 4

No one shall be held in slavery or servitude; slavery and the slave trade shall be prohibited in all their forms.

Article 5

No one shall be subjected to torture or to cruel, inhuman or degrading treatment or punishment.

Article 6

Everyone has the right to recognition everywhere as a person before the law.

Article 7

All are equal before the law and are entitled without any discrimination to equal protection of the law. All are entitled to equal protection against any discrimination in violation of this Declaration and against any incitement to such discrimination.

Article 8

Everyone has the right to an effective remedy by the competent national tribunals for acts violating the fundamental rights granted him by the constitution or by law.

Article 9

No one shall be subjected to arbitrary arrest, detention or exile.

Article 10

Everyone is entitled in full equality to a fair and public hearing by an independent and impartial tribunal, in the determination of his rights and obligations and of any criminal charge against him.

Article 11

1. Everyone charged with a penal offence has the right to be presumed innocent until proved guilty according to law in a public trial at which he has had all the guarantees necessary for his defence.
2. No one shall be held guilty of any penal offence on account of any act or omission which did not constitute a penal offence, under national or international law, at the time when it was committed. Nor shall a heavier penalty be imposed than the one that was applicable at the time the penal offence was committed.

Article 12

No one shall be subjected to arbitrary interference with his privacy, family, home or correspondence, nor to attacks upon his honor and reputation. Everyone has the right to the protection of the law against such interference or attacks.

Article 13

1. Everyone has the right to freedom of movement and residence within the borders of each State.
2. Everyone has the right to leave any country, including his own, and to return to his country.

Article 14

1. Everyone has the right to seek and to enjoy in other countries asylum from persecution.
2. This right may not be invoked in the case of prosecutions genuinely arising from nonpolitical crimes or from acts contrary to the purposes and principles of the United Nations.

Article 15

1. Everyone has the right to a nationality.
2. No one shall be arbitrarily deprived of his nationality nor denied the right to change his nationality.

Article 16

1. Men and women of full age, without any limitation due to race, nationality or religion, have the right to marry and to found a family. They are entitled to equal rights as to marriage, during marriage and at its dissolution.

2. Marriage shall be entered into only with the free and full consent of the intending spouses.
3. The family is the natural and fundamental group unit of society and is entitled to protection by society and the State.

Article 17

1. Everyone has the right to own property alone as well as in association with others.
2. No one shall be arbitrarily deprived of his property.

Article 18

Everyone has the right to freedom of thought, conscience and religion; this right includes freedom to change his religion or belief, and freedom, either alone or in community with others and in public or private, to manifest his religion or belief in teaching, practice, worship and observance.

Article 19

Everyone has the right to freedom of opinion and expression; this right includes freedom to hold opinions without interference and to seek, receive and impart information and ideas through any media and regardless of frontiers.

Article 20

1. Everyone has the right to freedom of peaceful assembly and association.
2. No one may be compelled to belong to an association.

Article 21

1. Everyone has the right to take part in the government of his country, directly or through freely chosen representatives.
2. Everyone has the right to equal access to public service in his country.
3. The will of the people shall be the basis of the authority of government; this will shall be expressed in periodic and genuine elections which shall be by universal and equal suffrage and shall be held by secret vote or by equivalent free voting procedures.

Article 22

Everyone, as a member of society, has the right to social security and is entitled to realization, through national effort and international co-operation and in accordance with the organization and resources of each State, of the economic, social and cultural rights indispensable for his dignity and the free development of his personality.

Article 23

1. Everyone has the right to work, to free choice of employment, to just and favorable conditions of work and to protection against unemployment.

2. Everyone, without any discrimination, has the right to equal pay for equal work.
3. Everyone who works has the right to just and favorable remuneration ensuring for himself and his family an existence worthy of human dignity, and supplemented, if necessary, by other means of social protection.
4. Everyone has the right to form and to join trade unions for the protection of his interests.

Article 24

Everyone has the right to rest and leisure, including reasonable limitation of working hours and periodic holidays with pay.

Article 25

1. Everyone has the right to a standard of living adequate for the health and well-being of himself and of his family, including food, clothing, and housing and medical care and necessary social services, and the right to security in the event of unemployment, sickness, disability, widowhood, old age or other lack of livelihood in circumstances beyond his control.
2. Motherhood and childhood are entitled to special care and assistance. All children, whether born in or out of wedlock, shall enjoy the same social protection.

Article 26

1. Everyone has the right to education. Education shall be free, at least in the elementary and fundamental stages. Elementary education shall be compulsory. Technical and professional education shall be made generally available and higher education shall be equally accessible to all on the basis of merit.
2. Education shall be directed to the full development of the human personality and to the strengthening of respect for human rights and fundamental freedoms. It shall promote understanding, tolerance and friendship among all nations, racial or religious groups, and shall further the activities of the United Nations for the maintenance of peace.
3. Parents have a prior right to choose the kind of education that shall be given to their children.

Article 27

1. Everyone has the right freely to participate in the cultural life of the community, to enjoy the arts and to share in scientific advancement and its benefits.
2. Everyone has the right to the protection of the moral and material interests resulting from any scientific, literary or artistic production of which he is the author.

Article 28

Everyone is entitled to a social and international order in which the rights and freedoms set forth in this Declaration can be fully realized.

Article 29

1. Everyone has duties to the community in which alone the free and full development of his personality is possible.
2. In the exercise of his rights and freedoms, everyone shall be subject only to such limitations as are determined by law solely for the purpose of securing due recognition and respect for the rights and freedoms of others and of meeting the just requirements of morality, public order and the general welfare in a democratic society.
3. These rights and freedoms may in no case be exercised contrary to the purposes and principles of the United Nations.

Article 30

Nothing in this Declaration may be interpreted as implying for any State, group or person any right to engage in any activity or to perform any act aimed at the destruction of any of the rights and freedoms set forth herein.

Annexure—6

Principles of Medical Ethics Relevant to the Role of Health Personnel, Particularly Physicians in the Protection of Prisoners and Detainees Against Torture and Other Cruel, Inhuman or Degrading Treatment or Punishment

ADOPTED BY GENERAL ASSEMBLY RESOLUTION 37/194 OF 18 DECEMBER, 1982

Principle 1

Health personnel, particularly physicians, charged with the medical care of prisoners and detainees have a duty to provide them with protection of their physical and mental health and treatment of disease of the same quality and standard as is afforded to those who are not imprisoned or detained.

Principle 2

It is a gross contravention of medical ethics, as well as an offence under applicable international instruments, for health personnel, particularly physicians, to engage, actively or passively, in acts, which constitutes participation in, complicity in, incitement to or attempts to commit torture or other cruel, inhuman or degrading treatment or punishment.

Principle 3

It is a contravention of medical ethics for health personnel, particularly physicians, to be involved in any professional relationship with prisoners or detainees the purpose of which is not solely to evaluate, protect or improve their physical and mental health.

Principle 4

It is a contravention of medical ethics for health personnel, particularly physicians:

a. To apply their knowledge and skills in order to assist in the interrogation of prisoners and detainees in a manner that may adversely affect the physical or mental health or conditions of such prisoners or detainees and which is not in accordance with the relevant international instruments;

b. To certify, or to participate in the certification of, the fitness of prisoners or detainees for any form of treatment or punishment that may adversely affect their physical or mental health, and which is not in accordance with the relevant international instruments, or to participate in any way in the infliction of any such treatment or punishment which is not in accordance with the relevant international instruments.

Principle 5

It is a contravention of medical ethics for health personnel, particularly physicians, to participate in any procedure for restraining a prisoner or detainee unless such a procedure is determined in accordance with purely medical criteria as being necessary for the protection of the physical or mental health or the safety of the prisoner or detainee himself, of his fellow prisoners or detainees, or of his guardians, and presents no hazard to his physical or mental health.

Principle 6

There may be no derogation from the foregoing principles on any ground whatsoever, including public emergency.

a. See Declaration on the protection of all persons from being subjected to torture and other cruel, inhuman or degrading treatment or punishment (resolution 3452 (XXX), annexure).
b. Particularly the Universal Declaration of Human Rights (resolution 217 A [III]), the International Covenants on Human Rights (resolution 2200 A [XXI]. annexure), the Declaration on the protection of All Persons from Being Subjected to Torture and Other Cruel, Inhuman or Degrading Treatment or Punishment [resolution 3452 (XXX), annexure] and the Standard Minimum Rules for the Treatment of Prisoners [First United Nations Congress on the Prevention of Crime and the Treatment of Offenders: report by the Secretariat (United Nations Publication, Sales No E 1956 IV 4, annexure IA)].

Annexure—7

Declaration of Geneva

Adopted by the 2nd General Assembly of the World Medical Association, Geneva, Switzerland, September 1948 and amended by the 22nd World Medical Assembly, Sydney, Australia, August 1968 and the 35th World Medical Assembly, Venice, Italy, October 1983 and the 46th WMA General Assembly, Stockholm, Sweden, September 1994 and editorially revised at the 170th Council Session, Divonne-les-Bains, France, May 2005 and the 173rd Council Session, Divonne-les-Bains, France, May 2006.

At the Time of Being Admitted as a Member of the Medical Profession

I Solemnly Pledge to consecrate my life to the service of humanity;

I Will Give to my teachers the respect and gratitude that is their due;

I Will Practise my profession with conscience and dignity;

The Health of My Patient will be my first consideration;

I Will Respect the secrets that are confided in me, even after the patient has died;

I Will Maintain by all the means in my power, the honor and the noble traditions of the medical profession;

My Colleagues will be my sisters and brothers;

I Will Not Permit considerations of age, disease or disability, creed, ethnic origin, gender, nationality, political affiliation, race, sexual orientation, social standing or any other factor to intervene between my duty and my patient;

I Will Maintain the utmost respect for human life;

I Will Not Use my medical knowledge to violate human rights and civil liberties, even under threat;

I Make These Promises solemnly, freely and upon my honor.

Annexure—8

Code of Medical Ethics

WORLD MEDICAL ASSOCIATION INTERNATIONAL CODE OF MEDICAL ETHICS

Adopted by the 3rd General Assembly of the World Medical Association, London, England, October 1949 and amended by the 22nd World Medical Assembly Sydney, Australia, August 1968 and the 35th World Medical Assembly, Venice, Italy, October 1983.

Duties of Physicians in General

A Physician shall	always maintain the highest standards of professional conduct
A Physician shall	not permit motives of profit to influence the free and independent exercise of professional judgment on behalf of patients
A Physician shall	in all types of medical practice, be dedicated to providing competent medical services in full technical and moral independence, with compassion and respect for human dignity
A Physician shall	deal honestly with patients and colleagues, and strive to expose those physicians deficient in character or competence, or who engage in fraud or deception

The Following Practices are Deemed to be Unethical Conduct

a. Self-advertising by physicians, unless permitted by the laws of the country and the code of ethics of the National Medical Association.
b. Paying or receiving any fee or any other consideration solely to procure the referral of a patient or for prescribing or referring a patient to any source.

A Physician shall	respect the rights of patients, of colleagues, and of other health professionals and shall safeguard patient confidences
A Physician shall	act only in the patient's interest when providing medical care which might have the effect of weakening the physical and mental condition of the patient
A Physician shall	use great caution in divulging discoveries or new techniques or treatment through non-professional channels
A Physician shall	certify only that which he has personally verified

Duties of Physicians to the Sick

A Physician shall	always bear in mind the obligation of preserving human life
A Physician shall	owe his patients complete loyalty and all the resources of his science. Whenever an examination or treatment is beyond the physician's capacity he should summon another physician who has the necessary ability
A Physician shall	preserve absolute confidentiality on all he knows his patient even after the patient has died
A Physician shall	give emergency care as a humanitarian duty unless he is assured that others are willing and able to give such care

Duties of Physicians to Each Other

A Physician shall	behave towards his colleagues as he would have them behave towards him
A Physician shall	entice patients from his colleagues
A Physician shall	observe the principles of the "Declaration of Geneva" approved by the World Medical Association

Indian Medical Council (Professional Conduct, Etiquette and Ethics) Regulations, 2002

Unethical Acts: A physician shall not aid or abet or commit any of the following acts which shall be construed as unethical.

Human Rights: The physician shall not aid or abet torture nor shall he be a party to either infliction of mental or physical trauma or concealment of torture inflicted by some other person or agency in clear violation of human rights.

Annexure—9

Declaration of Tokyo

Guidelines for Medical Doctors Concerning Torture and other Cruel, Inhuman or Degrading Treatment or Punishment in Relation to Detention and Imprisonment

(As adopted by the 29th World Medical Assembly, Tokyo, Japan, October 1975)

Preamble

It is the privilege of the medical doctor to practice medicine in the service of humanity, to preserve and restore bodily and mental health without distinction as to persons, to comfort and to ease the suffering of his or her patients. The utmost respect for human life is to be maintained even under threat, and no use made of any medical knowledge contrary to the laws of humanity.

For the purpose of this declaration, torture is defined as the deliberate, systematic of wanton infliction of physical or mental suffering by one or more persons acting alone or on the orders of any authority, to force another person to yield information, to make a confession, or for any other reason.

Declaration

1. The doctor shall not countenance, condone or participate in the practice of torture or other forms of cruel, inhuman or degrading procedures, whatever the offence of which the victim of such procedures is suspected, accused or guilty, and whatever the victim's beliefs or motives, and in all situations, including armed conflict and civil strife.
2. The doctor shall not provide any premises, instruments, substances or knowledge to facilitate the practice of torture or other forms of cruel, inhuman or degrading treatment or to diminish the ability of the victim to resist such treatment.
3. The doctor shall not be present during any procedure during which torture or other forms of cruel, inhuman or degrading treatment is used or threatened.
4. A doctor must have complete clinical independence in deciding upon the care of a person for whom he or she is medically responsible. The doctor's fundamental role is to alleviate the distress of his or her fellow men, and no motive whether personal, collective or political shall prevail against this higher purpose.
5. Where a prisoner refuses nourishment and is considered by the doctor as capable of forming an unimpaired and rational judgment concerning the consequences of such a voluntary refusal of nourishment, he or she shall not

be fed artificially. Me decision as to the capacity of the prisoner to form such a judgment should be confirmed by at least one other independent doctor. The consequences of the refusal of nourishment shall be explained by the doctor to the prisoner.

6. The World Medical Association will support, and should encourage the international community, the National Medical Associations and fellow doctors, to support the doctor and his or her family in the face of threats or reprisals resulting from a refusal to condone the use of torture or other forms of cruel, inhuman or degrading treatment.

Annexure—10

World Medical Association Declaration on Human Rights and Individual Freedom of Medical Practitioners

(Adopted by the 37th World Medical Assembly, Brussels, Belgium, October 1985)

The World Medical Association is in favor of equality of opportunity in medical society activities, medical education and training, employment, and all other aspects of medical professional endeavors regardless of race, color, religion, creed, ethnic affiliation, national origin, sex, age or political affiliation.

The World Medical Association is unalterably opposed to the denial of membership privileges and responsibilities in National Medical Associations to any duly registered physician because of race, color, religion, creed, ethnic affiliation, national origin, sex age or political affiliation.

The World Medical Association calls upon the medical profession and all individual members of National Medical Associations to exert every effort to end any instance in which such equal rights, privileges or responsibilities are denied.

Therefore, be it resolved that the 37th World Medical Assembly meeting in Brussels, Belgium, October 1985, hereby reaffirms its adherence to these principles.

Annexure—11

World Psychiatric Association (WPA) Cairo Declaration "Mass Violence and Mental Health"

THE GENERAL ASSEMBLY OF THE WORLD PSYCHIATRIC ASSOCIATION

- Emphasizing that the World Psychiatric Association, being the world's largest psychiatric association, comprising 130 societies from 113 countries, can speak on behalf of the profession.
- Conscious of the fact that violence is a major public health problem with important mental health implications. Concerned by the fact that mass violence such as war, terrorism, urban violence and similar acts causes many deaths, material losses and mental health problems in the lives of the survivors and in the population at large.
- Cognizant of the fact that violence does not help to solve problems but begets violence and brings with it poverty, hunger, disease and fear.
- Underlining that, unless properly addressed, the psychological consequences of violence affect future generations and can destroy the social cohesion that allows people to live together in harmony. Convinced that psychiatry and behavioral sciences can contribute to the understanding of the complex biological, psychological and social roots of violence and to the formulation of interventions that can prevent violence or alleviate its consequences.
- Recalling previous work of the World Psychiatric Association on alleviating consequences of disasters and the prevention of mental disorders.
- Recognizing that terrorism, by itself, is not a mental illness but a phenomenon often associated with oppression and absence of opportunities for free expression or redress.
- Considering that the alliance of mental health workers and leaders of religions that advocate mercy, compassion and forgiveness might help in the prevention of violence and in the alleviation of its consequences.

1. **Urges the WPA member societies**
   a. To develop and support research on the causes and consequences of violence and develop training programs that will help in the prevention of violence and in helping its victims.
   b. To invite their members to cooperate with other professionals and all those who are working for peace without any ideological or other prejudice.

2. **Request the scientific sections of the WPA to develop collaborative and multidisciplinary research on the origins of violence.**
3. **Request the executive committee of the WPA to:**
   a. Find ways to effectively collaborate with governmental and other agencies in the prevention of mass violence and the alleviation of its consequences.
   b. Invite the World Health Organization to strengthen its efforts to enhance the awareness of the public health importance of violence and to convey to its member states the need for research and action in this area.
   c. Undertake whatever is necessary to ensure that the scientific knowledge stemming from psychiatry and neurosciences and behavioral sciences is used in dealing with problems of violence.
   d. Create a special program on mental health aspects of violence to facilitate the above tasks and further stimulate research and action in this area of its work.
   e. Report on the steps taken in response to this declaration at the WPA General Assembly in 2008.

INDEX

Page numbers followed by *f* refer to figure and *t* refer to table, respectively.

D

E

F

G

H

I

Q

R

S